Empirical Likelihood Methods in Biomedicine and Health

Empirical Likelihood Methods in Biomedicine and Health

Albert Vexler

Jihnhee Yu

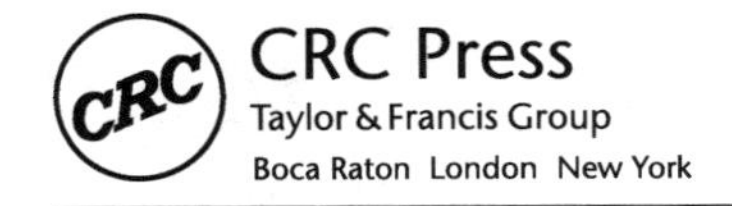

CRC Press is an imprint of the
Taylor & Francis Group, an **informa** business
A CHAPMAN & HALL BOOK

CRC Press
Taylor & Francis Group
6000 Broken Sound Parkway NW, Suite 300
Boca Raton, FL 33487-2742

Printed on acid-free paper

International Standard Book Number-13: 978-1-4665-5503-7 (Hardback)

Library of Congress Cataloging-in-Publication Data

Names: Vexler, Albert, author. | Yu, Jihnhee, author.
Title: Empirical likelihood methods in biomedicine and health / by Albert Vexler, The State University of New York at Buffalo, USA and Jihnhee Yu, The State University of New York at Buffalo, USA.
Description: Boca Raton, Florida : CRC Press, [2018] | Includes bibliographical references and index.
Identifiers: LCCN 2017060382| ISBN 9781466555037 (hardback : alk. paper) | ISBN 9781351001526 (e-book)
Subjects: LCSH: Medical informatics--Research--Methodology. | Bioethics--Research--Methodology.
Classification: LCC R858 .V49 2018 | DDC 610.285072--dc23
LC record available at https://lccn.loc.gov/2017060382

Visit the Taylor & Francis Web site at
http://www.taylorandfrancis.com

and the CRC Press Web site at
http://www.crcpress.com

To my parents, Octyabrina and Alexander, and my son, David

Albert Vexler

To Joonyeong

Jihnhee Yu

Contents

Preface

Empirical likelihood (EL) is a nonparametric likelihood approach that has been used frequently in recent statistical tool developments. The method tends to be more robust than purely parametric approaches and demonstrates its applicability in many data analytical problems. As distributions of data in the real world are commonly unknown, data-driven approaches such as the EL method should be more competitive than purely parametric approaches, given the lack of the knowledge of true distributions. As the EL methods are often comparatively efficient when compared to other existing approaches (such as t-test-based schemes) even with normal underlying distribution cases, more active use of the methods seems warranted. However, the method may be unfamiliar to some statistical researchers and potential end-users for data analysis, and thus it is difficult to find applications of the method in publications related to practical areas such as medicine and epidemiological research. For a more active use of the method, researchers need to convince the utility, accuracy, and efficiency of the method. We hope that this book will be truly successful toward that endeavor.

This book can be used as a textbook for a one or two-semesters advanced graduate course. The material in the book can be appropriate for use both as a text and as a reference. We hope that the mathematical level and breadth of examples will recruit students and teachers not only from statistics and biostatistics, but from a broad range of fields. We hope this book to be a connecting dot that leads interested readers to some technical details of subject areas more easily. The authors of this book have been working on the topics of the EL approaches to tackle problems related to clinical and epidemiological data. We believe that the research areas of EL are rich in yet-to-be-found applications and theoretical developments on many statistical problems and often those findings could provide better solutions than existing approaches. However, the concept of the EL may be foreign to people who do not have exposures to the approach and that fact would make new researchers hesitate considering EL for tool developments. In this regard, through this book, readers may be familiar with our developmental scheme of EL approach. Especially, Chapters 3 through 8 contain subject areas that the authors heavily worked on, and their contents will provide analytical issues and motivational questions, theoretical developments, software implementation, brief simulation results, and data applications, which pretty much sum up our procedures to develop *new* EL methods. For the theoretical developments in those chapters, readers will find recurring formal patterns almost similar to a "ceremony." In that patterns of developments, we tried to provide enough details of theoretical statements that cater the need of prospective EL method developers.

Chapter 1 offers the overview of statistical hypothesis tests and rational of using the EL approach. This chapter addresses the benefit of using the likelihood approach in details including the principal idea of the Neyman–Pearson Lemma, likelihood ratio tests, and maximum likelihood. Then the EL is introduced as a data-driven likelihood function that is nonparametric and comparatively powerful. This chapter further discusses the EL's benefits such as constructing efficient statistical tests using Bayesian methods in a similar manner to the parametric likelihood and setting up the EL statistics as composite semi- or nonparametric likelihoods. Chapter 2 focuses on the performance of EL constructs relative to ordinary parametric likelihood ratio-based procedures in the context of clinical experiments. This chapter first offers an overview of the classical EL methods. It explains the similarity between EL functions and parametric likelihood functions, detailed expressions of the Lagrange multipliers used in EL statements up to the fourth derivatives, and asymptotic properties of the EL likelihood functions. The chapter also touches the topics of extra estimating equation information, density-based EL methods, building composite hypotheses tests, Bayesian approaches, Bartlett correction, interpretation of the EL as an empirical goodness-of-fit test, and some comparison with bootstrap methods. Chapter 3 discusses how to incorporate EL in the Bayesian framework by showing a novel approach for developing the nonparametric Bayesian posterior expectation, the nonparametric analog of James–Stein estimation, and the nonparametric Bayesian confidence interval estimation. The chapter explains posterior expectations of general functionals. Chapter 4 discusses a general scheme to extend the conventional EL inference, considering the probability weighted moments (PWMs). The main task consists of forming constraints relevant to PWMs and showing that the developed EL test follows the classical asymptotic theories. The statistical test and confidence interval estimation of the PWMs are derived based on the proposed asymptotic proposition. Chapter 5 discusses methods to combine likelihood functions in parametric or empirical form in the setting of two-group comparison. It demonstrates an inference on incomplete bivariate data using a method that combines the parametric model and ELs. This chapter starts with discussions of two-group comparison of means where the EL ratio (ELR) test statistic carries out the mean-specific comparisons unlike other available nonparametric tests. It discusses comparison of multivariate means as a simple extension of univariate two-group comparison. Then, the likelihood ratio test based on the combined likelihood for the incomplete and complete data is developed to compare two treatment groups. Chapter 6 discusses the quantile estimation using the EL in the settings of testing one group and two groups. The Bahadur representation of the maximum EL estimator (MELE) of the quantile function is presented. Testing methods consist of the conventional EL method and the plug-in method. Chapter 7 discusses the ELR test with the constraints in the form of U-statistics. It first provides a general explanation of U-statistics including the variance estimation. Then, it discusses the EL test statistic with

U-statistic type constraints. The chapter discusses EL approaches for univariate and multivariate one-group and two-group U-statistics and provides some suitable examples including a multivariate rank statistic and an application to crossover designs. Chapter 8 starts with the general introduction of the receiver operating characteristic (ROC) curves and then discusses the construction of the EL statistic for the nonparametric estimator of the whole or partial area under the ROC curve (AUC) that has a form of the U-statistic. It discusses the best combinations of multiple biomarkers using ROC curve analysis. An important task of constructing the EL statistic is to incorporate the correct variance estimate to the EL statistic as discussed in Chapter 7. The problem is that the typical variance formula for U-statistics is inaccurate to estimate the variability of the estimator as plug-in estimators of the quantiles used. In this context, the chapter provides details of a correct variance estimation strategy. Finally, as an introductory manner, Chapter 9 presents several interesting topics that are discussed in the EL literature. This overview will demonstrate that the EL approach has a flexibility to be applied to various topics of interest as far as users can formulate a statistical question in a form of the estimating equations. Discussions of regression methods include incorporating validation data with error-prone covariates, analyzing longitudinal data, handling incomplete membership information, and regression with surrogate covariates. Discussions of censored data analyses include testing hazard functions, quantile function estimation, testing mean survival times, analyzing mean quality-adjusted lifetime (QAL) with censored data, and regression approach with censored data. Discussions of missing data include imputation, methods incorporating missing probabilities, and handling missing covariates. The chapter concludes introducing a pseudo-EL approach in survey sampling. The chapter provides some details in terms of describing analytical issues, building the constraints and relevant inferential results.

When we refer the Appendix in each chapter, it indicates the Appendix at the end of that chapter. In this book, we provide R codes that are readily usable and probably just enough to carry out the task we explained. We note that the software code mentioned in this book certainly can be improved, optimized, and extended.

As the statistical methodology has been continuously developed to tackle various data analytical issues, it is hard to cover all new developments; nevertheless, we hope that this book is a helpful introduction to show versatility and applicability of the EL method.

Authors

Albert Vexler obtained his PhD degree in Statistics and Probability Theory from the Hebrew University of Jerusalem, Israel, in 2003. His PhD advisor was Moshe Pollak, a fellow of the *American Statistical Association,* and Marcy Bogen Professor of Statistics at Hebrew University. Dr. Vexler was a postdoctoral research fellow in the Biometry and Mathematical Statistics Branch at the National Institute of Child Health and Human Development (National Institutes of Health, USA). Currently, Dr. Vexler is a tenured full professor at the State University of New York at Buffalo, Department of Biostatistics. Dr. Vexler has authored and coauthored various publications that contribute to both the theoretical and applied aspects of statistics in medical research. Many of his papers and statistical software developments have appeared in statistical/biostatistical journals, which have the top-rated impact factors and are historically recognized as the leading scientific journals, and include:
Biometrics, Biometrika, Journal of Statistical Software, The American Statistician, The Annals of Applied Statistics, Statistical Methods in Medical Research, Biostatistics, Journal of Computational Biology, Statistics in Medicine, Statistics and Computing, Computational Statistics and Data Analysis, Scandinavian Journal of Statistics, Biometrical Journal, Statistics in Biopharmaceutical Research, Stochastic Processes and their Applications, Journal of Statistical Planning and Inference, Annals of the Institute of Statistical Mathematics, The Canadian Journal of Statistics, Metrika, Statistics, Journal of Applied Statistics, Journal of Nonparametric Statistics, Communications in Statistics, Sequential Analysis, The STATA journal, American Journal of Epidemiology, Epidemiology, Paediatric and Perinatal Epidemiology, Academic Radiology, The Journal of Clinical Endocrinology & Metabolism, Journal of Addiction Medicine, Reproductive Toxicology, and *Human Reproduction.*

Dr. Vexler was awarded National Institutes of Health (NIH) grants to develop novel nonparametric data analysis and statistical methodology. Dr. Vexler's research interests are related to the following subjects: receiver operating characteristic curves analysis, measurement error, optimal designs, regression models, censored data, change point problems, sequential analysis, statistical epidemiology, Bayesian decision-making mechanisms, asymptotic methods of statistics, forecasting, sampling, optimal testing, nonparametric tests, empirical likelihoods, renewal theory, Tauberian theorems, time series, categorical analysis, multivariate analysis, multivariate testing of complex hypotheses, factor and principal component analysis, statistical biomarkers evaluations, and best combinations of biomarkers. Dr. Vexler is associate editor for *Biometrics* and the *Journal of Applied Statistics*. These journals belong to the first cohort of academic literature related to the methodology of biostatistical and epidemiological research and clinical trials.

Dr. Jihnhee Yu received her PhD degree in Statistics from Texas A&M University, College Station, Texas, in 2003. Her PhD advisor was Thomas E. Wehrly, PhD. Currently, Dr. Yu is a tenured associate professor at the State University of New York at Buffalo, New York, Department of Biostatistics. Also, Dr. Yu is the director of the Population Health Observatory, School of Public Health, and Health Professions at the State University of New York at Buffalo. Before her university carrier, she was a senior biostatistics consultant at Roswell Park Cancer Institute, Buffalo, New York. Dr. Yu has been working on cancer study designs; prospective clinical trials; retrospective data analysis; secondary data analyses; epidemiological studies; relevant statistical methodology development, and data analysis in epidemiology, psychology, pediatrics, oral biology, neurosurgery, and health behavior, and other population health- and medical-related areas. Her theoretical research interests are nonparametric tests and clinical trial methodologies. In particular, she has worked on group sequential designs, unbiased estimators associated with group sequential designs, exact methods, and few empirical likelihood approaches on several topics. She authored and coauthored many statistical and collaborative papers that were published in top-ranking journals. Dr. Yu was awarded National Institutes of Health (NIH) grants to develop novel nonparametric data analysis and statistical methodology. Dr. Yu is an associate editor for *Journal of Applied Statistics.*

1

Preliminaries

1.1 Overview: From Statistical Hypotheses to Types of Information for Constructing Statistical Tests

Most experiments in biomedicine and other health-related sciences involve mathematically formalized comparisons, employing appropriate and efficient statistical procedures in designing clinical studies and analyzing data. Decision making through formal rules based on mathematical strategies plays important roles in medical and epidemiological discovery, policy formulation, and clinical practice. In this context, the statistical discipline is commonly required to be applied to make conclusions about populations on the basis of samples from the populations.

The aim of methodologies in decision making is to maximize quantified gains and at the same time minimize losses to reach a conclusion. For example, statements of clinical experiments can target gains such as accuracy of diagnosis of medical conditions, faster healing, and greater patient satisfaction, while they minimize losses such as efforts, durations of screening for disease, and side effects and costs of the experiments.

There are generally many constraints and desirable characteristics for constructing a statistical test. An essential part of the test development is that statistical hypotheses should be clearly and formally set up with respect to objectives of clinical studies. Oftentimes, statistical hypotheses and clinical hypotheses are associated but stated in different forms and orders. In most applications, we are interested in testing characteristics or distributions of one or more populations. In such cases, the statistical hypotheses must be carefully formulated, and formally stated, depicting, e.g., the nature of associations in terms of quantified characteristics or distributions of populations. The term *Null Hypothesis*, symbolized H_0, commonly is used to point out our primary statistical hypothesis. For example, when one wants to test that a biomarker of oxidative stress has different circulating levels for patients with and without atherosclerosis (clinical hypothesis), the null hypothesis (statistical hypothesis) can be proposed corresponding to the *assumption* that levels of the biomarker in individuals with and without atherosclerosis are distributed equally. Note that the clinical hypothesis points out that we want to show the discriminating power of the biomarker, whereas H_0 says there are no significant associations between the disease and biomarker's levels. The reason of such null hypothesis specification lies in the ability to formulate H_0 clearly and unambiguously as well as to measure and calculate expected errors in decision making. Probably, if the null hypothesis would be formed in a similar manner to the clinical hypothesis, we could not unambiguously determine which sort of links between the disease and biomarker's levels should be tested.

The null hypothesis is usually a statement to be statistically tested. In the context of statistical testing that provides a formal test procedure and compares mathematical strategies to make a decision, algorithms for monitoring statistical test characteristics associated with the probability to reject a correct hypothesis should be considered. While developing and applying test procedures, the practical statistician faces a task to control the probability of the event that a test outcome rejects H_0 when in fact H_0 is correct, called a *Type I error* (TIE) rate.

Obviously, in order to construct statistical tests, we must review the corresponding clinical study, formalizing objectives of the experiments and making assumptions in hypothesis testing. A violation of the assumptions can pose incorrect results of the test and a vital malfunction of the TIE rate control procedure. Moreover, should the user verify that the assumptions are satisfied, errors of the verifications itself can affect the TIE rate control.

Interests of clinical investigators give rise to a mathematically express procedure or statistical decision rules that are based on sample from populations. When constructing decision rules, two additional information resources can be incorporated. The first is a defined function that consists of the explicit, quantified gains and losses and their relative weights to reach a conclusion. Frequently, this function defines the expected loss corresponding to each possible decision. This type of information can incorporate a *loss function* into the statistical decision-making process. The second information source is a prior knowledge. Commonly, in order to derive prior information, researches should consider past experiences about similar situations. The Bayesian methodology (e.g., Berger, 2010) formally provides clear technique manuals on how to construct efficient statistical decision rules with prior information in various complex problems related to clinical experiments, employing prior information.

1.2 Parametric Approach

In constructing decision rules, a statistician may use a sort of technical statements relevant to observed data. Some information used for test construction can give rise to technical statements that oftentimes are called assumptions regarding the distribution of data. The assumptions often define a fit of the data distribution to a functional form that is completely known or known up to parameters. A complete knowledge of the distribution of data can provide all the information that investigators need for efficient applications of statistical techniques. However, in many scenarios, the assumptions are reasonably guessed and very difficult to be proven or tested for their propriety. Widely used assumptions in biostatistics are that data derived via a clinical study follow one of the commonly used distribution functions such as the Normal, Lognormal, t, χ^2, Gamma, F, Binominal, Uniform, Wishart, and Poisson. The distribution function of the data can be defined including parameters. For example, the normal distribution $N(\mu,\sigma^2)$ has the shape of the famous bell curve, where the parameters μ and σ^2 representing a mean and variance of a population define the distribution. Values of the parameters may be assumed to be unknown. Mostly in such cases, assumed functional forms of the data distributions are involved to make statistical decision rules via the use of statistics from the sample, which we call *Parametric Statistics*. If certain key assumptions are met, parametric methods can yield very simple, efficient, and powerful inferences.

1.3 Warning—Parametric Approach and Detour: Nonparametric Approach

The statistical literature widely addresses an issue that parametric methods are often sensitive to moderate violations of parametric assumptions and hence are nonrobust (e.g., Freedman, 2009). In order to reduce a risk to apply an incorrect parametric approach, the parametric assumptions can be tested. In this case, statisticians can try to verify the assumptions while making decisions with respect to main objectives of the clinical study. This leads to complicated topics dealt with in multiple testing. Also, it turns out that a computation of an expected risk that may lead to a wrong decision strongly depends on errors that can be made by failing to reject the parametric assumptions. The complexity of this problem can increase when researchers examine various functional forms to fit the data distribution in order to apply parametric methods. A substantial theoretical and experimental literature has discussions of the pitfalls of multiple testing that places blame squarely on the shoulders of the many clinical investigators who examine their data before deciding how to analyze it or neglecting to report the statistical tests that may not have supported their theses (e.g., Austin et al., 2006). In this context, one can present various cases, both hypothetical and actual, to get to the heart of issues arising especially in the health-related sciences. Note also that in many situations, due to the wide variety and complex nature of problematic real data, e.g. incomplete data subject to instrumental limitations of studies (e.g., Vexler et al., 2008a,b), statistical parametric assumptions are hardly satisfied, and their relevant formal tests are complicated or oftentimes are not readily available. Unfortunately, even clinical investigators trained in statistical methods do not always verify the corresponding parametric assumptions and do not attend to probabilistic errors of the corresponding verification, when they use well-known basic parametric statistical methods, e.g., the *t*-test.

It is known that when the key assumptions are not met the parametric approach may be extremely biased and inefficient when compared to their robust nonparametric counterparts. Statistical inference under the nonparametric regime offers decision-making procedures, avoiding or minimizing the use of the assumptions regarding functional forms of the data distributions. In general, the choice between nonparametric and parametric approaches can boil down to expected efficiency versus robustness to assumptions. Thus, an important issue is to preserve efficiency of statistical techniques through the use of robust nonparametric likelihood methods, minimizing required assumptions about data distributions.

1.4 A Brief Ode to Likelihood

Testing statistical hypotheses based on the *t*-test or its modifications is one of the traditional instruments used in medical experiments and drug development. Despite the fact that these tests are straightforward with respect to their applications to clinical and medical settings, it should be noted that there has been a huge literature on the criticism of *t*-test type statistical tools. One major issue, which has been widely recognized, is with respect to the significant loss of efficiency of these procedures under different distributional assumptions. The legitimacy of *t*-test type procedures also comes into question in the context of inflated TIEs when data distributions differ from normal and the number of available observations is limited. The recent biostatistical literature has addressed the arguments well that values of biomarker measurements tend to follow skewed distributions, e.g. a lognormal distribution (Limpert et al., 2001), and hence the use of *t*-test type techniques in this setting is suboptimal and accompanied by difficulties to control the corresponding TIE rates.

Consider the following example based on data from a study evaluating biomarkers related to atherosclerotic coronary heart disease (Schisterman et al., 2001). A cross-sectional population-based sample of randomly selected residents (age 35–79) of Erie and Niagara counties of the state of New York, United States, was used for the analysis. The New York State Department of Motor Vehicles drivers' license rolls were employed as the sampling frame for adults between the ages of 35 and 65, whereas the elderly sample (age 65–79) was randomly selected from the Health Care Financing Administration database. Participants provided a 12-hour fasting blood specimen for biochemical analysis at baseline, and a number of characteristics were evaluated from fresh blood samples. Figure 1.1 depicts a screenshot, demonstrating the example though the use of R, a powerful and flexible statistical software language (e.g., Crawley, 2012 for its introduction).

The samples X and Y present 50 measurements (mg/dL) of the biomarker high-density lipoprotein (HDL) cholesterol obtained from healthy patients. These measurements were divided into the two groups (i.e., X and Y). Although one can reasonably expect the samples are from the same population, the t-test shows a significant difference of their distributions. Perhaps, the following issues may be taken into account to explain reasons of this incorrect output of the t-test. The histograms displayed in Figure 1.1 indicate that the distributions of the X and Y probably are skewed. In a non-asymptotic context, when the sample sizes are relatively small, one can show that the t-test-statistic is a product of likelihood ratio-type considerations based on normally distributed observations (e.g., Lehmann and Romano, 2005). That is, the t-test is a parametric test and the parametric assumption seems to be violated, in this example.

Thus, in many settings, it may be reasonable to propose an approach for developing statistical tests, attending data distributions, to provide procedures that are efficient as the t-test based on normally distributed observations. Toward this end the likelihood methodology can be employed.

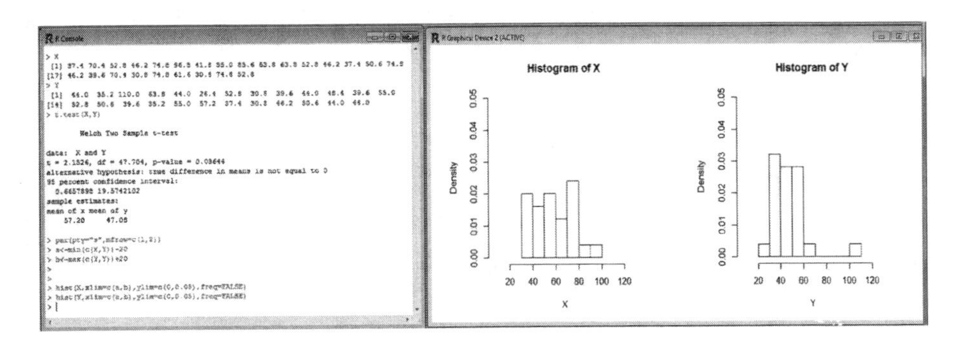

FIGURE 1.1
R data analysis output for measurements of HDL cholesterol levels in healthy individuals.

1.4.1 Likelihood Ratios and Optimality

Now we outline the likelihood principle. When the forms of data distributions are assumed to be known the likelihood principle is a central tenet for developing powerful statistical inference tools. The *likelihood method* or simply the *likelihood* is arguably the most important concept for inference in parametric modeling (Neyman and Pearson, 1992), and this fact equally applies when the underlying data are subjected to different problems and limitations related to medical and epidemiological studies, e.g. in the context of the analysis of survival data. Likelihood-based testing that we know was mainly found and formulated in a series of fundamental papers published in the period of 1928–1938 by Jerzy Neyman and Egon Pearson (Neyman and Pearson, 1928–1938). In 1928, the authors introduced the generalized likelihood ratio test and its association with chi-squared statistics. Five years later, the Neyman–Pearson Lemma (Neyman and Pearson, 1933) was introduced showing the optimality of the likelihood ratio test. These seminal works provided us with the familiar notions of simple and composite hypotheses and errors of the first and second kind, thus defining formal decision-making rules for testing. Without loss of generality, the principle idea of the proof of the Neyman–Pearson Lemma can be shown by using the trivial inequality

$$(A-B)\left(I\{A\geq B\}-\delta\right)\geq 0, \tag{1.1}$$

for any real numbers A, B, where $\delta\in[0,1]$ and $I\{\cdot\}$ denote the indicator function. For example, suppose we would like to classify independent identically distributed (i.i.d.) biomarker measurements $\{X_i, i=1,\ldots,n\}$ corresponding to hypotheses of the form H_0: X_1 is from a density function f_0 versus H_1: X_1 is from a density function f_1. In this context, to construct the likelihood ratio test statistic, we should consider the ratio between the joint density function of $\{X_1,\ldots,X_n\}$ obtained under H_1 and the joint density function of $\{X_1,\ldots,X_n\}$ obtained under H_0, and then define $\prod_{i=1}^n f_1(X_i)/\prod_{i=1}^n f_0(X_i)$ to be the likelihood ratio. In this case the likelihood ratio test is uniformly most powerful. This proposition directly follows from the expected value under H_0 of the inequality (1.1), where we define $A=\prod_{i=1}^n f_1(X_i)/f_0(X_i)$, B to be a test-threshold (i.e., the likelihood ratio test rejects H_0 if and only if $A\geq B$), and δ is assumed to represent any decision rule based on $\{X_i, i=1,\ldots,n\}$. The Appendix contains details of the proof. This simple proof-technique was used to show optimal aspects of different statistical decision-making policies based on the likelihood ratio concept applied in clinical experiments (e.g., Vexler, Wu, and Yu, 2008; Vexler and Wu, 2009; Vexler and Gurevich, 2011).

1.4.2 The Likelihood Ratio Based on the Likelihood Ratio Test Statistic Is the Likelihood Ratio Test Statistic

The Neyman–Pearson concept to test, fixing the probability of a TIE, comes under some criticism by epidemiologists. One of the critical points is related to the Type II error, the incorrect decision by failing to reject the null hypothesis when the alternative hypothesis is true. For example, Freiman et al. (1978) pointed out results of 71 clinical trials that reported no *significant* differences between the compared treatments. The authors found that in the great majority of these trials the strong effects of new treatment are reasonable. On failing to reject the null hypothesis, the investigators in such trials inappropriately accepted the null hypothesis as correct, which probably resulted in the Type II error. In the context of likelihood ratio-based tests, we present the following result that demonstrates an association between the probabilities of the Type I and II errors.

Suppose we would like to test for H_0 versus H_1, employing the likelihood ratio $L = f_{H_1}(D) / f_{H_0}(D)$ based on data D, where f_{H_i} defines a density function that corresponds to the data distribution under the hypothesis H_i. Say, for simplicity, we reject H_0 if $L > C$, where C is a presumed threshold. In this case, one can then show that

$$f_{H_1}^{L}(u) = u\, f_{H_0}^{L}(u), \tag{1.2}$$

where $f_{H}^{L}(u)$ is the density function of the test statistic L under the hypothesis H and $u > 0$. Details of the proof of this fact are shown in the Appendix. Thus, we can obtain the probability of a Type II error in the form of

$$\Pr\{\text{the test does not reject } H_0 \mid H_1 \text{ is true}\} = \Pr\{L \le C \mid H_1 \text{ is true}\}$$

$$= \int_0^C f_{H_1}^{L}(u)\,du = \int_0^C u f_{H_0}^{L}(u)\,du.$$

Now, if the density function $f_{H_0}^{L}(u)$ is assumed to be known to control the TIE rate, then the probability of the Type II error can be easily computed.

The likelihood ratio property $f_{H_1}^{L}(u) / f_{H_0}^{L}(u) = u$ can be applied to solve different issues related to performances of the likelihood ratio test. For example, in a term of the bias of the test, one can request to find a value of the threshold C that maximizes

$$\Pr\{\text{the test rejects } H_0 \mid H_1 \text{ is true}\} - \Pr\{\text{the test rejects } H_0 \mid H_0 \text{ is true}\},$$

where the probability Pr{the test rejects $H_0 \mid H_1$ is true} depicts the power of the test. This equation can be expressed as

$$\Pr\{L > C \mid H_1 \text{ is true}\} - \Pr\{L > C \mid H_0 \text{ is true}\} = \left(1 - \int_0^C f_{H_1}^L(u)\,du\right) - \left(1 - \int_0^C f_{H_0}^L(u)\,du\right).$$

Let the derivative of this notation equal zero and solve the equation:

$$\frac{d}{dC}\left[\left(1 - \int_0^C f_{H_1}^L(u)\,du\right) - \left(1 - \int_0^C f_{H_0}^L(u)\,du\right)\right] = -f_{H_1}^L(C) + f_{H_0}^L(C) = 0.$$

By virtue of property (1.2), this implies $-Cf_{H_0}^L(C) + f_{H_0}^L(C) = 0$ and then $C = 1$ that provides the maximum discrimination between the power and the probability of a TIE of the likelihood ratio test.

In words, an interesting fact is that the likelihood ratio $f_{H_1}^L / f_{H_0}^L$ *based on the likelihood ratio* $L = f_{H_1} / f_{H_0}$ *becomes to be the likelihood ratio, that is,* $f_{H_1}^L(L) / f_{H_0}^L(L) = L$. *We leave interpretations of this statement, may be in terms of information, to the reader's imagination.*

1.5 Maximum Likelihood: Is It the Likelihood?

Various real-world data problems require considerations of statistical hypotheses with structures, which depend on unknown parameters. In this case, the maximum likelihood method proposes to approximate the most powerful likelihood ratio, employing a proportion of the maximum likelihoods, where the maximizations are over values of the unknown parameters belonging to distributions of observations under the corresponding hypotheses. We shall assume the existence of essential maximum likelihood estimators. The influential theorem of Wilks (1938) provides the basic rational as to why the maximum likelihood ratio approach has had tremendous success in statistical applications. Wilks showed that under regularity conditions, asymptotic null distributions of maximum likelihood ratio test statistics are independent of nuisance parameters. That is, the TIE rates of the maximum likelihood ratio tests can be controlled asymptotically and approximations of the corresponding p-values can also be computed.

Thus, if certain key assumptions are met one can show that parametric likelihood methods are very powerful and efficient statistical tools. We should emphasize that the discovery related to the likelihood ratio methodology in statistical developments may be comparable with the development of the assembly line technique of mass production. The likelihood ratio principle gives clear instructions and technique manuals on how to construct efficient statistical decision rules in various complex problems related to clinical experiments. For example, Vexler et al. (2011c) developed a maximum likelihood ratio test for comparing populations based on incomplete longitudinal data subjected to instrumental limitations.

Although many statistical publications continue to contribute to the likelihood paradigm and are very important in the statistical discipline (an excellent account can be found in Lehmann and Romano, 2005), several significant questions arise naturally about the general applicability of the maximum likelihood approach. Conceptually, there is an issue specific to classifying maximum likelihoods in terms of likelihoods that are given by joint density (or probability) functions based on data. Integrated likelihood functions, with respect to arguments related to data points, are equal to one; however, accordingly integrated maximum likelihood functions often have values that are indefinite. Thus, although likelihoods present full information regarding the data, the maximum likelihoods might lose information conditional on the observed data. Consider the simple example: Suppose we observe X_1, that is assumed to be from a normal distribution $N(\mu,1)$ with mean parameter μ. In this case the likelihood has the form $(2\pi)^{-0.5}\exp(-(X_1-\mu)^2/2)$ and correspondingly $\int(2\pi)^{-0.5}\exp(-(X_1-\mu)^2/2)dX_1=1$, whereas the maximum likelihood, i.e., the likelihood evaluated at estimated $\mu, \hat{\mu}=X_1$, is $(2\pi)^{-0.5}$, which clearly does not represent the data and is not a proper density. This demonstrates that as the Neyman–Pearson lemma is fundamentally found on the use of the density-based constitutions of likelihood ratios, maximum likelihood ratios cannot be optimal in general. That is, the likelihood ratio principle is in general not robust when the hypothesis tests have corresponding nuisance parameters to consider, e.g. testing a hypothesized mean given an unknown variance. An additional inherent difficulty of the likelihood ratio test occurs when a clinical experiment is associated with an infinite-dimensional problem with the number of unknown parameters being relatively large. In this case, Wilks theorem should be re-evaluated and nonparametric approaches can be considered in the contexts of reasonable alternatives to the parametric likelihood methodology (e.g., Fan et al., 2001).

The ideas of likelihood and maximum likelihood ratio testing may not be fiducial and applicable in general nonparametric function estimation/testing settings. It is also well known that when key assumptions are not met, parametric approaches may be suboptimal or biased as compared to their robust counterparts across the many features of statistical inferences. For example, in a biomedical application, Ghosh (1995) proved that the maximum likelihood estimators for the Rasch model are inconsistent as the number of nuisance parameters increases to infinity (Rasch models are often utilized in clinical trials that deal with psychological measurements, e.g., abilities, attitudes, personality traits). Due to the structure of likelihood functions based on products of densities or conditional density functions, relatively nonsignificant errors of classifications of data distributions can lead to vital problems related to applications of likelihood ratio-type tests (e.g., Gurevich and Vexler, 2010). Moreover, one can note that given the wide variety and complex nature of biomedical data, e.g. incomplete data subject to instrumental limitations or complex correlation structures, parametric assumptions are rarely satisfied. The respective formal tests are complicated or oftentimes are not readily available.

1.6 Empirical Likelihood

The empirical likelihood (EL) approach is based on a data-driven likelihood function, thus is intrinsically nonparametric and comparatively powerful (Lazar and Mykland, 1998). An advantage of using the EL method is that it does not require the distribution assumption. The EL is able to incorporate known constraints on parameters in an inferential setting under both the null and alternative hypotheses. EL hypothesis tests maintain a prespecified TIE rate relatively well with various underlying distributions. In two group comparisons, they offer robust testing procedures under violations of the exchangeability assumptions (e.g., Yu et al., 2011). Historically the EL method was first introduced for the analysis of censored data (Thomas and Grunkemeier, 1975; Owen, 1991). Owen (1988) introduced the empirical likelihood ratio (ELR) approach to construct confidence intervals. Since being introduced into the statistical literature, the EL approach has demonstrated its practical applicability via extensions to a variety of statistical problems (e.g., Yang and Zhao, 2007; Vexler and Gurevich, 2010; Wang et al., 2010). The EL method incorporates information or assumptions regarding the parameters and translates those to the distribution-free likelihood estimation; thus the method can be used to combine additional information about parameters of interest (Qin and Lawless, 1994).

In comparison with classical testing methods based on normal approximations, the EL ratio test statistic does not rely on symmetric rejection regions, thus giving rise to more accurate tests (Hall and La Scala, 1990). Owen (1990) showed that the EL ratio provides confidence intervals less affected by the skewness of distribution comparing with methods based on the central limit theorem. DiCiccio et al. (1991) demonstrated that the EL method can achieve an excellent coverage rate for confidence intervals by applying some parametric techniques such as the Bartlett correction. The EL method for constructing confidence regions for parameters has comparable sampling properties of the bootstrap. Although the bootstrap uses resampling, the EL method computes the profile likelihood of a general multinomial distribution based on data points. The property that EL produces regions that reflect emphasis in the observed dataset and involves no predetermined assumptions about the shape has considerable potential in the construction of confidence bands for curve estimators. Chen (1994) compared the powers of EL ratios and bootstrap tests for a mean parameter against a series of local alternative hypotheses (see Chapter 2 for details). It is shown that the EL ratio test can be more powerful than the bootstrap test depending on the population skewness parameter.

Versatility of the EL method is demonstrated in many different data analytical settings. Researchers have worked in the area specifically related to quantiles using the EL method; e.g., Chen and Hall (1993) used a smoothed EL approach to estimate confidence intervals for quantiles using kernel functions. They showed that the coverage accuracy may be improved from order $n^{-1/2}$ to order n^{-1} by appropriately smoothing the EL method. The improvement is available for a wide range of choices of the smoothing parameter so that accurate choice of an *optimal* value of the parameter is not necessary. Chen and Chen (2000) investigated the properties of EL quantile estimation in large samples; Zhou and Jing (2003a) proposed an alternative smoothed EL approach where the EL ratio has an explicit form based on the concept of the M-estimators; and Lopez et al. (2009) investigated testing general parameters that are determined by the expectation of non-smooth functions. No distributional assumptions of EL allow the method to be used for analyzing data with complicated underlying distributions. The EL provides better performance with the confidence interval for the mean of a population with many zeros comparing with the method using parametric likelihood, whereas overall coverage properties are similar for both methods under various distribution assumptions (Chen et al., 2003; Kang et al., 2010). Qin and Leung (2005) used a semiparametric likelihood approach to estimate the distribution of the malaria parasite level, which is a mixture distribution where a component of the mixture distribution was again the mixture of discrete and continuous distributions. Qin (2000) showed an inference on incomplete bivariate data using a method that combines the parametric model and ELs. His work was extended to the group comparison using the EL by Yu et al. (2010). The EL method also incorporates auxiliary information of variables in a form of constraints, which can be obtained from reliable resources such as census reports (e.g., Qin and Lawless, 1994; Chen and Qin, 1993).

We conclude this section emphasizing the following important aspects: (1) The EL concept can provide efficiently nonparametric approximations to optimal (e.g., most powerful) parametric statistical schemes; (2) the EL methodology yields robust algorithms to solve a variety of complex problems related to clinical trials; (3) EL functions can be easily combined with parametric and semiparametric likelihood functions to develop statistical procedures that demonstrate attractive properties in complicated model settings. These factors adduce evidence that EL techniques have great potentials to be adopted as primary statistical tools employed by clinical investigators.

1.7 Why Empirical Likelihood?

1.7.1 The Necessity and Danger of Testing Statistical Hypothesis

The ubiquitous use of statistical decision-making procedures in the current medical literature displays the vital role that statistical hypothesis testing plays in different branches of biomedical sciences. The benefits and fruits of statistical tests based on mathematical-probabilistic techniques, in epidemiology or other health-related disciplines, strongly depend on successful formal presentations of statements of problems and a description of nature. Oftentimes, certain assumptions about the observations used for the tests provide the probability statements that are required for the statistical tests. These assumptions do not come for free and ignoring their appropriateness can cause serious bias or inconsistency of statistical inferences, even when the test procedures thyself are carried out without mistakes. The sensitivity of the probabilistic properties of a test to the assumptions is referred to as the lack of robustness of the test (e.g., Wilcox, 1998).

Various statistical techniques require parametric assumptions that are to define forms of data distributions to be known up to parameters' values. For example, in the conventional t-test, the assumptions are that the observations of different individuals are realizations of independent, normally distributed, random variables, with the same expected value and variance for all individuals within the investigated group. Such assumptions are not automatically satisfied, and for some assumptions it may be doubted whether they are ever satisfied exactly. The null hypothesis H_0 and alternative hypothesis H_1 are statements which, strictly speaking, imply these assumptions, and which therefore are not each other's complement. There is a possibility that the assumptions are invalid, and neither H_0 nor H_1 is true. Thus, we can reject a statement related to clinical trials' interests just because the assumptions are not met. This issue is an impetus to departure from parametric families of data distributions, employing nonparametric test strategies.

One of the advantages of EL techniques lies in their generality and an assessment of their performance lies under conditions that are commonly unrestricted by parametric assumptions.

1.7.2 The Three Sources That Support the Empirical Likelihood Methodology for Applying in Practice

When in doubt about the best strategy to make statistical decision rules, the following arguments can be accepted in favor of EL methods:

1. The EL methodology employs the likelihood concept in a simple non-parametric fashion to approximate optimal parametric procedures. The benefit of using this approach is that the EL techniques are often robust and highly efficient. In this context, we also may apply EL functions to replace parametric likelihood functions in known and well-developed constructions. Consider the following example. The statistical literature widely suggests applying Bayesian methods for various tasks of clinical experiments, for example, when data are subjected to complex missing data problems, e.g. parts of data are not manifested as numerical scores (Daniels and Hogan, 2008). Commonly, to apply a Bayesian approach, one needs to assume functional forms corresponding to the distribution of the underlying data and parameters of interest. Lazar (2003) demonstrated potentials of constructing nonparametric Bayesian inference based on ELs that take the role of model-based likelihoods. This research demonstrated that the EL is a valid function for Bayesian inference. Vexler et al. (2013a) recommended applying EL functions to create Bayes Factor (BF)-type nonparametric procedures. The BF, a practical tool of applied biostatistics, has been dealt with extensively in the literature in the context of hypothesis testing (e.g., Carlin and Louis, 2000). The EL concept was shown to be very efficient when it is employed for modifying BF-type procedures to the nonparametric setting.
2. Similar to the parametric likelihood concept including Bayesian approaches, the EL methodology gives relatively simple systematic directions for constructing efficient statistical tests that can be applied in various complex clinical experiments.
3. Perhaps, the extreme generality of EL methods and their wide scope of usefulness partly follow on abilities to easily set up EL statistics as components of composite parametric/semi- and nonparametric likelihood-based systems, efficiently attending any observed data and relevant information. Parametric, semiparametric, and EL methods play roles complementary to one another, providing powerful statistical procedures for complicated practical problems.

In conclusion, we note that EL-based methods are employed in much of modern statistical practice, and we cannot describe all relevant theory and examples. In the following sections, we will outline several specific research problems, their motivation, and application.

The interested reader will find many pertinent articles in various statistical journals. This book is a systematic compendium of typical EL methods applied in practical studies. With examples and data from biomedical studies, this book explains newly advanced EL techniques applied to problems encountered in practical areas.

Implementation of tests introduced in this book may not be difficult to scientists who are new to the research area, including those who may not have a strong statistical background and also help to attract statisticians interested in learning more about advanced topics.

This book shows important nonparametric and semiparametric problems in the area of multiple comparisons encountered in practical fields including medical and epidemiological applications and explains how to solve them in a *real-time* fashion, that is, we describe relevant EL-based statistical methodology, illustrate the methodology using real-life examples, and provide software code for solving the problems.

We aim to present general and powerful methods for constructing nonparametric/semiparametric procedures with properties that are approximate to those of optimal parametric techniques. We hope that these EL applications introduced in this book demonstrate the versatility and flexibility of the method to solve different problems in various data forms and statistical issues.

We would like to draw attentions of theoretical statisticians and practitioners in epidemiology or medicine to the necessity of new developments, extensions, and investigations related to the EL methodology and its applications.

Appendix

The Most Powerful Test

As discussed in Section 1.4, the most powerful statistical decision rule is to reject H_0 if and only if $\prod_{i=1}^{n} f_1(X_i)/f_0(X_i) \geq B$. The term *most powerful* induces to formally define how to compare statistical tests. Without loss of generality, as the ability to control the TIE rate of statistical tests has an essential role in statistical decision making, we compare tests with equivalent probabilities of the TIE, $\Pr_{H_0}\{\text{test rejects } H_0\} = \alpha$, where the subscript H_0

indicates that we consider the probability given that the hull hypothesis is correct. The level of significance α is the probability of making a TIE. In practice, the researcher should choose a value of α, e.g., $\alpha = 0.05$, before performing the test. Thus, we should compare the likelihood ratio test with δ, any decision rule based on $\{X_i, i = 1,\ldots,n\}$, setting up $\Pr_{H_0}\{\delta \text{ rejects } H_0\} = \alpha$, and $\Pr_{H_0}\left\{\prod_{i=1}^{n} f_1(X_i)/f_0(X_i) \geq B\right\} = \alpha$. This comparison is with respect to the power $\Pr_{H_1}\{\text{test rejects } H_0\}$. Note that to derive the mathematical expectation, in the context of a problem related to testing statistical hypotheses, one must define under H_0- or H_1-regime the expectation should be conducted. For example,

$$E_{H_1}\phi(X_1, X_2, \ldots X_n) = \int \phi(x_1, x_2, \ldots x_n) f_1(x_1, x_2, \ldots x_n) dx_1 dx_2 \ldots dx_n$$

$$= \int \phi(x_1, x_2, \ldots x_n) \prod_{i=1}^{n} f_1(x_i) \prod_{i=1}^{n} dx_i,$$

where the expectation is considered under the alternative hypothesis. The indicator $I\{C\}$ of the event C can be considered as a random variable with values 0 and 1. By virtue of the definition, the expected value of $I\{C\}$ is $EI\{C\} = 0 \times \Pr\{I\{C\} = 0\} + 1 \times \Pr\{I\{C\} = 1\} = \Pr\{I\{C\} = 1\} = \Pr\{C\}$. Taking into account the comments mentioned above, we derive the expectation under H_0 of the inequality (1.1), where $A = \prod_{i=1}^{n} f_1(X_i)/f_0(X_i)$, B is a test threshold, and δ represents any decision rule based on $\{X_i, i = 1,\ldots,n\}$. One can assume that $\delta = 0,1$ and when $\delta = 1$, we reject H_0. Thus, we obtain

$$E_{H_0}\left[\prod_{i=1}^{n} \frac{f_1(X_i)}{f_0(X_i)} I\left\{\prod_{j=i}^{n} \frac{f_1(X_i)}{f_0(X_i)} \geq B\right\}\right] - BE_{H_0}\left[I\left\{\prod_{i=1}^{n} \frac{f_1(X_i)}{f_0(X_i)} \geq B\right\}\right]$$

$$\geq E_{H_0}\left\{\prod_{i=1}^{n} \frac{f_1(X_i)}{f_0(X_i)} \delta\right\} - BE_{H_0}(\delta),$$

where $E_{H_0}(\delta) = E_{H_0}(I\{\delta = 1\}) = \Pr_{H_0}\{\delta = 1\} = \Pr_{H_0}\{\delta \text{ rejects } H_0\}$.

And hence

$$E_{H_0}\left[\prod_{i=1}^{n} \frac{f_1(X_i)}{f_0(X_i)} I\left\{\prod_{j=i}^{n} \frac{f_1(X_i)}{f_0(X_i)} \geq B\right\}\right] \geq E_{H_0}\left\{\prod_{i=1}^{n} \frac{f_1(X_i)}{f_0(X_i)} \delta\right\}, \quad \text{(A.1.1)}$$

Since we compare the tests with the fixed level of significance

$$E_{H_0}\left(I\left\{\prod_{i=1}^{n}\frac{f_1(X_i)}{f_0(X_i)}\geq B\right\}\right)=Pr_{H_0}\left\{\prod_{i=1}^{n}\frac{f_1(X_i)}{f_0(X_i)}\geq B\right\}=Pr_{H_0}\{\delta \text{ rejects } H_0\}=\alpha,$$

Consider

$$\begin{aligned}E_{H_0}\left(\prod_{i=1}^{n}\frac{f_1(X_i)}{f_0(X_i)}\delta\right)&=E_{H_0}\left(\prod_{i=1}^{n}\frac{f_1(X_i)}{f_0(X_i)}\delta(X_1,\ldots,X_n)\right)\\&=\int\prod_{i=1}^{n}\frac{f_1(x_i)}{f_0(x_i)}\delta(x_1,\ldots,x_n)f_0(x_1,\ldots,x_n)dx_1\ldots dx_n\\&=\int\frac{\prod_{i=1}^{n}f_1(x_i)}{\prod_{i=1}^{n}f_0(x_i)}\delta(x_1,\ldots,x_n)\prod_{i=1}^{n}f_0(x_i)dx_1\ldots dx_n\\&=\int\delta(x_1,\ldots,x_n)\prod_{i=1}^{n}f_1(x_i)dx_1\ldots dx_n\\&=E_{H_1}(\delta)=\Pr_{H_1}\{\delta \text{ rejects } H_0\}.\end{aligned}\tag{A.1.2}$$

Since δ represents any decision rule based on $\{X_i, i=1,\ldots,n\}$ including the likelihood ratio-based test, Equation (A.1.2) implies

$$E_{H_0}\left(\prod_{i=1}^{n}\frac{f_1(X_i)}{f_0(X_i)}I\left\{\prod_{j=1}^{n}\frac{f_1(X_i)}{f_0(X_i)}\geq B\right\}\right)=Pr_{H_1}\left\{\prod_{j=1}^{n}\frac{f_1(X_j)}{f_0(X_j)}\geq B\right\}.$$

Applying this equation and (A.1.2) to (A.1.1), we complete to prove that the likelihood ratio test is a most powerful statistical decision rule.

The Likelihood Ratio Property $f_{H_1}^{L}(u)=f_{H_0}^{L}(u)u$

In order to obtain this property, we consider

$$\begin{aligned}\Pr_{H_1}\{u-s\leq L\leq u\}&=E_{H_1}I\{u-s\leq L\leq u\}=\int I\{u-s\leq L\leq u\}f_{H_1}\\&=\int I\{u-s\leq L\leq u\}\frac{f_{H_1}}{f_{H_0}}f_{H_0}=\int I\{u-s\leq L\leq u\}Lf_{H_0}.\end{aligned}$$

This implies the inequalities

$$\Pr_{H_1}\{u-s\le L\le u\}\le\int I\{u-s\le L\le u\}uf_{H_0}=u\Pr_{H_0}\{u-s\le L\le u\}$$

and

$$\Pr_{H_1}\{u-s\le L\le u\}\ge\int I\{u-s\le L\le u\}(u-s)f_{H_0}=(u-s)\Pr_{H_0}\{u-s\le L\le u\}.$$

Dividing these inequalities by s and employing $s\to 0$, we get $f_{H_1}^{L}(u)=f_{H_0}^{L}(u)u$, where $f_{H_0}^{L}(u)$ and $f_{H_1}^{L}(u)$ are the density functions of the statistic $L=f_{H_1}/f_{H_0}$ under H_0 and H_1, respectively.

2

Basic Ingredients of the Empirical Likelihood

2.1 Introduction

As mentioned in Chapter 1, when using robust statistical testing methods, which minimize the assumptions regarding the underlying data distributions, it is important to still maintain a high level of efficiency when compared to their parametric counterparts. Toward this end, the recent biostatistical literature has shifted focus toward robust and efficient nonparametric and semiparametric developments of various "artificial" or *approximate* likelihood techniques. These methods have a wide variety of applications related to clinical experiments. Many nonparametric and semiparametric approximations to powerful parametric likelihood (PL) procedures have been used routinely in both statistical theory and practice. Well-known examples include the quasi-likelihood method, which are approximations of PLs via orthogonal functions, techniques based on quadratic artificial likelihood functions, and the local maximum likelihood methodology (Wedderburn, 1974; Fan et al., 1998; Claeskens and Hjort, 2004; Wang, 2006). Various studies have shown that "artificial" or approximate likelihood-based techniques efficiently incorporate information expressed through the data and have many of the same asymptotic properties as those derived from the corresponding PLs. The empirical likelihood (EL) method is one of a growing array of "artificial" or approximate likelihood-based methods currently in use in statistical practice (Owen, 1990). Interest and the resulting impact in EL methods continue to grow rapidly. Perhaps more importantly, EL methods now have various vital applications in expanding numbers of areas of clinical studies.

In this chapter we discuss the properties and performance of the EL methods relative to ordinary PL ratio-based procedures or other methods. Our desire to incorporate several recent developments and applications in these areas in an easy-to-use manner provides one of the main impetuses for this chapter. Also, toward the end of this chapter, we include brief discussions of some asymptotic properties of EL regarding bias and high-order power, interpretation of EL as a class of empirical goodness of fit tests, and comparison with bootstrapping. Finally, we conclude this chapter by introducing commonly used R functions and packages (R Development Core Team, 2014).

2.2 Classical Empirical Likelihood Methods

As background for the development of EL-type techniques, we first outline the classical EL approach. The classical EL takes the form $\prod_{i=1}^{n}(F(X_i)-F(X_i-))$, which is a functional of the cumulative distribution function F and independent identically distributed (i.i.d.) observations X_i, $i=1,\ldots,n$. This EL technique is *distribution function-based* (Owen, 1990). In the distribution-free setting, an empirical estimator of the likelihood takes the form of $L_p=\prod_{i=1}^{n}p_i$, where the components p_i, $i=1,\ldots,n$, are the probability weights. Values of pi, i = 1, n, can be found maximizing the likelihood L_p, provided that $\sum_{i=1}^{n}p_i=1$ and empirical constraints based on $X_1,\ldots,X_n$. For example, suppose we would like to test the hypothesis

$$H_0: Eg(X_1,\theta)=0 \text{ and } H_1: Eg(X_1,\theta)\neq 0. \tag{2.1}$$

where $g(.,.)$ is a given function and θ is a parameter. Then, in a nonparametric fashion, we define the EL function of the form

$$\mathrm{EL}(\theta)=L(X_1,\ldots,X_n\mid\theta)=\prod_{i=1}^{n}p_i, \tag{2.2}$$

where $\sum_{i=1}^{n}p_i=1$. Under the null hypothesis, the maximum likelihood approach requires one to find the values of the p_i's that maximize EL, given the empirical constraints $\sum_{i=1}^{n}p_i=1$ and $\sum_{i=1}^{n}p_i g(X_i,\theta)=0$ that present an empirical version of the condition under H_0 that $Eg(X_1,\theta)=0$ (the null hypothesis is assumed to be rejected when there are no $0<p_1,\ldots,p_n<1$ to satisfy the empirical constraints). In this case, using Lagrange multipliers, one can show that

$$\mathrm{EL}(\theta)=\sup_{0<p_1,p_2,\ldots,p_n<1,\sum p_i=1,\sum p_i g(X_i,\theta)=0}\prod_{i=1}^{n}p_i=\prod_{i=1}^{n}\left(n+\lambda g(X_i,\theta)\right)^{-1}, \tag{2.3}$$

where λ is a root of $\sum g(X_i,\theta)\left(n+\lambda g(X_i,\theta)\right)^{-1}=0$ (Owen, 1988; Also see Chapter 5 for a two-group approach for this type of derivations). As under H_1, the only constraint under consideration is $\sum p_i=1$, we have

$$\mathrm{EL}=\sup_{0<p_1,p_2,\ldots,p_n<1,\sum p_i=1}\prod_{i=1}^{n}p_i=\prod_{i=1}^{n}n^{-1}=(n)^{-n}. \tag{2.4}$$

Combining Equations (2.3) and (2.4), we obtain the EL ratio (ELR) test statistic $\mathrm{ELR}(\theta)=\mathrm{EL}/\mathrm{EL}(\theta)$ for the hypothesis test of H_0 versus H_1. For example, when the function $g(u,\theta)=u-\theta$, the null hypothesis corresponds to the expectation given above.

Owen (1990) showed that the nonparametric test statistic $2\log ELR(\theta)$ has an asymptotic chi-square distribution under the null hypothesis. This result illustrates that Wilks' Theorem-type results continue to hold in the context of this infinite-dimensional problem. Consequently, there are techniques for correcting forms of ELRs to improve the convergence rate of the null distributions of ELR test statistics to chi-square distributions. These techniques are similar to those applied in the field of parametric maximum likelihood ratio procedures (Vexler et al., 2009). The statement of the above-mentioned hypothesis testing can easily be inverted with respect to providing nonparametric confidence interval estimators.

In terms of the accessibility of this method, it should be noted that the number of EL software packages continues to expand, particularly the R-based software packages. For example, see the links to `library(emplik)` and `library(EL)`, R packages that include the R function `el.test()` and `EL.test()`. These simple R functions can be very useful for the EL analysis of data from clinical studies.

For an illustrative example, we revisit the high-density lipoprotein (HDL) cholesterol data shown in Figure 1.1 in Chapter 1. Now, we use the ELR test for means. The following R output shows the result of the empirical likelihood comparison between the means of the groups: X and Y. Note that the function `EL.means` in R package `EL` carries out a two-sample EL test.

```
library(EL)
EL.means(X,Y)
       Empirical likelihood mean difference test
data: X and Y
-2 * LogLikelihood = 3.547, p-value = 0.05965
95 percent confidence interval:
-0.4900842 19.0138090
sample estimates:
Mean difference
       10.17393
```

Perhaps, in this example, the ELR test outperforms the *t*-test that claims to reject the hypothesis E(X) = E(Y), when X and Y are the measurements related to the same group of patients.

The classical EL methodology has been shown to have properties that make it attractive for testing hypotheses regarding parameters (e.g., moments) of distributions (e.g., Owen, 1988; Qin and Lawless, 1994). However, practicing statisticians working on clinical experiments, e.g. case-control studies, commonly face a variety of distribution-free comparisons and/or evaluations over all distribution functions of complete and incomplete data subjected to different types of measurement errors. In this framework, the *density-based* empirical likelihood methodology figures prominently (Section 2.6).

For example, assume that we have a sample of i.i.d. measurements $X_1,\ldots,X_{25}$ simulated from the following schemes: (1) $X_i \sim N(0,1)$ and (2) $X_i = Z_i - 1$, where $Z_i \sim Exp(1)$, $i = 1,\ldots,n$. We would like to test $H_0: EX = 0$ versus $H_1: EX \neq 0$ at the $\alpha = 0.05$ significance level. For both scenarios, we fail to reject H_0 based on either the EL methodology or the t-test. However, in the latter case, the result of the t-test is not valid as the distributional assumption is not satisfied. The following code implements the procedures: Herein, we use function `el.test` in R package `emplik`.

```
library(emplik)
n<-25
## (1) generating the data from N(0,1)
X<-rnorm(n,0,1)
el.obj<-el.test(X,mu=0)
el.obj$Pval
[1] 0.1673519                    # p-value of one group EL test
t.test(X,mu=0)$p.value                     # p-value of t-test
[1] 0.2019836

## (2) generating the data from exp(1)-1
X<-rexp(n,rate=1)-1
el.obj<-el.test(X,mu=0)
el.obj$Pval
[1] 0.2043935
t.test(X,mu=0)$p.value
[1] 0.1463612
```

2.3 Techniques for Analyzing Empirical Likelihoods

In this section, we consider the hypothesis described at (2.1) and the simple form of the ELR test statistic defined previously via (2.3) and (2.4). The analysis is relatively clear and has the basic ingredients for more general cases. We posit that the following results can be associated with deriving different properties of EL-type procedures including the power and Type I error (TIE) rate analysis of the ELR test statistics.

Properties of many statistical quantities based on PLs can be studied by using the fact that PL functions are often highly peaked about their maximum values (e.g., DasGupta, 2008). The modern biostatistical literature considers a variety of semi- and nonparametric procedures created by proposing to use EL functions in efficient parametric schemes instead of PLs. For example, in this context, the results of Qin and Lawless (1994) have a remarkable utility with respect to operations with ELs in a similar manner to that of those related to parametric maximum likelihoods. The following lemma illustrates a strong similarity between behaviors of empirical and PL functions. Suppose the function $g(x,\theta)$ appeared in (2.3) and (2.4) is one differentiable with respect to the second argument θ, then we have the following result:

Lemma 2.1

Let θ_M be a root of the equation $n^{-1}\sum_{i=1}^{n} g(X_i,\theta_M)=0$, where $\partial g(X_i,\theta)/\partial\theta<0$ (or $\partial g(X_i,\theta)/\partial\theta>0$), for all i = 1, 2, …, n. Then the argument θ_M is a global maximum of the function

$$\text{EL}(\theta)=\max\left\{\prod_{i=1}^{n} p_i:\ 0<p_i<1, \sum_{i=1}^{n} p_i=1, \sum_{i=1}^{n} p_i g(X_i,\theta)=0\right\},$$

follows from the fact that it increases and decreases monotonically for $\theta<\theta_M$ and $\theta>\theta_M$, respectively.

The proof scheme of this fact is presented in Section 3.2.1.

For example, when $g(u,\theta)=u-\theta$, we obtain $\theta_M=\bar{X}=n^{-1}\sum_{i=1}^{n}(X_i)$; if, for a given function $z(u)$, $g(u,\theta)=z(u)-\theta^2, \theta>0$ then $\theta_M{}^2=n^{-1}\sum_{i=z}^{n} z(X_i)$.

2.3.1 Illustrative Comparison of Empirical Likelihood and Parametric Likelihood

Let $\mathbf{x}=\{X_1,\dots,X_n\}$ denote a random sample from the following distributions: (1) normal distribution $N(\theta,1)$, and (2) exponential (θ), where θ is the rate parameter. Define, in the normal case, the minus maximum log-likelihood ratio test statistic as

$$-\log \text{MLR}(\theta)=-\sum_{i=1}^{n}(X_i-\theta)^2/2+\sum_{i=1}^{n}\left(X_i-\bar{X}\right)^2/2$$

and the minus log-ELR test statistic for $E\left(X_1\right)=\theta$ as

$$-\log \text{ELR}(\theta)=-\sum_{i=1}^{n}\log\{1+\lambda(X_i-\theta)/n\},$$

where λ is a root of $\sum_{i=1}^{n}(X_i-\theta)\left(n+\lambda(X_i-\theta)\right)^{-1}=0$ and $\bar{X}=n^{-1}\sum_{i=1}^{n}X_i$. In the case of the exponential distribution, the minus maximum log-likelihood ratio test statistic is

$$-\log \text{MLR}(\theta)=n\log\theta-n\theta\bar{X}+n\log\bar{X}+n$$

and the minus log-ELR test statistic for $E\left(X_1\right)=(\theta)^{-1}$ is

$$-\log \text{ELR}(\theta)=-\sum_{i=1}^{n}\log\{1+\lambda(X_i-1/\theta)/n\},$$

where λ satisfies $\sum_{i=1}^{n}\left(X_i-1/\theta\right)\left(n+\lambda(X_i-1/\theta)\right)^{-1}=0$. Generating, $\mathbf{x}=\{X_1,\ldots,X_n\}$ from the distributions with $\theta=1$, we obtain Figure 2.1 that presents the plot of the parametric log-likelihood ratio and the log-ELRs versus the parameter θ based on samples of sample sizes $n=25,\ 50,\ 150$, where the solid line and the dashed line correspond to the log-ELR and the log-likelihood ratio when the underlying distribution is normal, respectively, whereas the dotted line and the dotted dash line represent the minus log-ELR and the minus log-likelihood ratio when the underlying distribution is exponential, respectively. Figure 2.1 illustrates Lemma 2.1. The figure shows that the ELR behaves in a similar manner to the PL ratio and approaches to the PL ratio asymptotically. Furthermore, as the sample size n increases, the log-ELR approximates the log-likelihood ratio well in the neighborhood of the maximum likelihood

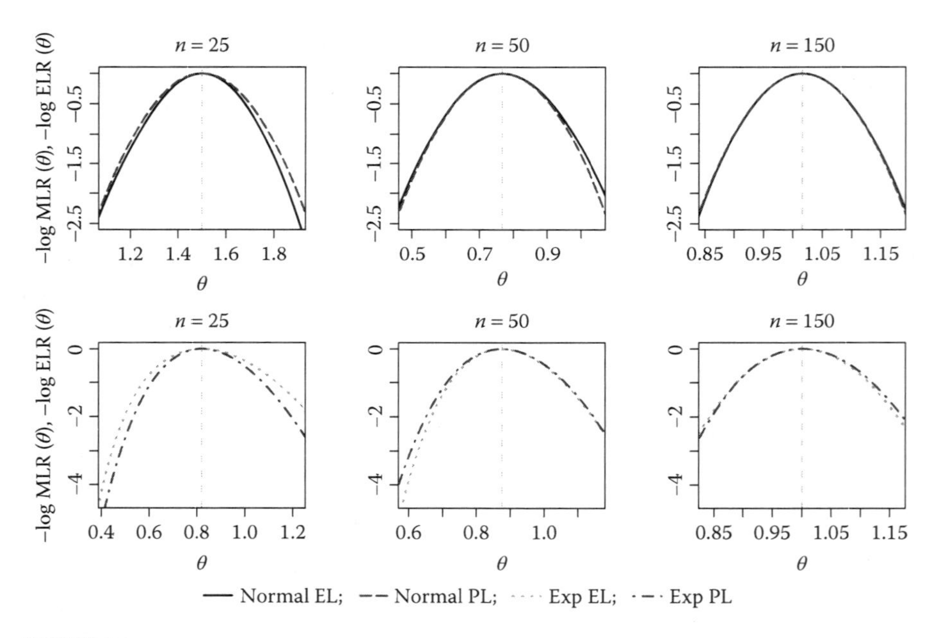

FIGURE 2.1
The log-empirical likelihood ratios (ELR) and the parametric log-likelihood ratios (PL) based on samples of sample sizes $n=25, 50$, and 150, where the solid line and the dashed line represent the log-empirical likelihood ratios and the log-likelihood ratios when the underlying distribution is normal, respectively, whereas the dotted line and the dotted dash line represent the log-empirical likelihood ratio and the log-likelihood ratio when the underlying distribution is exponential, respectively.

estimator. The log-empirical likelihood (ratio) increases monotonically up to the maximum likelihood estimator and then decreases monotonically. The R code for implementation of the procedure is provided in the Appendix.

Turning to task of developing asymptotic evaluations of methods based on ELs, we provide the following proposition. Without loss of generality and for simplicity of notation, we set $g(u,\theta) = u - \theta$ in the definition of the function $\mathrm{ELR}(\theta)$ via (2.2) and (2.3). Thus, $\mathrm{EL}(\theta) = \prod_{i=1}^{n} p_i$, $\log \mathrm{ELR}(\theta) = \sum_{i=1}^{n} \log\{1 + \lambda(X_i - \theta)/n\}$ with $p_i = \{n + \lambda(X_i - \theta)\}^{-1}$, where λ is a root of

$$\sum_{i=1}^{n} (X_i - \theta)\left(n + \lambda(X_i - \theta)\right)^{-1} = 0. \tag{2.5}$$

Note that $\lambda = \lambda\ (\theta)$ is a function of θ. Then, by defining $\lambda' = d\lambda(\theta)/d\theta$, $\lambda'' = d^2\lambda(\theta)/d\theta^2$, $\lambda^{(k)} = d^k\lambda(\theta)/d\theta^k$, $k = 3,4$ and using Equation (2.5), one can show:

Proposition 2.1

We have the following expressions:

$$d \log \mathrm{ELR}(\theta)/d\theta = -\lambda(\theta).$$

$$\lambda' = -n\sum_{i=1}^{n} p_i^2 \Big/ \sum_{i=1}^{n} (X_i - \theta)^2 p_i^2,$$

$$\lambda'' = -\left\{2\lambda'^2 \sum_{i=1}^{n} (X_i - \theta)^3 p_i^3 + 4n\lambda' \sum_{i=1}^{n} (X_i - \theta) p_i^3 - 2n\lambda \sum_{i=1}^{n} p_i^3\right\} \Big/ \sum_{i=1}^{n} (X_i - \theta)^2 p_i^2,$$

$$\lambda^{(3)} = \left\{6\lambda'\lambda'' \sum_{i=1}^{n} (X_i - \theta)^3 p_i^3 + 6n\lambda'' \sum_{i=1}^{n} (X_i - \theta) p_i^3 - 6\lambda'^3 \sum_{i=1}^{n} (X_i - \theta)^4 p_i^4 - 18n\lambda'^2 \sum_{i=1}^{n} (X_i - \theta)^2 p_i^4 + 12n\lambda' \sum_{i=1}^{n} p_i^3 - (18n^2\lambda' + 6n\lambda^2) \sum_{i=1}^{n} p_i^4\right\} \Big/ \sum_{i=1}^{n} (X_i - \theta)^2 p_i^2,$$

$$\lambda^{(4)} = \Big\{ \big(8\lambda'\lambda^{(3)} + 6\lambda''^2\big) \sum_{i=1}^{n} (X_i - \theta)^3 p_i^3 + 8n\lambda^{(3)} \sum_{i=1}^{n} (X_i - \theta) p_i^3$$

$$- 36\lambda'^2\lambda'' \sum_{i=1}^{n} (X_i - \theta)^4 p_i^4 - 72n\lambda'\lambda'' \sum_{i=1}^{n} (X_i - \theta)^2 p_i^4$$

$$- (36n^2\lambda'' - 18n\lambda\lambda') \sum_{i=1}^{n} p_i^4 + 24n\lambda'' \sum_{i=1}^{n} p_i^3 + 24\lambda'^4 \sum_{i=1}^{n} (X_i - \theta)^5 p_i^5$$

$$+ 96n\lambda'^3 \sum_{i=1}^{n} (X_i - \theta)^3 p_i^5 - 72n\lambda' \sum_{i=1}^{n} (X_i - \theta) p_i^4$$

$$+ (144n^2\lambda'^2 + 24n\lambda^2\lambda') \sum_{i=1}^{n} (X_i - \theta) p_i^5 - (72n^2\lambda\lambda' + 24n\lambda^3) \sum_{i=1}^{n} p_i^5 \Big\} \Big/$$

$$\sum_{i=1}^{n} (X_i - \theta)^2 p_i^2.$$

This proposition can support a variety of evaluations of $\mathrm{ELR}(\theta)$ type procedures. To show the relevant examples, we should note that $\log \mathrm{ELR}(\theta_M) = 0$, as, in this case, $p_i = 1/n$, for all i, and $\mathrm{EL}(\theta_M) = \mathrm{EL}$. It is also clear that, when $\theta = \theta_M$, $\lambda(\theta) = 0$, as $p_i = 1/n$, $i = 1, \ldots, n$ maximize $\mathrm{EL} \geq \mathrm{EL}(\theta)$, for all θ and satisfy automatically the constraint $\sum p_i g(X_i, \theta) = 0$, when $\theta = \theta_M$, by virtue of the definition of θ_M. Thus, one can use Proposition 2.1 to obtain the Taylor expansion for the function $\log \mathrm{ELR}(\theta)$ at argument $\theta_M = \bar{X}$, in the form of

$$\log \mathrm{ELR}(\theta)$$

$$\approx \log \mathrm{ELR}(\bar{X}) + (\theta - \bar{X}) \left.\frac{d \log \mathrm{ELR}(\bar{X})}{d\theta}\right|_{\theta = \bar{X}} + \frac{(\theta - \bar{X})^2}{2!} \left.\frac{d^2 \log \mathrm{ELR}(\bar{X})}{d\theta^2}\right|_{\theta = \bar{X}}$$

$$+ \frac{(\theta - \bar{X})^3}{3!} \left.\frac{d^3 \log \mathrm{ELR}(\bar{X})}{d\theta^3}\right|_{\theta = \bar{X}}$$

$$= \frac{1}{2}\left(n^{0.5}(\theta - \bar{X})\right)^2 \Big/ \left[\frac{1}{n} \sum_{i=1}^{n} (X_i - \bar{X})^2\right] + \frac{1}{3} n(\theta - \bar{X})^3 \Big/ \left[\frac{1}{n} \sum_{i=1}^{n} (X_i - \bar{X})^2\right]^3.$$

This approximation depicts Wilks's Theorem when $\theta = EX_1$. (In the case of $\theta = EX_1$ and $n \to \infty$, $n^{0.5}(\theta - \bar{X})$ has a normal distribution, $n(\theta - \bar{X})^3 \xrightarrow{p} 0$ and $\sum_{i=1}^{n} ((X_i - \bar{X})^2 / n \to \mathrm{var}(X_1))$. Using Proposition 2.1 to figure more terms in the Taylor expansion can provide high-order approximations to the null distribution of the ELR test, e.g., to obtain the Bartlett correction of the ELR structure (e.g., Vexler et al., 2009). Under the alternative hypothesis $\theta \neq EX_1$, the approximation above shows the power of the ELR test.

Lazar and Mykland (1998) considered a general form of ELRs and the case where $|\theta - EX_1| \sim O(n^{-0.5})$. The authors compared the local power of EL to that of an ordinary PL. Their notable research shows that there is no loss of efficiency in using EL model up to a second-order approximation.

In a similar manner to Proposition 2.1, more complicated ELR structures can be evaluated. For example, one can consider the null hypothesis: $H_0 : E(X_1) = \theta_1$ and $E(X_1^2) = \theta_2$. In this case, under the null hypothesis, the EL function is given as

$$\mathrm{EL}(\theta_1, \theta_2) = \max\left\{\prod_{i=1}^{n} p_i : \quad \sum\nolimits_{i=1}^{n} p_i = 1, \sum\nolimits_{i=1}^{n} p_i X_i = \theta_1, \sum\nolimits_{i=1}^{n} p_i X_i^2 = \theta_2\right\}.$$

Then using the Lagrangian

$$\Lambda = \sum\nolimits_{i=1}^{n} \log p_i + \lambda\left(1 - \sum\nolimits_{i=1}^{n} p_i\right) + \lambda_1\left(\theta_1 - \sum\nolimits_{i=1}^{n} p_i X_i\right) + \lambda_2\left(\left(\theta_2 - \sum\nolimits_{i=1}^{n} p_i X_i^2\right),\right.$$

we obtain $p_i = \{n + \lambda_1(X_i - \theta_1) + \lambda_2(X_i^2 - \theta_2)\}^{-1}$, where λ_1 and λ_2 are roots of $\sum(X_i - \theta_1)p_i = 0$ and $\sum(X_i^2 - \theta_2)p_i = 0$. The Appendix presents several results that are similar to those related to the evaluations of ELR(θ) mentioned above.

2.4 In Case of the Presence of Extra Estimating Equation Information

Qin and Lawless (1994) considered a case that p-dimensional parameter θ is of interest, yet the information about θ consists of r ($\geq p$) distinctive independent estimating functions in a form of

$$E\{g_j(x, \theta)\} = 0, \ j = 1, \ldots, r,$$

where g_j, $j = 1,\ldots,r$, are is continuous in θ and at least two times differentiable. The EL is obtained by maximizing $\prod_{i=1}^{n} p_i$ under the constraints

$$0 < p_i < 1, \ \sum\nolimits_{i=1}^{n} p_i = 1, \ \sum\nolimits_{i=1}^{n} p_i g(X_i, \theta) = 0,$$

where $g(X_i, \theta) = (g_1(X_i, \theta), \ldots, g_r(X_i, \theta))^T$. We find p_i using the Lagrange formula,

$$\sum_i \log p_i + \lambda\left(1 - \sum_i p_i\right) - nt^T \sum_i p_i g(x_i, \theta),$$

where λ and t are the Lagrange multipliers. This leads to $p_i = 1/\{n(1+t^T g(x_i,\theta))\}$ Thus, the ELR statistic is

$$l_E(\theta) = \sum_{i=1}^{n} \log[1 + t^T(\theta)\, g(x_i, \theta)], \tag{2.6}$$

where $t = t(\theta)$. Using the fact $\sum p_i = 1$ and $p_i = 1/\{n(1+t^T g(x_i,\theta))\}$, the Lagrange multiplier can be expressed as

$$t(\theta) \simeq \left[\frac{1}{n}\sum_{i=1}^{n} g(x_i,\theta) g^T(x_i,\theta)\right]^{-1} \left[\frac{1}{n}\sum_{i=1}^{n} g(x_i,\theta)\right] \text{ as } n \to \infty. \tag{2.7}$$

Using (2.7) and the Taylor expansion of the first two terms of $l_E(\theta)$, we can show that

$$l_E(\theta) \simeq \frac{n}{2}\left[\frac{1}{n}\sum_{i=1}^{n} g(x_i,\theta)\right]^T \left[\frac{1}{n}\sum_{i=1}^{n} g(x_i,\theta) g^T(x_i,\theta)\right]^{-1} \left[\frac{1}{n}\sum_{i=1}^{n} g(x_i,\theta)\right]. \tag{2.8}$$

Suppose that the maximum EL estimator (MELE) $\tilde{\theta}$ maximizes $l_E(\theta)$. Qin and Lawless (1994) showed that

$$\sqrt{n}(\tilde{\theta} - \theta_0) \to N(0, V), \tag{2.9}$$

where

$$V = \left[E\left(\frac{\partial g}{\partial \theta}\right)(Egg^T)^{-1} E\left(\frac{\partial g}{\partial \theta}\right)\right]^{-1}.$$

The following is the sketch of the proof. More details can be found in Qin and Lawless (1994).

2.4.1 Sketch of the Proof of Equation (2.9)

Say, the estimators $\tilde{\theta}$ and $\tilde{t}$ maximize $l_E(\theta)$ in $\|\theta - \theta_0\| \le n^{-1/3}$. Based on $\sum_{i=1}^{n} p_i g(X_i, \theta) = 0$ and Equation (2.6), we can show

$$Q_{1n}(\tilde{\theta}, \tilde{t}) = \frac{1}{n}\sum_i \frac{1}{1 + \tilde{t}^T(\tilde{\theta})\, g(x_i, \tilde{\theta})} g(x_i, \tilde{\theta}) = 0,$$

$$Q_{2n}(\tilde{\theta}, \tilde{t}) = \frac{1}{n}\sum_i \frac{1}{1 + \tilde{t}^T(\tilde{\theta})\, g(x_i, \tilde{\theta})} \left(\frac{\partial g(x_i, \tilde{\theta})}{\partial \tilde{\theta}}\right)^T \tilde{t} = 0.$$

Expanding $Q_{1n}(\tilde{\theta},\tilde{t})$ and $Q_{2n}(\tilde{\theta},\tilde{t})$ using the Taylor expansion, we have

$$
\begin{aligned}
0 &= Q_{1n}(\tilde{\theta},\tilde{t}) = Q_{1n}(\theta_0,0) + \frac{\partial Q_{1n}(\theta_0,0)}{\partial\theta}(\tilde{\theta}-\theta_0) + \frac{\partial Q_{1n}(\theta_0,0)}{\partial t^T}(\tilde{t}-0) + o_p(\delta_n),\\
0 &= Q_{2n}(\tilde{\theta},\tilde{t}) = Q_{2n}(\theta_0,0) + \frac{\partial Q_{2n}(\theta_0,0)}{\partial\theta}(\tilde{\theta}-\theta_0) + \frac{\partial Q_{2n}(\theta_0,0)}{\partial t^T}(\tilde{t}-0) + o_p(\delta_n),
\end{aligned}
\tag{2.10}
$$

where $\delta_n = \left\|\tilde{\theta}-\theta_0\right\| + \left\|\tilde{t}\right\|$ and

$$
\frac{\partial Q_{1n}(\theta,0)}{\partial\theta} = \frac{1}{n}\sum_i \frac{\partial g(x_i,\theta)}{\partial\theta},\quad \frac{\partial Q_{1n}(\theta,0)}{\partial t^T} = -\frac{1}{n}\sum_i g(x_i,\theta)g(x_i,\theta)^T,
$$

$$
\frac{\partial Q_{2n}(\theta,0)}{\partial\theta} = 0,\ \frac{\partial Q_{2n}(\theta,0)}{\partial t^T} = \frac{1}{n}\sum_i \left(\frac{\partial g(x_i,\theta)}{\partial\theta}\right)^T.
$$

The system of Equations (2.10) can be expressed as

$$
\begin{pmatrix} \tilde{t} \\ \tilde{\theta}-\theta_0 \end{pmatrix} = S_n^{-1}\begin{pmatrix} -Q_{1n}(\theta_0,0)+o_p(\delta_n) \\ o_p(\delta_n) \end{pmatrix},
\tag{2.11}
$$

where

$$
S_n = \begin{pmatrix} \dfrac{\partial Q_{1n}}{\partial t^T} & \dfrac{\partial Q_{1n}}{\partial\theta} \\ \dfrac{\partial Q_{2n}}{\partial t^T} & 0 \end{pmatrix}_{(\theta_0,0)} \to \begin{pmatrix} -E(gg^T) & E\left(\dfrac{\partial g}{\partial\theta}\right) \\ E\left(\dfrac{\partial g}{\partial\theta}\right)^T & 0 \end{pmatrix} \triangleq \begin{pmatrix} S_{11} & S_{12} \\ S_{21} & 0 \end{pmatrix} \triangleq S \text{ as } n\to\infty.
$$

The relationship (2.11) leads to

$$
\sqrt{n}(\tilde{\theta}-\theta_0) = S^{21}\sqrt{n}Q_{1n}(\theta_0,0) + o_p(1),
$$

where S^{21} is the component corresponding to S_{21} in the block inverse matrix of S. Using the central limit theorem, we have the result (2.9).

Under $H_0:\theta=\theta_0$, using (2.8) and (2.9), Qin and Lawless (1994) showed the ELR test can be expressed as

$$
W(\theta_0) = 2l_E(\theta_0) - 2l_E(\tilde{\theta}) \simeq nQ_{1n}^T(\theta_0,0)S_{11}^{-1}S_{12}(S_{21}S_{11}^{-1}S_{12})^{-1}S_{21}S_{11}^{-1}Q_{1n}^T(\theta_0,0),
$$

where $-\sqrt{n}\,S_{11}^{-1/2}Q_{1n}^T(\theta_0,0)$ converges to a standard multivariate normal distribution and $S_{11}^{-1/2}S_{12}(S_{21}S_{11}^{-1}S_{12})^{-1}S_{21}S_{11}^{-1/2}$ is symmetric and idempotent matrix. This result leads to the fact that $W(\theta_0)$ converges to χ_p^2 distribution as

$n \to \infty$. In addition, Qin and Lawless (1984) showed that, if $H_0 : \theta_1 = \theta_{1,0}$ where θ_1 is the parameter that consists of $q\ (< p)$ elements of $\theta = (\theta_1^T, \theta_2^T)^T$,

$$W(\theta_{1,0}) = 2l_E\left((\theta_{1,0}, \tilde{\theta}_{2,0})\right) - 2l_E(\tilde{\theta}),$$

has χ_q^2 distribution as $n \to \infty$.

Lopez et al. (2009) proved that $W(\theta_0)$ converges to χ_p^2 distribution as $n \to \infty$ when the estimating equation functions may not be smooth functions.

2.5 Some Helpful Properties

In this section we show several simple propositions that can assist in analyzing empirical likelihood-type procedures. For example, the remainder term in the approximation

$$\log\{\text{ELR}(\theta)\} \approx \frac{1}{2}\left(n^{0.5}(\theta - \bar{X})\right)^2 \Big/ \left[\frac{1}{n}\sum\nolimits_{i=1}^{n}(X_i - \bar{X})^2\right] + \frac{1}{3}n(\theta - \bar{X})^3 \Big/ \left[\frac{1}{n}\sum\nolimits_{i=1}^{n}(X_i - \bar{X})^2\right]^3,$$

when $\text{ELR}(\theta) = n^{-n}\left(\text{EL}(\theta)\right)^{-1}$,

$$\text{EL}(\theta) = \sup_{0<p_1,p_2,\ldots,p_n<1, \sum p_i = 1, \sum p_i g(X_i,\theta)=0} \prod_{i=1}^{n} p_i = \prod_{i=1}^{n}\left(n + \lambda(X_i - \theta)\right)^{-1}, g(u,\theta) = u - \theta$$

with $\lambda = \lambda(\theta)$, which is a root of $\sum (X_i - \theta)\left(n + \lambda(X_i - \theta)\right)^{-1} = 0$, can be evaluated using the propositions presented in this section. The analysis is relatively clear and has the basic ingredients for more general cases.

Proposition 2.2

Assume $E\left(|X_1|^3\right) < \infty$. *Then* $\max_{i=1,\ldots,n}|X_i| = o_p\left(n^{1/3+\varepsilon}\right)$, *for all* $\varepsilon > 0$.

Proof

Chebyshev's inequality provides

$$\Pr\left(\max_{i=1,\ldots,n}|X_i| \geq n^{1/3+\varepsilon}\right) \leq \sum_{i=1}^{n}\Pr\left(|X_i| \geq n^{1/3+\varepsilon}\right) \leq \sum_{i=1}^{n}\frac{E|X_i|^3}{n^{1+3\varepsilon}} = \frac{E|X_1|^3}{n^{3\varepsilon}} \xrightarrow[n\to\infty]{} 0.$$

This completes the proof.

In many cases, while analyzing EL-type procedures, we need to evaluate forms similar to $\lambda(\theta)X_i, \lambda'(\theta)X_i = X_i(d\lambda(\theta)/d\theta)$ etc., for all θ. Proposition 2.2 shows $X_i = o_p(n^{1/3+\varepsilon}), i = 1,...,n$. The following results examine $\lambda(\theta)$. Suppose we would like to test the hypothesis

$$H_0 : E\{g(X_1,\theta)\} = 0 \quad \text{versus} \quad H_1 : E\{g(X_1,\theta)\} \neq 0,$$

where $g(.,.)$ is a given differentiable function and θ is a parameter. In this case, the empirical likelihood is

$$\text{EL}(\theta) = \sup_{0<p_1,p_2,...,p_n<1, \sum p_i = 1, \sum p_i g(X_i,\theta)=0} \prod_{i=1}^{n} p_i = \prod_{i=1}^{n} \left(n + \lambda g(X_i,\theta)\right)^{-1},$$

where λ is a root of $\sum g(X_i,\theta)\left(n + \lambda g(X_i,\theta)\right)^{-1} = 0$. Then we obtain the following propositions.

Proposition 2.3

We have that $\lambda \geq 0$ if and only if $\sum_{i=1}^{n} g(X_i,\theta) \geq 0$ and $\lambda < 0$ if and only if $\sum_{i=1}^{n} g(X_i,\theta) < 0$.

Proof

The forms $p_i = \{n + \lambda g(X_i,\theta)\}^{-1}$, $i = 1,..,n$, and $n^{-n} \geq \prod_{i=1}^{n} p_i$ $(p_i = n^{-1}, i = 1,..,n,$ maximize $\prod_{i=1}^{n} p_i$ provided that $0 < p_1,...,p_n < 1, \sum p_i = 1)$ imply that

$$0 \leq \log\left(n^{-n} \Big/ \prod_{i=1}^{n} p_i\right) = \sum_{i=1}^{n} \log\{1 + \lambda g(X_i,\theta)/n\}.$$

Using the inequality $\log(1+s) \leq s$ for $s > -1$, we obtain

$$0 \leq \sum_{i=1}^{n} \log\{1 + \lambda g(X_i,\theta)/n\} \leq \sum_{i=1}^{n} \lambda g(X_i,\theta)/n = \lambda \sum_{i=1}^{n} g(X_i,\theta)/n.$$

This completes the proof.

Proposition 2.4

The Lagrange multiplier λ satisfies $\lambda = \sum_{i=1}^{n} g(X_i,\theta) / \sum_{i=1}^{n} \{g(X_i,\theta)\}^2 p_i$.

Proof

The constraint $\sum_{i=1}^{n} g(X_i,\theta)p_i = 0$ with $p_i = \{n+\lambda g(X_i,\theta)\}^{-1}, i=1,...,n,$ implies that

$$\begin{aligned}\sum_{i=1}^{n} g(X_i,\theta) &= \sum_{i=1}^{n}\{g(X_i,\theta)(1-p_i)\}+\sum_{i=1}^{n}\{g(X_i,\theta)p_i\}\\ &=\sum_{i=1}^{n} g(X_i,\theta)(1-p_i)\\ &=\sum_{i=1}^{n} g(X_i,\theta)\left\{\frac{n+\lambda g(X_i,\theta)-1}{n+\lambda g(X_i,\theta)}\right\}\\ &= n\sum_{i=1}^{n} g(X_i,\theta)p_i+\lambda\sum_{i=1}^{n} g(X_i,\theta)^2 p_i-\sum_{i=1}^{n} g(X_i,\theta)p_i\\ &=\lambda\sum_{i=1}^{n}\{g(X_i,\theta)\}^2 p_i.\end{aligned}$$

This completes the proof.

Proposition 2.5

If $\lambda \ge 0$, *we have* $0 \le \lambda \le n\sum_{i=1}^{n} g(X_i,\theta)\left[\sum_{i=1}^{n}\{g(X_i,\theta)\}^2 I\{g(X_i,\theta)<0\}\right]^{-1}$; *if* $\lambda < 0$, *we have* $n\sum_{i=1}^{n} g(X_i,\theta)\left[\sum_{i=1}^{n}\{g(X_i,\theta)\}^2 I\{g(X_i,\theta)>0\}\right]^{-1} \le \lambda < 0$, *where* $I\{.\}$ *is the indicator function.*

Proof

Having $\lambda \ge 0$, we obtain

$$\begin{aligned}\sum_{i=1}^{n}\{g(X_i,\theta)\}^2 p_i &\ge \sum_{i=1}^{n}\left[g(X_i,\theta)^2 p_i I\{g(X_i,\theta)<0\}\right]\\ &=\sum_{i=1}^{n}\left[\{g(X_i,\theta)\}^2\frac{I\{g(X_i,\theta)<0\}}{n+\lambda g(X_i,\theta)}\right]\\ &\ge\sum_{i=1}^{n}\left[\{g(X_i,\theta)\}^2\frac{1}{n}I\{g(X_i,\theta)<0\}\right],\end{aligned}$$

where $p_i = \{n+\lambda g(X_i,\theta)\}^{-1}, i = 1,\ldots,n.$

Applying this result and Proposition 2.3 to Proposition 2.4 yields

$$0 \le \lambda < n\sum_{i=1}^{n} g(X_i,\theta)\left[\sum_{i=1}^{n}\{g(X_i,\theta)\}^2 I(g(X_i,\theta)<0)\right]^{-1}.$$

It follows similarly that when $\lambda < 0$,

$$n\sum_{i=1}^{n} g(X_i,\theta)\left[\sum_{i=1}^{n}\{g(X_i,\theta)\}^2 I\{g(X_i,\theta)>0\}\right]^{-1} < \lambda < 0.$$

This completes the proof.

Proposition 2.5 provides the exact non-asymptotic bounds for λ. Owen (1988) used very complicated considerations to obtain the approximate bounds for λ as $n \to \infty$. Proposition 2.5 immediately demonstrates that, for all $\varepsilon > 0$, $\lambda = o_p\left(n^{1/2+\varepsilon}\right)$ under H_0, as the bounds presented in Proposition 2.5 are based on the sums of i.i.d. random variables. The above propositions can be useful in the context of numerical computations of ELs, providing, e.g., the exact bounds for λ that is a numerical solution of $\sum g(X_i,\theta)\left(n+\lambda g(X_i,\theta)\right)^{-1} = 0$.

Proposition 2.6

Since the probability weighs $p_i = \left(n+\lambda g(X_i,\theta)\right)^{-1}, i = 1,\ldots,n$, *we have the properties*

$$\sum g(X_i,\theta)^2 p_i^2 = -\frac{n}{\lambda^2} + \frac{n^2}{\lambda^2}\sum p_i^2 \text{ and } \sum_{i=1}^{n} p_i^2 \ge n^{-1}.$$

Proof

By virtue of $\sum p_i = 1$, it is clear that

$$0 \le \sum g(X_i,\theta)^2 p_i^2 = \frac{1}{\lambda^2}\sum \frac{\lambda^2 g(X_i,\theta)^2}{\{n+\lambda g(X_i,\theta)\}^2} = \frac{1}{\lambda^2}\sum \frac{\lambda^2 g(X_i,\theta)^2 + 2n\lambda g(X_i,\theta) + n^2}{\{n+\lambda g(X_i,\theta)\}^2}$$

$$-\frac{1}{\lambda^2}\sum \frac{2n\lambda g(X_i,\theta)+n^2}{\{n+\lambda g(X_i,\theta)\}^2} = \frac{n}{\lambda^2} - \frac{1}{\lambda^2}\sum \frac{2n\lambda g(X_i,\theta)+n^2}{\{n+\lambda g(X_i,\theta)\}^2},$$

where

$$\frac{n}{\lambda^2} - \frac{1}{\lambda^2}\sum \frac{2n\{\lambda g(X_i,\theta)+n\} - 2n^2 + n^2}{\{n+\lambda g(X_i,\theta)\}^2} = \frac{n}{\lambda^2} - \frac{2n}{\lambda^2}\sum p_i + \frac{n^2}{\lambda^2}\sum p_i^2 \text{ and } \sum p_i = 1.$$

Thus, we obtain $-\frac{n}{\lambda^2}+\frac{n^2}{\lambda^2}\sum p_i^2 \geq 0$. This completes the proof.

For example, consider the equation $\sum g(X_i,\theta)\left(n+\lambda g(X_i,\theta)\right)^{-1}=0$. We have

$$\frac{d}{d\theta}\sum \frac{g(X_i,\theta)}{\left(n+\lambda g(X_i,\theta)\right)}=0$$

which implies

$$\sum \frac{g'(X_i,\theta)\left(n+\lambda g(X_i,\theta)\right)-\lambda' g(X_i,\theta)^2-\lambda g'(X_i,\theta)g'(X_i,\theta)}{\left(n+\lambda g(X_i,\theta)\right)^2}=0.$$

Then

$$\sum \frac{g'(X_i,\theta)n-\lambda' g(X_i,\theta)^2}{\left(n+\lambda g(X_i,\theta)\right)^2}=0.$$

This result leads to

$$\lambda' = \frac{n\sum_{i=1}^{n} g'(X_i,\theta)p_i^2}{\sum_{i=1}^{n} g(X_i,\theta)^2 p_i^2}.$$

In the case with $g(u,\theta)=u-\theta$, one can use Proposition 2.6 to obtain the inequality:

$$\lambda' = -\frac{n\sum_{i=1}^{n} p_i^2}{\sum_{i=1}^{n}(X_i-\theta)^2 p_i^2} \leq -\frac{1}{\sum_{i=1}^{n}(X_i-\theta)^2 p_i^2}.$$

2.6 Density-Based Empirical Likelihood Methods

According to the Neyman–Pearson Lemma, density-based likelihood ratios can provide uniformly most powerful tests. Using this as a starting point, Vexler et al. (2010, 2013b) proposed an alternative to the *distribution function-based* EL methodology. The authors employed the approximate density-based likelihood, which has the following form:

$$L_f=\prod_{i=1}^{n} f(X_i)=\prod_{i=1}^{n} f_i,\quad f_i=f(X_{(i)}),$$

where $X_{(1)} \leq X_{(2)} \leq \ldots \leq X_{(n)}$ are the order statistics based on $X_1,\ldots,X_n$, and $f_1,\ldots,f_n$ take on the values that maximize L_f given empirical constraints corresponding to $\int f(u)du = 1$. This density-based EL approach was used successfully to construct efficient entropy-based goodness of fit test procedures (Vexler and Gurevich, 2010; Vexler et al., 2011b; Vexler and Yu, 2011). The density-based EL methodology has been satisfactorily applied to develop a test for symmetry based on paired data. This test significantly outperforms classical procedures. Vexler and Yu (2011) extended the density-based EL approach to a two-sample nonparametric likelihood ratio test. Vexler et al. (2012a) used the density-based EL concept to present two-group comparison principles based on bivariate data with a missing pattern as a consequence of data collection procedures. The density-based EL methods were used to efficiently address nonparametric problems of complex composite hypothesis testing in children, in social/behavioral studies based on randomized prospective experiments (e.g., Gurevich and Vexler, 2011). In many practical settings, the density-based ELRs can provide simple and exact tests. Some distinctive characteristics of the density-based EL method test statistic as compared to the typical EL approach are summarized in Table 2.1 (Owen, 1988; Yu et al., 2011).

We note that Table 2.1 cannot reflect all relevant EL constructions. For example, Hall and Owen developed large-sample methods for constructing *distribution function-based* EL confidence bands in problems of nonparametric density estimation (Hall and Owen, 1993). Einmahl and McKeague (2003) proposed to localize the *distribution function-based* EL approach using one or more *time* variables implicit in the given null hypothesis. Integrating the log-likelihood ratio over those variables, the authors constructed exact-test procedures for detecting a change in distribution, testing for symmetry about zero, testing for exponentiality, and testing for independence.

TABLE 2.1

The comparison of the classical EL and density-based EL approaches

Characteristics	**The Classical EL Method**[a]	**The Density-Based EL Method**
Construction of the likelihood function	Distribution-based	Density-based
Usage of Lagrange multipliers method	Yes	Yes
Usage of constraints for maximization	Yes	Yes
Common focus of the test	Parameters (e.g., moments)	Overall distributions
Critical value	Asymptotic	Exact
The form of the test statistic	Numeric approach is required for calculate values of Lagrange multipliers	No numeric approach

[a] Owen (1988); Yu et al. (2011).

It is a common practice to conduct medical trials to compare a new therapy with a standard of care based on paired data consisting of pre- and post-treatment measurements. In such cases, there is often a great interest in identifying treatment effects within each therapy group and in detecting a between-group difference. Nonparametric comparisons between distributions of new therapy and control groups, as well as detecting treatment effects within each group, may be based on multiple-hypothesis tests. For this purpose, one can create relevant tests combining, e.g., the Kolmogorov–Smirnov test and the Wilcoxon signed-rank test. The use of the classical procedures commonly requires complex considerations about combining the known nonparametric tests, preserving the TIE rate control, and maintaining reasonable power of the resulting test. Alternatively, the density-based ELR technique provides a direct distribution-free approach for efficiently analyzing a variety of tasks occurring in clinical trials. The density-based EL method can easily be applied to test nonparametrically for different composite hypotheses. In this case, the density-based EL approach implies a standard scheme to develop highly efficient procedures, approximating nonparametrically the most powerful Neyman–Pearson test rules, given aims of clinical studies. For example, Vexler et al. (2012a) developed a density-based ELR methodology that was efficiently used to compare two therapy strategies for treating children's attention deficit/hyperactivity disorder and severe mood dysregulation. It was demonstrated that various composite hypotheses in a paired data setting (e.g., before vs. after treatment) can be tested with the density-based ELR tests, which give more emphasis to the overall distributional difference rather than to certain location parameter differences.

The R software can be employed to implement a computer program that realizes a density-based EL strategy. For example, programs of this type are presented in the *Statistics in Medicine* journal's Web domain:

http://onlinelibrary.wiley.com/doi/10.1002/sim.4467/suppinfo

Miecznikowski et al. (2013) developed the R package "dbEmpLikeGOF" for nonparametric density-based likelihood ratio tests for goodness of fit and two-sample comparisons. See also

http://cran.r-project.org/web/packages/dbEmpLikeNorm/

for the R package "dbEmpLikeNorm: Test for joint assessment of normality," developed by Drs. Shepherd, Tsai, Vexler, and Miecznikowski. The group of coauthors Vexler et al. (2014) presented a package entitled "Novel and Efficient Density Based Empirical Likelihood procedures for Symmetry and K-sample Comparisons" in STATA, a general-purpose statistical software language. It is available over the web at

http://sphhp.buffalo.edu/biostatistics/research-and-facilities/software/stata.html

In order to exemplify the density-based empirical likelihood method, we employ the data of measurements of HDL cholesterol levels mentioned in Section 2.2. This study was designed as a case–control study of biomarkers for coronary heart disease. In accordance with the biomedical literature, the HDL biomarker has been suggested as having strong discriminatory ability for myocardial infarction (MI). To define cases, we consider the sample Y that consists of 25 measurements of the HDL biomarker on individuals who recently survived an MI. To represent controls, 25 HDL biomarker measurements on healthy subjects are denoted as the sample X. The following R code inputs the data and constructs the histograms of the data, as shown in Figure 2.2:

```
x<-c(96.8,57.2,37.4,44.0,55.0,41.8,46.2,41.8,41.8,59.4,44.0,
52.8,33.0,52.8,41.8,44.0,52.8,59.4,37.4,77.0,39.6,57.2,57.2,
41.8,39.6)
y<-c(26.4,33.0,30.8,35.2,44.0,48.4,61.6,41.8,26.4,28.6,55.0,
61.6,63.8,24.2,37.4,48.4,52.8,46.2,57.2,68.2,46.2,37.4,46.2,
52.8,35.2)
a<-min(c(x,y))-20
b<-max(c(x,y))+20
par(pty="s",mfrow=c(1,2),oma=c(0,0,0,0),mar=c(0,4,0,0))
hist(x,xlim=c(a,b),ylim=c(0,0.05),freq=FALSE)
hist(y,xlim=c(a,b),ylim=c(0,0.05),freq=FALSE)
```

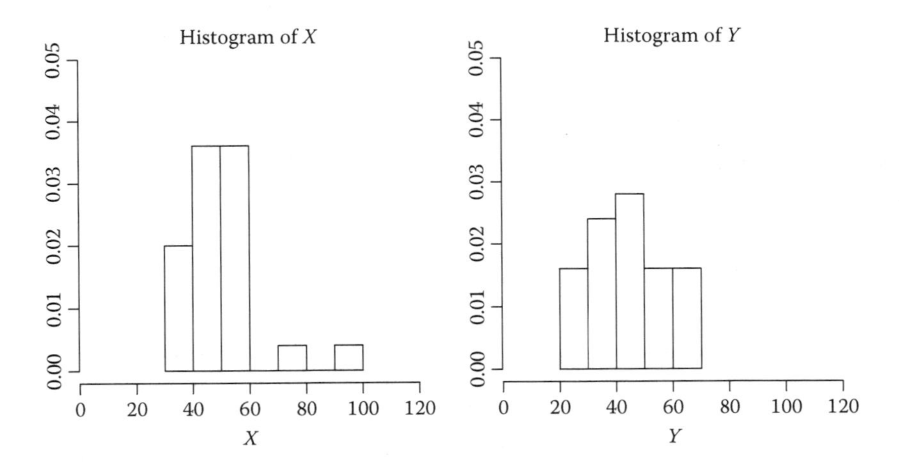

FIGURE 2.2
The R data analysis output based on measurements of the HDL cholesterol levels, X and Y, related to individuals with and without the disease, respectively.

The classical ELR test can be conducted via the R function EL.means. With a p-value of 0.101 as shown in the following, we fail to reject that $E(X) = E(Y)$ at the 0.05 significance level.

```
EL.means(x,y)
      Empirical likelihood mean difference test
data: x and y
-2 * LogLikelihood = 2.6898, p-value = 0.101
95 percent confidence interval:
-1.066513 13.850197
sample estimates:
Mean difference
      5.720065
```

Thus, in this example, the ELR test cannot be used to demonstrate the discriminatory ability of the HDL biomarker with respect to the MI disease. In this case, the two-sample density-based ELR test proposed by Gurevich and Vexler (2011) shows the p-value <0.043, supporting rejection of the hypothesis regarding equivalency of distributions of X and Y. For the sake of completeness, we present in the Appendix an example of R procedures for executing the two-sample density-based ELR test. For the critical values relevant to the size of the test, the outcome statistic can be compared against the corresponding table provided in Gurevich and Vexler (2011) (we provide the part of the table in the Appendix, Table 2.2). We note that Vexler, Tsai, and Hutson (2014) proposed a simple, but very efficient, density-based ELR test for independence and provided the R code to run the procedure.

2.7 Flexible Likelihood Approach Using Empirical Likelihood

Strictly speaking, *distribution-function/density-based* EL techniques and PL methods are closely related concepts. This provides the impetus for an impressive expansion in the number of EL developments, based on combinations of likelihoods of different types (e.g., Qin and Zhang, 2005).

Consider a simple example, where we assume to observe independent bivariate data given as (X,Y). In this case, the likelihood function can be denoted as $L(X,Y)$. Suppose the data points of X's are observed completely, whereas a proportion of the observed data for the Y's is incomplete. Assume a model of Y given X, i.e. $Y \mid X$, is well defined, e.g., $Y_i = \beta X_i + \varepsilon_i$, where β denotes the model parameter and ε_i is a normally distributed error term, for $i = 1,\ldots,n$. Then, we refer to Bayes' theorem to represent $L(X,Y) = L(Y \mid X)L(X)$, where $L(X)$ can be substituted by EL to avoid parametric assumptions regarding distributions of X's. In this context, Qin (2000) showed an inference on incomplete bivariate data using a method that combines the parametric model and ELs. This method also incorporates auxiliary information from variables in the form of constraints, which can be obtained from reliable resources such as census reports. This approach makes it possible to use all available bivariate data, whether completely or incompletely observed. More of this type of examples, theoretical discussion, and expansion will be found in Chapter 5.

In semi- and nonparametric contexts, Qin and Leung (2005) and Qin and Zhang (2005) showed that the full likelihood can be decomposed into the product of a conditional likelihood and a marginal likelihood in a similar manner to the PL considerations, and EL can be incorporated to construct the likelihood function. These techniques augment the study's power by enabling researchers to use any observed data and relevant information. Consider the example by Qin and Leung (2005). In endemic areas of malaria, an individual may have symptoms attributable either to malaria or to other causes. From a clinical viewpoint, it is important to correctly diagnose an individual who has developed symptoms so that the appropriate treatments can be given and to determine the proportion of malaria-affected cases in individuals who have symptoms so that policies on intervention program can be developed. Once symptoms have developed in an individual, the diagnosis of malaria can be based on the analysis of the parasite levels in blood samples. However, even a blood test is not conclusive because in endemic areas, many healthy individuals can have parasites in their blood slides. Therefore, data from this type of study can be viewed as coming from a mixture distribution, with the components corresponding to malaria and nonmalaria cases. By letting X to indicate a variable of parasite levels, its density function can be expressed as a mixture distribution

$$f(x) = p(1-\lambda)I(x=0) + \{(1-\lambda)(1-p)f_1(x) + \lambda f_2(x)\}I(x>0),$$

where $f_1(x)$ and $f_2(x)$ are density functions for nonmalaria parasites and true malaria parasites, λ is the proportion of people with true malaria, and p is the proportion of people without any parasites among nonmalaria subjects.

Say that $z_1,\ldots,z_m$ indicate an available training dataset consisting of the nonmalaria observations including zeros and $x_1,\ldots,x_n$ are the separately observed mixture data, respectively. Also assume that there are m_0 zeros and m_1 non-zeros among m z_i values, and n_0 zeros and n_1 non-zeros among n x_i values. The log likelihood consists of two parts

$$l = l_1 + l_2, \tag{2.12}$$

where l_1 is the marginal likelihood of the number of zeros

$$l_1 = m_0 \log p + m_1 \log(1-p) + n_0 \log\{(1-\lambda)p\} + n_1 \log\{1-(1-\lambda)p\},$$

and l_2 is the conditional likelihood of the parasite level, given the positive parasite level (both malaria and nonmalaria):

$$l_2 = \sum_{i=1}^{m_1} \log f_1(z_i) + \sum_{j=1}^{n_1} \log\{(1-\lambda^*)f_1(x_j) + \lambda^* f_2(x_j)\}. \quad (2.13)$$

Note that $\lambda^* = \lambda / \{1-p(1-\lambda)\}$ in Equation (2.13) indicates the probability of malaria given non-zero data. In addition, Qin and Leung (2005) defined the relationship $f_2(x) = \exp(\alpha + \beta x) f_1(x)$. The EL is implemented to the log likelihood (2.13) where the density $f_1(x_i)$ and $f_1(z_i)$ are replaced by probability masses (say q_i, $i = 1,\ldots,n_1$ for x_i, $i = n_1+1,\ldots,n_1+m_1$ for the training dataset) and optimized when subjected to the constraint

$$\sum_{i=1}^{n_1+m_1} q_i = 1, \; \sum_{i=1}^{n_1} q_i \{\exp(\alpha + \beta x_i) - 1\} = 0. \quad (2.14)$$

This task is conducted using the Lagrange multiplier method. The second constraint of (2.14) is based on the fact $\int f_2(x)dx = \int \exp(\alpha+\beta x) f_1(x)\,dx = 1$. The full likelihood function (2.12) is maximized with respect to $(p, \lambda^*, \alpha, \beta)$ and the Lagrange multiplier. Qin and Leung (2005) showed that the resulting likelihood ratio test of λ asymptotically has χ_1^2 distribution.

2.8 Bayesians and Empirical Likelihood: Are They Mutually Exclusive?

The statistical literature has shown that Bayesian methods can be applied for various tasks of clinical experimentations, e.g., when data are subject to complex missing data problems, e.g., parts of data are not manifested as numerical scores (Daniels and Hogan, 2008). Commonly, the application of a Bayesian approach requires assumption of functional forms corresponding to the distribution of underlying data and parameters of interest. However, in cases with data subjected to complex missing data problems, parametric estimation is complicated and formal tests for the relevant goodness-of-fit are often not available. The statistical literature has shown that tests derived from empirical likelihood methodology possess many of the same asymptotic properties as those that are based on PLs. This leads naturally to the idea of using empirical likelihood instead of PL as the basis for Bayesian inference.

Lazar (2003) demonstrated the potential for constructing nonparametric Bayesian inference based on ELs. The key idea is to substitute the parametric likelihood (PL) with EL in the Bayesian likelihood construction relative to the component of the likelihood that is used to model the observed data. It is demonstrated that the EL function is a proper likelihood function and can serve as the basis for robust and accurate Bayesian inference. This Bayesian empirical likelihood method provides a robust nonparametric data-driven alternative to the more classical Bayesian procedures. Furthermore, Vexler et al. (2013a) recommended applying EL functions to create Bayes Factor (BF)-type nonparametric procedures. The EL concept was shown to be very efficient when it is employed for modifying BF-type procedures to the nonparametric setting.

Vexler et al. (2014b) developed the nonparametric Bayesian posterior expectation by incorporating the EL methodology into the posterior likelihood construction. The asymptotic forms of the EL-based Bayesian posterior expectation are shown to be similar to those derived in the well-known parametric Bayesian and frequentist statistical literature. In the case when the prior distribution function depends on unknown hyperparameters, a nonparametric version of the empirical Bayesian method, which yields double empirical Bayesian estimators, can be obtained. This approach yields a nonparametric analog of the well-known James–Stein estimation that has been well addressed in the literature dealing with multivariate-normal observations. Note that when the data are normally distributed the non-parametric estimator is comparable to the maximum likelihood estimator (MLE). When informative priors are used and the data are generated from either a normal or lognormal distribution the estimator provides significantly smaller variances as compared to the classical estimators $\bar{X}$ and the MLE. This in turn yields much narrower confidence intervals. The asymptotic approximations to the EL-based posterior expectations are shown to be quite accurate.

The EL Bayesian procedures can serve as a powerful approach to incorporating external information into the inference process about given data, in a distribution-free manner. Let $X_1,...X_n$ be i.i.d. observations from some unknown distribution F, which has a d-dimensional mean vector μ and a nonsingular $d \times d$ covariance matrix Σ. Suppose that we are interested in inference concerning some functional of F, say $\theta(F)$. For simplicity we assume that $d = 1$. To proceed with the Bayesian analysis, the profile empirical likelihood function may serve as the likelihood part of Bayes' theorem. Lazar (2003) considered to put a prior on θ, the functional of interest, focusing on the specific case of the mean, μ. Consider an alternative likelihood, L_a, to the data likelihood, built for a functional θ of the underlying unspecified distribution. A definition of validity of an alternative likelihood L_a with which to perform Bayesian inference is suggested based on the coverage properties of posterior sets, along with a numerical technique that may be used to invalidate certain likelihoods (Lazar, 2003). A posterior density based on L_a is valid by coverage for the model $f(y \mid t)$ if and only if $\Pr\{\theta \in S_\alpha(y)\} = \alpha$ for every $S_\alpha(y)$, a posterior coverage set function of level α under the measure $p(t)f(y \mid t)$, where $p(t)$ is the prior. The *likelihood* L_a is proper in terms of coverage if and only if the posterior $p_a(t \mid y)$ is valid by coverage for every absolutely continuous prior. To verify properness, one can calculate, in the one-dimensional case,

$$H = \int_{-\infty}^{\theta} p_a(t \mid y)dt.$$

This corresponds to posterior coverage set functions of the form $(-\infty, t_a^\alpha)$, where t_a^α is the a-th percentile point of the posterior density $p_a(t \mid y)$. If $p_a(t \mid y)$ is valid by coverage, then H is distributed as Uniform(0,1). Moreover, if there exists a prior for which the distribution of H is not uniform, then $L_a(y \mid t)$ is not a proper likelihood for Bayesian inference.

When $\theta(F)$ can be determined by equation $Eg(X_1,\theta)=0$, following Section 2.2, the EL function is defined as $\mathrm{EL}(\theta) = \prod_{i=1}^{n}(n + \lambda(g(X_i,\theta))^{-1}$, where λ is a root of $\sum_{i=1}^{n}(X_i - \theta)\left(n + \lambda g(X_i,\theta)\right)^{-1}$. Then by setting $L_a = \mathrm{EL}(\theta)$,one can calculate the statistic H. It is demonstrated that even for the most diffuse of the priors, the distribution of H calculated from EL lies very close to the quantiles of the uniform distribution, confirming that EL gives valid posterior intervals. Furthermore, EL is robust to the choice of prior to a certain extent and is reasonable to use within the Bayesian paradigm.

2.8.1 Nonparametric Posterior Expectations of Simple Functionals

Suppose we have i.i.d. observations $X_1,...X_n$ from a density function $f(x \mid \theta)$, where θ is the parameter to be evaluated. For convenience of exposition and without loss of generality, we assume the parameter θ is one-dimensional and consider nonparametric posterior expectations of simple functionals here; for the case of general functionals, we refer the reader to Vexler et al. (2014b). When the form of the density function f is assumed to be known, the Bayesian point estimator of θ can be defined as the posterior expectation

$$\hat{\theta} = \frac{\int \theta \prod_{i=1}^{n} f(X_i \mid \theta)\pi(\theta)d\theta}{\int \prod_{i=1}^{n} f(X_i \mid \theta)\pi(\theta)d\theta},$$

where $\pi(\theta)$ is the prior distribution. In the case where the density function f is unknown, instead of the PLs, one can use the EL function. Following Section 2.2, the simple EL function with respect to the mean of $X_1,...X_n$ can be defined as $EL(\theta) = \prod_{i=1}^{n}(n + \lambda(X_i - \theta))^{-1}$ and the ELR has the form of $ELR(\theta) = EL(\theta)n^n$, where λ is a root of $\sum_{i=1}^{n}\left(X_i - \theta\right)\left(n + \lambda(X_i - \theta)\right)^{-1}$. Thus the nonparametric posterior expectation is

$$\hat{\theta} = \frac{\int_{X_{(1)}}^{X_{(n)}} \theta e^{\log \mathrm{EL}(\theta)} \pi(\theta) d\theta}{\int_{X_{(1)}}^{X_{(n)}} e^{\log \mathrm{EL}(\theta)} \pi(\theta) d\theta} = \frac{\int_{X_{(1)}}^{X_{(n)}} \theta e^{\log \mathrm{ELR}(\theta)} \pi(\theta) d\theta}{\int_{X_{(1)}}^{X_{(n)}} e^{\log \mathrm{ELR}(\theta)} \pi(\theta) d\theta},$$

where $X_{(1)},...X_{(n)}$ are the order statistics based on the sample $X_1,...X_n$. Vexler et al. (2014b) showed that the posterior expectation based on EL gives rise to a nonparametric analog of the James–Stein estimator and has better efficiency than classical nonparametric procedures. Bayesian adaptation of EL will be discussed in detail in Chapter 3.

2.9 Bartlett Correction

The chi-squared approximation to the ELR statistic is typically of order n^{-1}, that is, for testing q-dimensional parameter $\theta = \theta(\mu_0) = (\theta^1,...,\theta^q)^T$ as a function of true mean $\mu_0 = (\mu_{0_1},..., \mu_{0_r})^T$,

$$P_r(W_0 \le z) = P_r(\chi_q^2 \le z) + O(n^{-1}),$$

where W_0 is the ELR under the null hypothesis. However, $E\{W_0\} \ne q$. In fact, $E\{W_0\} = q\{1 + c/n + O(n^{-2})\}$ for a constant c (Hall and La Scala, 1990). DiCiccio et al. (1988) showed that empirical likelihood intervals are Bartlett adjustable such that the order of coverage error in two-sided intervals is n^{-2}. To show this, they obtained the q-dimensional signed root R that satisfies $n^{-1}W_0 = R^T R + O_p(n^{-5/2})$. The ratio $\{E(nR^T R)/q\}^{-1}$ can be expanded as

$$\{E(nR^T R)/q\}^{-1} = 1 - an^{-1} + O(n^{-2}), \tag{2.15}$$

for a fixed constant a. Adjusting W_0 by $\{E(nR^T R)/q\}^{-1}$ reduces the order of error, that is,

$$P_r(W_0\{E(nR^T R)/q\}^{-1} \le z) = P_r(\chi_q^2 \le z) + O(n^{-2}).$$

Say $Y = (Y_1,...,Y_r)^T$ is a standardized r-dimensional variable (zero-mean and identity matrix as the variance). Let $\theta^u_{j1...jr} = \partial\theta^u / \partial\mu_{j1}...\partial\mu_{jr}|_{\mu=0}$. Also, define a $q \times r$ matrix $\Theta = (\theta^u_j)$ and define matrices $Q = (\Theta\Theta^T)^{-1}$,

$M = \Theta^T(\Theta\Theta^T)^{-1}\Theta$, and $N = \Theta^T(\Theta\Theta^T)^{-1}$. In addition, define $\alpha^{j1...jk} = E(Y_{j1}...Y_{jk})$ and $A^{j1...jk} = n^{-1}\sum_{i=1}^{n}(Y_{j1}...Y_{jk} - \alpha^{j1...jk})$. Then, it can be shown

$$E(nR^TR) = q + n^{-1}\left(\frac{5}{3}t_1 - 2t_2 + \frac{1}{2}t_3 - \frac{1}{4}t_4 + \frac{1}{4}t_5\right) + O(n^{-2}),$$

where

$$\begin{aligned} t_1 &= \alpha^{jkl}\alpha^{mno}M^{jm}M^{kn}M^{lo},\ t_2 = \alpha^{jkl}\alpha^{mno}M^{jk}M^{lm}M^{no}, \\ t_3 &= \alpha^{jklm}M^{jk}M^{lm},\ t_4 = \alpha^{jkl}N^{ju}\theta^{u}_{mn}(I-M)^{mk}(I-M)^{nl}, \\ t_5 &= Q^{uv}\theta^{u}_{jk}\theta^{v}_{lm}\{(I-M)^{jk}(I-M)^{lm} + 2(I-M)^{jl}(I-M)^{km}\}. \end{aligned} \tag{2.16}$$

Note that superscripts in (2.16) indicate summation convention over repeated indices (DiCiccio et al., 1991). For the detailed derivation, we refer the paper by DiCiccio et al. (1991) and the accompanying technical report (1988). The corresponding correction term in (2.15) is

$$\frac{1}{E(nR^TR)/q} = 1 - (qn)^{-1}\left(\frac{5}{3}t_1 - 2t_2 + \frac{1}{2}t_3 - \frac{1}{4}t_4 + \frac{1}{4}t_5\right) + O(n^{-2}). \tag{2.17}$$

In case of testing the univariate mean with the standardized variable, formula (2.17) gives $(E(nR^2/q))^{-1} = 1 - n^{-1}(-\alpha_3^2/3 + \alpha_4/2) + O(n^{-2})$. Hall and La Scala (1990) suggested that (2.17) can be best estimated using the bootstrap. Based on B bootstrap EL statistics $W^*_{0\,b}(\hat{\theta})$, $b = 1,\ldots,B$ where $\hat{\theta}$ is the bootstrap estimator of θ, we obtain $\hat{c}$, an estimate of c satisfying the relationship:

$$B^{-1}\sum_{b=1}^{B} W^*_{0\,b}(\hat{\theta}) = q(1 + \hat{c}/n).$$

Then, the EL statistic is corrected to be $W_0/(1+\hat{c}/n)$.

2.10 Empirical Likelihood in a Class of Empirical Goodness of Fit Tests

Baggerly (1998) suggested that the empirical likelihood method can be considered as a new class of nonparametric likelihood ratio tests that allocate probabilities to an n-cell contingency table in a manner that a goodness-of-fit criterion known as the Cressie–Read power-divergence statistic (Cressie and Read, 1984) is minimized. When considering the empirical likelihood for the mean, common constraints are $\sum p_i = 1$ and $\sum p_i X_i = u_0$. The Cressie–Read power-divergence statistic is defined as

$$\mathrm{CR}(\lambda) = \frac{2}{\lambda(\lambda+1)} \sum_{i=1}^{n} o_i \left\{ \left(\frac{o_i}{e_i} \right)^{\lambda} - 1 \right\} \quad (-\infty < \lambda < \infty),$$

where n is the number of distinct cells in the table, o_i and e_i are the observed and expected cell counts, respectively, and λ is a user-specified parameter. When λ is 0 or −1, by continuity, we use.

$$\lim_{\lambda \to 0} \mathrm{CR}(\lambda) = 2\sum\nolimits_i^n o_i \log(o_i / e_i), \quad \lim_{\lambda \to -1} \mathrm{CR}(\lambda) = 2\sum\nolimits_i^n e_i \log(e_i / o_i).$$

When the Cressie–Read power-divergence statistic is used as a criterion, it can express several popular statistics, including $\lambda = -1$, maximum entropy; $\lambda = 0$, maximum likelihood statistic; and $\lambda = 1$, Pearson's χ^2 statistic. Now, if we assign the probability value for each observation instead of using the data value (o_i becomes 1 and e_i becomes np_i), the Cressie–Read statistic has form

$$\mathrm{CR}(\lambda) = \frac{2}{\lambda(\lambda+1)} \sum_{i=1}^{n} \left\{ (np_i)^{-\lambda} - 1 \right\}. \tag{2.18}$$

When λ is 0 in Equation (2.18), it is equivalent to maximize $2\sum_i^n \log(np_i)$ or $\sum_i^n \log p_i$, the log of EL. The result of the EL confidence region (Owen, 1990) can be generalized for the Cressie–Read statistics, that is, the empirical goodness-of-fit regions can be constructed using χ^2 cut-off levels in large samples (Baggerly, 1998). Empirical goodness-of-fit regions may not be accurate when asymptotic χ^2 cut-off levels are used with relatively small samples, and various relevant strategies have been suggested such as bootstrap (Owen, 1988). Let R denote indicate the q-dimensional signed root of the empirical goodness of fit statistic, i.e., $nR^T R = \mathrm{CR}(\lambda) + O_p(n^{-5/2})$. Baggerly (1998) showed that $E(nR^T R)$ is expressed as $q + f(\lambda)/n + O(n^{-2})$, where $f(\lambda)$ is a quadratic polynomial of λ.This fact describes that the class of goodness-of-fit tests based on Cressie–Read statistic is not Bartlett correctable in general, as the term $f(\lambda)$ does not allow simple scaling of $nR^T R$ to match the expectation of χ_q^2 distribution. On the other hand, when λ is 0, $f(\lambda)$ reduces to a constant, indicating that the ELR is Bartlett correctable.

Bravo (2003) further investigated the local unbiasedness condition and second-order power property of the class of goodness-of-fit tests based on the Cressie–Read statistic under fairly general conditions such as existence of moments up to a certain order and Cramér's condition. Consider q-dimensional random vectors $X_1, \ldots, X_n$ with mean μ and covariance matrix Σ. The local alternative to the null hypothesis $H_0 : \mu = \mu_0$ is set as $H_n : \mu = \mu_0 + n^{-1/2}\Sigma^{1/2}\gamma$ using a Pttman drift, where $0 < \gamma^T \gamma < \infty$. Using the Edgeworth expansion, under H_n, it is shown that class of the goodness-of-fit statistic converges to a noncentral χ_q^2 distribution with the noncentrality parameter $\gamma^T \gamma \ (= \tau)$ and the fact that no $\mathrm{CR}(\lambda)$ with specific λ is uniformly superior in terms of the second-order (i.e., expansion with terms of $o(n^{-1/2})$) power comparison. To achieve the local unbiasedness, it is shown that the general class of the goodness-of-fit tests needs to be modified, e.g., $\mathrm{CR}_0(\lambda)+c_\lambda(\mu_0)=W_{\lambda,b}(\mu_0)$, where $\mathrm{CR}_0(\lambda)$ is the Cressie–Read statistic under $H_0 : \mu = \mu_0$, $W_{\lambda,b}(\mu_0)$ satisfies the local unbiasedness test conditions, that is,

$$P_r\{W_{\lambda,b}(\mu_{r0}) \ge c_\alpha\} = \alpha,\ \partial P\{W_{\lambda,b}(\mu_0 - n^{-1/2}\Sigma^{1/2}\gamma) \ge c_\alpha\} / \partial\gamma\Big|_{\gamma=0} = 0,$$

and $c_\lambda(\mu_0)$ is a corresponding $o(n^{-1/2})$ correction. It is shown that $c_0(\mu_0)=0$ indicating that EL is the only test to achieve local unbiasedness without modification of the statistic. In univariate cases, $c_\lambda(\mu_0)$ becomes 0 regardless of different λ values. It is also noted that the class of goodness-of-fit tests using the Cressie–Read statistic has a size of $\alpha + o(n^{-1/2})$. It is shown that the class of goodness-of-fit tests has the second-order average power over the values $\{\gamma : \gamma^T\gamma = \tau\}$ to be 0, that is, no second-order power discrimination is possible with the average power criterion. However, Bravo (2003) further noted that the minimum of the second-order power term of $c_\lambda(\mu_0)$ is greatest when $\lambda = 0$, that is, the ELR statistic enjoys the second-order optimality property of local maximinity (Mukerjee, 1994).

2.11 Empirical Likelihood as a Competitor of the Bootstrap

Bootstrapping is a nonparametric method to approximate the distribution of an estimator through resampling, thus it is used for estimating the variance, confidence regions, and hypothesis testing. The bootstrap confidence regions can be obtained by the Monte Carlo simulation from an approximated distribution (e.g., empirical distribution function) unlike EL that requires maximization subjected to constraints. Bootstrapping is quite versatile so that it can be used for various statistics with little modification, whereas an application of EL may be difficult for very complex problems. On the other hand, in hypothesis testing, the shape of the rejection region of the EL test for multidimensional cases is determined automatically by the sample itself, whereas the rejection region of the bootstrap may be the complement region of a predetermined shape such as an ellipsoid (Chen, 1994).

For the direct power comparison, consider $X_1,\ldots,X_n$, p-dimensional i.i.d. sample with the mean μ and the variance matrix Σ. Let the null hypothesis $H_0 : \mu = \mu_0$, and a series of local alternatives $H_n : \mu = \mu_0 + n^{-1/2}\Sigma^{1/2}\tau$ for some constant vector τ. In this hypothesis setting, the bootstrap test and the EL test have the same asymptotic power depending on τ (Chen, 1994).

Thus, the comparison of the power needs to consider higher order expansion of the power function. Note that, as previously mentioned, the Bartlett-corrected EL test has the TIE rate of order n^{-2}, whereas the EL test without the Bartlett correction has the TIE rate of order n^{-1}. The bootstrap test has the TIE rate of order n^{-2} (Hall and La Scala, 1992), which is same as that of the Bartlett-corrected EL test. Thus, Chen (1994) compared the power properties of the bootstrap method and the Bartlett-corrected EL method. Under some regularity conditions, the power functions of the Bartlett-corrected EL and the bootstrap test based on the test statistic $n(\bar{x}-\mu)^T\hat{\Sigma}^{-1}(\bar{x}-\mu)$ are asymptotically same, and the difference is shown in higher order terms. $\bar{x}=\sum_{i=1}^{n} X_1$ and $\hat{\Sigma}$ denotes the sample estimator of Σ. In particular, the difference of the second-order terms between the EL and bootstrap methods is $E_2 - F_2$ (Chen, 1994), where

$$E_2 = \int_D \left\{\left(\tfrac{1}{3}\alpha^{jlm}\tau^l\tau^m - \tfrac{1}{6}\alpha^{jkk}\right)v_j + \tfrac{1}{6}\alpha^{jkl}\tau^l\left(v_jv_k - \delta^{jk}\right)\right\}\phi(v)dv,$$

$$F_2 = -\int_D \left\{\tfrac{1}{2}\alpha^{jkk}v_j + \tfrac{1}{2}\alpha^{jkl}\tau^l\left(v_jv_k - \delta^{jk}\right) + \tfrac{1}{3}\alpha^{jkl}H_3(v_j,v_k,v_l)\right\}\phi(v)dv, \tag{2.19}$$

where δ^{ik} is the Kronecker delta, D is the relevant rejection region of v under the alternative hypotheses $\phi(v)$ is the standard normal density function and $H_3(\cdot)$ is the third order Hermite polynomials (Barndorff-Nielson and Cox, 1989), $\alpha^{tjk} = E(Z_i^t Z_i^j Z_i^k)$ with $Z_i = \Sigma^{-1/2}(X_i - \mu)$.

Notice that superscripts in (2.19) indicate summation convention over repeated indices. In particular, for the univariate case, Chen (1994) showed

$$E_2 - F_2 = \tfrac{1}{3}\alpha^{111}c_\alpha\left\{\phi(\sqrt{c_\alpha}-\tau) - \phi(\sqrt{c_\alpha}+\tau)\right\}, \tag{2.20}$$

where c_α is the critical value from the χ^2 distribution with the dimension of μ under H_0. For a positive τ, the second-order power difference (2.20) shows that the EL test can have a larger power with the positively skewness. Chen (1994) offered the following rule for the univariate test with $\hat{\alpha}$, the estimate of α:

- With reasonably large sample sizes, it is recommended to use
  - The EL test if $\hat{\alpha}_3\tau > 0$.
  - Any of the two tests if $\hat{\alpha}_3\tau = 0$.
  - The bootstrap test if $\hat{\alpha}_3\tau < 0$.

The similar rule for the multivariate tests can be obtained depending on the sample version of $E_2 - F_2$ based on formula (2.20).

2.12 Convex Hull

An important requirement for constructing the EL is that the parameter of interest should be in the convex hull of the sample. For n independent p-variate observations $X_1,\ldots,X_n$, consider a constraint $E(g(X\mid\boldsymbol{\theta}))=0$, where $g(X\mid\boldsymbol{\theta})=(g_1(X\mid\theta),\ldots,g_q(X\mid\theta))^T$ and $\theta=(\theta_1,\ldots,\theta_q)^T$. The corresponding empirical constraint is $\sum_{i=1}^{n}p_i g(X_i\mid\boldsymbol{\theta})=\mathbf{0}$. Then, the convex hull composed of the points $\{g(X_i\mid\boldsymbol{\theta}), i=1,\ldots,n\}$ should contain $\mathbf{0}$. This condition is related to the existence of p_i that satisfies the empirical constraint. Using the Lagrange multiplier method, we have $p_i=\{n(1+\lambda^T g(X_i\mid\boldsymbol{\theta})\}^{-1}$, where λ is obtained to solve a nonlinear equation,

$$\sum_{i=1}^{n}\frac{g(X_i\mid\theta)}{1+\lambda^T g(X_i\mid\boldsymbol{\theta})}=\mathbf{0}. \tag{2.21}$$

The value of $1+\lambda^T g(X_i\mid\boldsymbol{\theta})$ should be greater than 0, thus the Equation (2.21) cannot be satisfied if 0 is not in the interval $\left(\min(g_k(X_i\mid\theta_k)),\max(g_k(X_i\mid\theta_k))\right)$ for $i=1,\ldots,n$ and $k=1,\ldots,q$. For example, consider a simple constraint $E(X)=0$, where X is a univariate random variable. The empirical constraint is $\sum_{i=1}^{n}p_iX_i=0$. Suppose that all $X_i>0$, thus 0 is not in the interval of $(\min(x_i),\max(x_i))$. It is immediate that there are no p_i's that satisfies $\sum_{i=1}^{n}p_iX_i=0$. This simple example demonstrates that, if 0 is the true mean of the population and we have a reasonable size of sample, the problem associated with the convex hull would rarely happen. The convex hull problem can be more serious when the dimension of $g(X\mid\theta)$ is much larger than the dimension of $\boldsymbol{\theta}$. If $E(g(X\mid\theta))$ is not in the convex hull, $\mathbf{0}$ would not be a plausible value of $g(X\mid\theta)$; thus we may consider that the ELR statistic has an extremely large value.

One may apply an alternative approach such as the adjusted EL (Chen et al., 2008), which adds a pseudodata point to prevent the problem with the convex hull. With the constraint $E(g(X\mid\theta))=\mathbf{0}$, the added data point is

$$g_{n+1}=-\frac{a_n}{n}\sum_{i=1}^{n}g(X_i\mid\theta)$$

for some positive constant $a_n=o_p(n^{2/3})$. The EL is obtained subject to the constraints

$$\sum_{i=1}^{n+1}p_i=1,\quad \sum_{i=1}^{n+1}p_i g(X_i\mid\theta)=\mathbf{0}.$$

Chen et al. (2008) showed that the resulting -2log-ELR test converges to a χ_m^2 distribution with $m=\dim(\mathbf{0})$.

2.13 Empirical Likelihood with Plug-In Estimators

The concept of the plug-in approach is to replace unknown nuisance parameters by sample statistics in the construction of the EL function. Some statistics require incorporating the other parameter estimates. An example is the sample variance,

$$S^2 = \sum_{i=1}^{n} \frac{(X_i - \bar{X})^2}{n-1}, \tag{2.22}$$

where $\bar{X}$ is to estimate the population mean. Compare (2.22) to the following statistic,

$$S_\mu^2 = \sum_{i=1}^{n} \frac{(X_i - \mu)^2}{n-1}, \tag{2.23}$$

where μ is the population mean. Both Equations (2.22) and (2.23) converge to the population variance, the target parameter. However, the respective variances are

$$\text{Var}(S_\mu^2) = \frac{n(\mu_4 - \mu_2^2)}{(n-1)^2} \tag{2.24}$$

and

$$\text{Var}(S^2) = \frac{(n-1)\mu_4 - (n-3)\mu_2^2}{n(n-1)}, \tag{2.25}$$

where μ_k is k-th central moment. Although the variances (2.24) and (2.25) are similar with a large n, we can see the relationship

$$\text{Var}(S_\mu^2) = \frac{n(\mu_4 - \mu_2^2)}{(n-1)^2} > \frac{(n-1)(\mu_4 - \mu_2^2)}{n(n-1)} > \frac{(n-1)\mu_4 - (n-3)\mu_2^2}{n(n-1)} = \text{Var}(S^2). \tag{2.26}$$

Inequality (2.26) clearly shows that $\text{Var}(S^2)$ is smaller than $\text{Var}(S_\mu^2)$ although the magnitude of the difference decreases when n increases. The sample variance example demonstrates that the plug-in estimator changes the variance profile of a statistic and the asymptotic behavior of the EL statistic.

Several articles in the literature discuss the plug-in approaches in the construction of EL (e.g., Qin and Jing, 2001; Wang and Jing, 2001; Li and Wang, 2003). In general, when the plug-in approach is used, EL test statistics do not converge to the standard χ^2 distribution. In the context of one sample problem, Hjort et al. (2009) showed that the limit distribution of −2 log ELR test is a sum of a weighted χ^2 distribution, where the weights are often intractable because of the complexity of the asymptotics. As the asymptotic distribution of the plug-in ELR test is intractable, the ELR's limiting distribution is approximated by the bootstrap method. Recently, for median comparisons between two groups, Yu et al. (2011) obtained the analytic form of the asymptotic distribution of −2 log ELR test based on the plug-in EL approach, which indeed has a weighted χ^2 distribution. They also showed that both classical and plug-in ELR tests outperform the other alternative tests (e.g., Wilcoxon rank sum test) in terms of the TIEs when the underlying distributions of two groups are seemingly different. Some relevant discussions are found in Chapters 6 through 8.

2.14 Implementation of Empirical Likelihood Using R

As a data-driven method, EL requires to estimate the distribution depending on the data. The procedure always requires maximizing the nonparametric likelihood such as (2.2) subjected to certain constraints unless a closed asymptotic solution (e.g., ELR in Proposition 6.1, Chapter 6) is available. A few functions are available in software R for this purpose (http://cran.r-project.org). The maximization can be carried out using other software as well, but in this book, we use R that is freely downloadable and has specialized functions and packages for EL.

The maximization can be carried out using optimization functions. The following are some of the available optimization functions in R:

1. `optimize`: The function `optimize` is suitable to find a single parameter solution to minimize the object. It minimizes an object of a function at default. The object of the function indicates the value to be returned as a result of carrying out the function.

   It basically searches the optimal value in a one-dimensional boundary that is set by users. Thus, it is suitable for EL with one constraint on one parameter as obtaining the Lagrange multiplier requires solving a nonlinear function. As `optimize` minimizes the object, we need to change the default to maximization or modify the object for maximization. The examples of using `optimize` function are found in Chapters 4, 6, and 7.

2. `uniroot`: It can be used for the similar purpose to `optimize` function. Unlike `optimize` function that finds the solution minimizing

the object, `uniroot` solves an equation itself. An equation can be defined as a separate function. For an application to EL, a function that contains the nonlinear equation for the Lagrange multiplier such as (2.5) needs to be created. The solution of the equation is searched through a given boundary provided by users.

3. `optim`: It carries out the minimization as `optimize` function does but with multiple parameters to look for. This function can be used with EL subjected to multiple constraints. Instead of the boundary given, the function requires an initial value. The function minimizes the object at default. The parameters to be searched should be provided as a list form. The examples of using `optim` function are found in Chapters 3, 4, and 8.
4. `solnp`: It is a convenient function to find the solution for the general Lagrange method. It incorporates multiple constraints simultaneously. For the application of EL, `solnp` provides the point masses consisting of EL. The initial values of the point masses and their suitable boundaries need to be provided. The examples of using `solnp` are found in Chapter 5.

Now, we conclude this section briefly naming R packages for the EL methods. Incorporating available functions in existing packages can make complicated EL maximization problem simple. In this book, we sometimes incorporate and implement some R functions in the following packages to obtain the numerical solutions easily.

1. `emplik`: This R package is equipped with one-group mean test for censored/truncated and fully observed data. For censored data, it also provides the EL test for discrete hazard function. The package also provides the functions to carry out the linear regression for censored response.
2. `emplik2`: This is an R package for two sample means. It has functions to compute p-values for a single mean-type or multiple mean-type hypotheses. The package handles censored data as well.
3. `EL`: This R package specialized for two sample comparisons. The package contains the functions for obtaining two-group EL test for means and for plotting the quantile–quantile plots, receiver operating characteristic (ROC) curves and quantile differences, and their confidence interval bands.

In addition, R package called `dbEmpLikeGOF` provides the density-based empirical likelihood approach (Vexler and Gurevich, 2010) as introduced in Section 2.6.

Appendix

ELR (θ_1,θ_2): Several Results That Are Similar to Those Related to the Evaluations of ELR(θ)

One can show that the logarithm of the ELR test statistic for the null hypothesis $H_0: E(X_1)=\theta_1$ and $E(X_1^2)=\theta_2$ has the form of $\log \mathrm{ELR}(\theta_1,\theta_2)=\sum_{i=1}^n \log\{1+\lambda_1(X_i-\theta_1)/n+\lambda_2(X_i^2-\theta_2)/n\}$. In this case, $\partial \log \mathrm{ELR}/\partial\theta_1=-\lambda_1$ and $\partial \log \mathrm{ELR}/\partial\theta_2=-\lambda_2$. At point $\left(\theta_1=\sum_{i=1}^n X_i/n,\ \theta_2=\overline{X}^2=\sum_{i=1}^n X_i^2/n\right)$, we have $\log \mathrm{ELR}(\theta_1,\theta_2)=\lambda_1=\lambda_2=0$, $p_i=1/n$, and the following derivatives' values:

$$\frac{\partial\lambda_1}{\partial\theta_1}=\frac{n^2\sum_{i=1}^n (X_i^2-\overline{X}^2)^2}{\Delta},$$

$$\frac{\partial\lambda_2}{\partial\theta_2}=\frac{n^2\sum_{i=1}^n (X_i-\overline{X})^2}{\Delta},$$

$$\frac{\partial\lambda_1}{\partial\theta_2}=\frac{\partial\lambda_2}{\partial\theta_1}=\frac{n^2\sum_{i=1}^n (X_i-\overline{X})(X_i^2-\overline{X}^2)}{\Delta},$$

$$\frac{\partial^2\lambda_1}{\partial\theta_1^2}=\frac{1}{n\Delta}[2\sum_{i=1}^n (X_i^2-\overline{X}^2)\{\frac{\partial\lambda_1}{\partial\theta_1}(X_i-\overline{X})+\frac{\partial\lambda_2}{\partial\theta_1}(X_i^2-\overline{X}^2)\}^2$$
$$\sum_{i=1}^n (X_i-\overline{X})(X_i^2-\overline{X}^2)-2\sum_{i=1}^n (X_i-\overline{X})\{\frac{\partial\lambda_1}{\partial\theta_1}(X_i-\overline{X})$$
$$+\frac{\partial\lambda_2}{\partial\theta_1}(X_i^2-\overline{X}^2)\}^2\sum_{i=1}^n (X_i^2-\overline{X}^2)^2],$$

$$\frac{\partial^2\lambda_2}{\partial\theta_1^2}=\frac{1}{n\Delta}[2\sum_{i=1}^n (X_i-\overline{X})\{\frac{\partial\lambda_1}{\partial\theta_1}(X_i-\overline{X})+\frac{\partial\lambda_2}{\partial\theta_1}(X_i^2-\overline{X}^2)\}^2\sum_{i=1}^n (X_i-\overline{X})(X_i^2-\overline{X}^2)$$
$$-2\sum_{i=1}^n (X_i^2-\overline{X}^2)\{\frac{\partial\lambda_1}{\partial\theta_1}(X_i-\overline{X})+\frac{\partial\lambda_2}{\partial\theta_1}(X_i^2-\overline{X}^2)\}^2\sum_{i=1}^n (X_i-\overline{X})^2],$$

$$\frac{\partial^2\lambda_1}{\partial\theta_2^{\,2}} = \frac{\partial^2\lambda_2}{\partial\theta_1\partial\theta_2} = \frac{1}{n\Delta}[2\sum_{i=1}^{n}(X_i^{\,2}-\bar{X}^2)\{\frac{\partial\lambda_1}{\partial\theta_2}(X_i-\bar{X})+\frac{\partial\lambda_2}{\partial\theta_2}(X_i^{\,2}-\bar{X}^2)\}^2$$

$$\sum_{i=1}^{n}(X_i-\bar{X})(X_i^2-\bar{X}^2)-2\sum_{i=1}^{n}(X_i-\bar{X})\{\frac{\partial\lambda_1}{\partial\theta_2}(X_i-\bar{X})$$

$$+\frac{\partial\lambda_2}{\partial\theta_2}(X_i^{\,2}-\bar{X}^2)\}^2\sum_{i=1}^{n}(X_i^{\,2}-\bar{X}^2)^2],$$

$$\frac{\partial^2\lambda_2}{\partial\theta_1^{\,2}} = \frac{\partial^2\lambda_1}{\partial\theta_1\partial\theta_2} = \frac{1}{n\Delta}[2\sum_{i=1}^{n}(X_i-\bar{X})\{\frac{\partial\lambda_1}{\partial\theta_1}(X_i-\bar{X})+\frac{\partial\lambda_2}{\partial\theta_1}(X_i^{\,2}-\bar{X}^2)\}^2$$

$$\sum_{i=1}^{n}(X_i-\bar{X})(X_i^2-\bar{X}^2)-2\sum_{i=1}^{n}(X_i^{\,2}-\bar{X}^2)\{\frac{\partial\lambda_1}{\partial\theta_1}(X_i-\bar{X})$$

$$+\frac{\partial\lambda_2}{\partial\theta_1}(X_i^{\,2}-\bar{X}^2)\}^2\sum_{i=1}^{n}(X_i-\bar{X})^2],$$

where $\Delta = \left\{\sum_{i=1}^{n}(X_i-\bar{X})(X_i^2-\bar{X}^2)\right\}^2 - \sum_{i=1}^{n}(X_i-\bar{X})^2\sum_{i=1}^{n}(X_i^2-\bar{X}^2)^2.$

R Code to Produce Figure 2.1

```
library(emplik)
theta0<-1
n.seq<-c(25, 50, 150)

#Function to plot for the normal distribution cases.
plot.norm<-function(X){
       get.elr<-function(theta) sapply(theta,
       function(pp) el.test(X,mu=pp)$'-2LLR'/(-2)) #log EL
       get.plr<-function(theta) sapply(theta,
       function(pp) sum(-(X-pp)^2/2)+sum((X-mean(X))^2/2))
       #log(PL)
       rg<-6/sqrt(length(X))
       curve(get.elr,xlim=c(max(0,mean(X)-rg),mean(X)+rg),
       type ="l",lty=1,lwd=2,add=TRUE,col=1)
       curve(get.plr,xlim=c(max(0,mean(X)-rg),mean(X)+rg),
       type ="l",lty=2,lwd=2,add=TRUE,col=2)}
```

```
#Function to plot for the exponential distribution cases.
plot.exp<-function(X){
       get.elr.exp<-function(theta) sapply(theta,
       function(pp) el.test(X,mu=1/pp)$'-2LLR'/(-2)) #log EL
       get.l.exp<-function(theta) sum(log(dexp(X,rate=theta)))
       get.plr.exp<-function(theta) sapply(theta,
       function(pp) get.l.exp(pp)-get.l.exp(1/mean(X)))
       #log(PL)
       rg<-6/sqrt(length(X))
       curve(get.elr.exp,xlim=c(max(0.1,1/mean(X)-rg),
       1/mean(X)+rg),type="l",lty=3,lwd=2,add=TRUE,col=3)
       curve(get.plr.exp,xlim=c(max(0.1,1/mean(X)-rg),
       1/mean(X)+rg),type="l",lty=4,lwd=2,add=TRUE,col=4)
}

#Function to add legend for the plot
add_legend <- function(...) {
       opar <- par(fig=c(0, 1, 0, 1), oma=c(0, 0, 0, 0),
       mar=c(0, 0, 0, 0), new=TRUE)
       on.exit(par(opar))
       plot(0, 0, type='n', bty='n', xaxt='n', yaxt='n')
       legend(...)}

#The R code to produce Figure 2.1.
par(mar=c(5.5, 4, 3.5, 1.5),mfrow=c(2,3),mgp=c(2,1,0))

for (n in n.seq){                      #for normal distribution
       rg<-2/sqrt(n)
       X<-rnorm(n,theta0,1)
       plot(theta0,1,xlim=c(max(0,mean(X)-rg),mean(X)+rg),
       xlab=expression(theta), ylim=c(- 2.5,0.005),
       ylab=expression(paste("log-EL(log-PL) ratio
       (",theta,")")), main=paste0("n=",n),cex.axis=1.2)
       plot.norm(X)
       abline(v=mean(X),lty=2,col="grey")}

for (n in n.seq){                 #for exponential distribution
       rg<-2/sqrt(n)
       X<-rexp(n,rate=theta0)
       plot(theta0,1,xlim=c(max(0,1/mean(X)-rg),1/mean(X)+rg),
       xlab=expression(theta), ylim=c(-4.5,0.005),
       ylab=expression(paste("log-EL(log-PL) ratio
       (",theta,")")), main=paste0("n=",n),cex.axis=1.2)
       plot.exp(X)
       abline(v=1/mean(X),lty=2,col="grey")
}

add_legend("bottom", legend=c("Normal, EL","Normal, PL","Exp,
EL","Exp, PL"), lwd=2, lty=1:4, col=1:4, horiz=TRUE, bty='n',
cex=1.1)
```

R Procedures for Executing the Two-Sample Density-Based Empirical Likelihood Ratio Test

```
###########sample data with the sample sizes n1=n2=25###########
n1=25
n2=25

delta<-0.1    #a control value. See Gurevich and Vexler (2011)
z<-c(x,y)                        #x and y are from Section 2.6
sx<-sort(x)
sy<-sort(y)
sz<-sort(z)

#################################################
#######obtaining the ELR based on the sample X###
#################################################

m<-c(round(n1^(delta+0.5)):min(c(round((n1)^(1-delta)),
round(n1/2)))) ###generate a vector of "m"
a<-replicate(n1,m)    #store repeated values of the vector "m"
rm<-as.vector(t(a))
L<-c(1:n1)- rm                       #order from (1-m) to (n1-m)
LL<-replace(L, L <= 0, 1 )
#replace values that are <=0 with 1 when (1-m) <=0
U<-c(1:n1)+ rm                       #order from (1+m) to (n1+m)
UU<-replace(U, U > n1, n1)
#replace values that are n1 with n1 when (n1+m)>n1

xL<-sx[LL] #obtain x(i-m)
xU<-sx[UU] #obtain x(i+m)
F<-ecdf(z)(xU)-ecdf(z)(xL) #the empirical distribution function
F[F==0]<-1/(n1+n2)
I<-2*rm/(n1*F)
#a (n1*length(m)) vector of (2*m)/(n1*empirical
#distribution function)
ux<-array(I, c(n1,length(m))
#make the previous vector as a n1*length(m) matrix
tstat1<-log(min(apply(ux,2,prod)))
#part of the test statistic based on X

#################################################
#######obtaining the ELR based on the sample Y###
#################################################

m<-c(round(n2^(delta+0.5)):min(c(round
((n2)^(1-delta)),round(n2/2))))
a<-replicate(n2,m)    #store repeated values of the vector "m"
rm<-as.vector(t(a))
#rm<-rep(m, each = n2)
#repeat the vector of "m" n2 times
```

```
L<-c(1:n2)-rm                          #order from (1-m) to (n2-m)
LL<-replace(L, L <= 0, 1 )
#replace values that are <=0 with 1 when (1-m) <=0
U<-c(1:n2)+ rm                         #order from (1+m) to (n2+m)
UU<-replace(U, U > n2, n2)
#replace values that are>n2 with n2 when (n2+m)>n2
yL<-sy[LL] #obtain y(i-m)
yU<-sy[UU] #obtain y(i+m)


F<-ecdf(z)(yU)-ecdf(z)(yL) #the empirical distribution function
F[F==0]<-1/(n1+n2)

I<-2*rm/(n2*F)
#(n2*length(m)) vector of (2*m)/(n2*empirical distribution
#fuction)
uy<-array(I, c(n2,length(m)))
tstat2<-log(min(apply(uy,2, prod)))                    #get ELR_Y

finalts<-tstat1+tstat2        #the final test statistic log(V)
```

TABLE 2.2

The critical values of the density-based test (Gurevich and Vexler, 2011) at the different significance levels α

Group 1 Sample Size	α	Group 2 Sample Size						
		10	15	20	25	50	100	200
10	0.01	11.535	12.222	12.912	13.712	15.940	19.986	24.955
	0.03	10.482	11.242	11.958	12.695	14.933	18.83	23.824
	0.05	9.763	10.497	11.223	11.910	14.120	17.975	22.988
	0.1	9.042	9.748	10.464	11.123	13.250	17.083	22.092
15	0.01		12.899	13.517	14.161	16.567	20.443	25.597
	0.03		11.880	12.531	13.199	15.509	19.406	24.501
	0.05		11.128	11.779	12.432	14.670	18.524	23.629
	0.1		10.406	11.066	11.721	13.853	17.680	22.728
20	0.01			14.072	14.724	17.135	21.139	26.238
	0.03			13.146	13.785	16.064	19.997	25.151
	0.05			12.424	13.071	15.259	19.167	24.301
	0.1			11.724	12.381	14.490	18.317	23.388
25	0.01				15.485	17.525	21.650	26.797
	0.03				14.473	16.540	20.577	25.728
	0.05				13.741	15.808	19.765	24.885

(*Continued*)

TABLE 2.2 (*Continued*)

The critical values of the density-based test (Gurevich and Vexler, 2011) at the different significance levels α

Group 1 Sample Size	α	Group 2 Sample Size 10	15	20	25	50	100	200
	0.1				13.050	15.107	18.961	23.996
50	0.01					19.593	23.454	28.810
	0.03					18.621	22.522	27.793
	0.05					17.935	21.807	27.002
	0.1					17.220	21.061	26.221
100	0.01						27.389	32.602
	0.03						26.438	31.720
	0.05						25.729	30.970
	0.1						25.004	30.220
200	0.01							37.930
	0.03							37.025
	0.05							36.295
	0.1							35.509

3

Empirical Likelihood in Light of Nonparametric Bayesian Inference

3.1 Introduction

The Bayesian approach defines probability as a measure of an individual's objective view of scientific truth based on his or her current state of knowledge. The state of knowledge, given as a probability measure, is then updated through new observations. We take the approach that both the Bayesian and frequentist methods are useful and that in general there should not be much disagreement between the approaches in the practical setting. In general, Bayesian techniques are more computationally intensive than frequentist approaches, hence this limited their use historically. However, due to the advances in computing power, Bayesian methods have emerged as an increasingly effective and practical alternative to the corresponding frequentist methods. Recently, there have been some interests in the empirical likelihood (EL) approach in the Bayesian framework. For example, Zhong and Ghosh (2016) successfully developed asymptotic expansion of posterior cumulative distributions that incorporate the various forms of ELs with a general class of priors. Vexler et al. (2016) developed an EL technique for incorporating prior information into the equal-tailed (ET) and highest posterior density (HPD) confidence interval (CI) estimators in the Bayesian manner. Chib et al. (2018) developed a Bayesian semiparametric analysis of moment condition models by casting the problem within the EL framework. This chapter provides a basic introduction to the Bayesian view on statistical testing strategies and the adaptation of the EL in the Bayesian fashion.

As an introduction to the Bayesian approach as it contrasts to frequentist methods, first consider the simple hypothesis test $H_0 : \theta = \theta_0$ versus $H_1 : \theta = \theta_1$, where the parameters θ_0 and θ_1 are known. Given an observed random sample $\mathbf{x} = \{x_1, \ldots, x_n\}$, we can then construct the likelihood ratio test statistic

$$L = f(x \mid \theta_1)/f(x \mid \theta_0)$$

for the purpose of determining which hypothesis is more probable. The decision-making procedure is to reject H_0 for large values of L. In this case, the decision-making rule based on the likelihood ratio test is uniformly most powerful. Although this classical hypothesis testing approach continues to be popular among practitioners, it can be applied straightforward only in the case of a simple hypothesis, that is, the parameter under the alternative hypothesis, θ_1, is known.

Various practical hypothesis testing problems involve the consideration of the scenarios where the parameter under the alternative, θ_1, is unknown, e.g., testing the composite hypothesis $H_0 : \theta = \theta_0$ versus $H_1 : \theta \neq \theta_0$. In general, when the alternative parameter is unknown, the parametric likelihood ratio test is not applicable as it is not well-defined. When a hypothesis is composite, Neyman and Pearson suggested replacing the density at a single parameter value with the maximum of the density over all parameters in that hypothesis. In practice we rely on the function $f(x \mid \hat{\theta})$ ($\hat{\theta}$ is the estimate of θ) in place of $f(x \mid \theta)$, which technically does not yield a likelihood function, that is, it is not a proper density function. Therefore, the maximum likelihood ratio test may lose efficiency as compared to the likelihood ratio test of interest.

Alternatively, one can provide testing procedures substituting the unknown alternative parameter by variables that do not depend on the observed data. Such approaches can be extended to provide test procedures within a Bayes Factor (BF)-type framework. We can integrate test statistics through variables that represent the unknown parameters with respect to a function commonly called a *prior* distribution. This approach can be generalized to more complicated hypotheses and models. (e.g., Vexler and Hutson, 2018).

In the following sections, we introduce two EL adaptations to Bayesian methods. First, we discuss the nonparametric posterior expectation incorporating the EL. Its asymptotic approximations using the Laplace method provide very efficient nonparametric procedures. Second, we discuss the confidence interval incorporating the prior information, where a data-driven EL function replaces the parametric likelihood function.

We hope that this chapter provides an insight that the EL method can be easily workable in the framework of the Bayesian methods.

3.2 Posterior Expectation Incorporating Empirical Likelihood

Bayesian posterior expectations are commonly used to characterize posterior and predictive distributions (Tierney et al., 1989) and serve as Bayes analogs of frequentist point estimators based on parametric statistical models (Carlin and Louis, 2000). The posterior expectation efficiently incorporates information from prior distributions and likelihood functions based on the observed data. Oftentimes the posterior estimators are more accurate than those constructed in classical approaches relative to standard criteria such as the mean-squared error, even when noninformative prior distributions are utilized.

Commonly, when forms of data distributions are unknown, the posterior expectation cannot be presented using the well-established conventional Bayesian-based methods. The traditional Bayesian-based methodology assumes a parametric form for the likelihood based on data. When the choice of distributions used to model the underlying data is misspecified within the parametric likelihood, the parameter estimation, such as the posterior expectation, may be critically inaccurate as compared to their sample counterparts found in the frequentist setting. Hence, it may be desirable in the Bayesian framework to develop a more robust nonparametric approach relative to the traditional likelihood construction. In this case we should require that the posterior distribution, based on a nonparametric likelihood, preserves a context of the probability measure.

The statistical literature displays that in the general case, parametric-based posterior expectations are difficult to calculate analytically (e.g., Tierney and Kadane, 1986; Polson, 1991; Kass and Vaidyanathan, 1992; Lieberman, 1994; Newton and Raftery, 1994; Sweeting, 1995; Diciccio et al., 1997). In some elementary cases, e.g., the exponential family of data distributions given a set of conjugate priors, the integrals used in the posterior expectation calculations might be evaluable analytically. However, this is typically not the case. In general, the relevant integrals of interest are intractable and therefore need to be evaluated using numerical methods (e.g., Tierney et al., 1989; Erkanli, 1994; Diciccio et al., 1997; Miyata, 2004). In the case involving integrals of posterior distributions that incorporate EL functions the integrants have no analytical forms and must be computed using numerical methods at each value of the functions' arguments. (Regarding the EL functional forms, see, e.g., Lazar and Mykland, 1998; Owen, 2001; Vexler et al., 2009, 2012b; Yu et al., 2011). This increases the complexity of calculations related to the proposed estimators, especially when the nonparametric procedures are based on relatively large samples.

Tierney and Kadane (1986) developed an easily computable asymptotic approximation for the parametric posterior expectation using the Laplace method. If we assume that the posterior density is unimodal or at least dominated by a single mode, then it is highly peaked about its maximum, which is the posterior mode. In this case, expanding the log-likelihood as a quadratic about the maximum likelihood estimator (MLE) of the parameter and then exponentiating it yields normal-density-type approximations to the integrants of posterior expectation. We derive asymptotic approximations to the proposed nonparametric posterior expectations. We demonstrate that the asymptotic propositions are very accurate and have a direct analogy to those of parametric posterior-based procedures.

In various Bayesian scenarios, prior functions are known up to a given set of parameters. The empirical Bayes method uses the observed data to estimate the prior parameters, e.g., by maximizing the marginal distributions, and then proceeds as though the prior is known (e.g., Carlin and Louis, 2000). Herein, we propose to use ELs as substitutes for corresponding parametric likelihoods (PL) in the empirical Bayesian posterior procedures. The distribution-free estimators obtained via this manner are denoted as *double empirical Bayesian point estimators.*

In the case of multivariate normally distributed data, Stein (1956) proved that when the dimension of the observed vectors is greater than or equal to three, the MLEs are inadmissible estimators of the corresponding parameters. James and Stein (1961) provided another estimator that yields the frequentist risk (MSE) no larger than that of the MLEs. Efron and Morris (1972) showed that the James–Stein estimator belongs to a class of parametric empirical Bayes (PEB) point estimators in the Gaussian/Gaussian model. In this context, we infer and illustrate that the proposed double empirical Bayesian point estimators can lead to nonparametric versions of the James–Stein estimators when normal priors with unknown parameters are used.

3.2.1 Nonparametric Posterior Expectations of Simple Functionals

Suppose we have independent identically distributed observations $X_1,\ldots,X_n$ from a density function $f(x\,|\,\theta)$, where θ is the parameter to be evaluated. For simplicity of the notation, let us assume the parameter θ is one dimensional. The Bayesian point estimator of θ can be defined as the posterior expectation

$$\hat{\theta} = \frac{\int \theta \prod_{i=1}^{n} f(X_i\,|\,\theta)\pi(\theta)d\theta}{\int \prod_{i=1}^{n} f(X_i\,|\,\theta)\pi(\theta)d\theta}, \tag{3.1}$$

where f is the density function of X_i and $\pi(\theta)$ is the prior distribution. The estimator at Equation (3.1) uses the parametric likelihood (PL), $\prod_{i=1}^{n} f(X_i\,|\,\theta)$, provided that the form of f is known. The posterior expectation based on using the PL approach is well addressed in the statistical literature (e.g., Johnson, 1970; Tierney and Kadane, 1986; Evans and Swartz, 1995; Yee et al., 2002; DasGupta, 2008). In some elementary cases, e.g., the exponential family of data distributions with conjugate priors, the integrals used in the posterior expectation may be evaluated analytically (e.g., Consonni and Veronese, 1992). In general, the integrals used for calculating the posterior mean are intractable and need to be evaluated numerically (e.g., Tierney and Kadane, 1986; Polson, 1991; Kass and Vaidyanathan, 1992; Lieberman, 1994; Newton and Raftery, 1994; Sweeting, 1995; Diciccio et al., 1997). A useful and accurate approximation for analyzing integrals necessary for Bayesian calculations can be achieved by assuming the posterior density is unimodal or at least dominated by a single mode, such that it is highly peaked about its maximum, which is the posterior mode. In this instance we can expand the log-PL, $\log \prod f(X_i\,|\,\theta)$, as a quadratic about the MLE of θ. Then, exponentiating it yields approximations to the integrants at Equation (3.1) that have the normal density-type forms (e.g., Vexler and Hutson, 2018). This method is based on the Laplace method (e.g., Tierney and Kadane, 1986; Bleistein and Handelsman, 2010).

Lazar (2003) showed that the EL technique can provide proper nonparametric likelihoods that can serve as the basis for Bayesian inference. Following the EL literature (e.g., Owen, 1988; Lazar and Mykland, 1998; Vexler et al., 2009; Yu et al., 2011) we define the simple EL function with respect to the mean of $X_1, ..., X_n$ as

$$\mathrm{EL}_1(\theta) = \max_{0<p_1,...,p_n<1}\left\{\prod_{i=1}^{n} p_i : \sum_{i=1}^{n} p_i = 1, \sum_{i=1}^{n} p_i X_i = \theta\right\}.$$

Thus the nonparametric posterior expectation has the form of

$$\hat{\theta} = \frac{\int_{X_{(1)}}^{X_{(n)}} \theta e^{\log \mathrm{EL}_1(\theta)} \pi(\theta) d\theta}{\int_{X_{(1)}}^{X_{(n)}} e^{\log \mathrm{EL}_1(\theta)} \pi(\theta) d\theta} = \frac{\int_{X_{(1)}}^{X_{(n)}} \theta e^{\log \mathrm{ELR}_1(\theta)} \pi(\theta) d\theta}{\int_{X_{(1)}}^{X_{(n)}} e^{\log \mathrm{ELR}_1(\theta)} \pi(\theta) d\theta}, \tag{3.2}$$

where $X_{(1)}, ..., X_{(n)}$ are the order statistics based on the sample $X_1, ..., X_n$, $\mathrm{ELR}_1(\theta) = \mathrm{EL}_1(\theta) n^n$ is the EL ratio (ELR) (e.g., Vexler et al., 2014b). In our application, the integrants at Equation (3.2) involve the EL function that has no analytical form and henceforth must be computed using numerical methods at each value of the function's argument (e.g., Owen, 2001). This analytical shortcoming increases the complexity of calculations related to the proposed estimator. Note also that the behavior of the EL function is not well addressed in literature when the arguments of the EL function are not asymptotically near the expectation EX_1, whereas the integrals at Equation (3.2) can be considered on the support $(X_{(1)}, X_{(n)})$. Interestingly, nonparametric marginal distributions based on the EL approach behave similarly to those based on parametric likelihoods, that is, $\mathrm{EL}_1(\theta)$ is highly peaked about its maximum value. That is, we can approximate integrals of the forms of $\int \theta \mathrm{EL}_1(\theta)\pi(\theta)d\theta$ and $\int \mathrm{ELR}_1(\theta)\pi(\theta)d\theta$ in a similar manner to the approximations related to the parametric posterior expectations. Toward this end we introduce the following lemma that can be considered as a nonasymptotic alternative to the result (Lemma 1) presented in Qin and Lawless (1994).

Lemma 3.1

Define θ_M to be a root of the equation $n^{-1}\sum_{i=1}^{n} G(X_i, \theta_M) = 0$, where $\partial G(X_i, \theta)/\partial\theta < 0$ (or $\partial G(X_i, \theta)/\partial\theta > 0$), for all $i = 1, 2, \ldots, n$. Then the argument θ_M is a global maximum of the function

$$W(\theta) = \max\left\{\prod_{i=1}^{n} p_i : 0 < p_i < 1, \sum_{i=1}^{n} p_i = 1, \sum_{i=1}^{n} p_i G(X_i, \theta) = 0\right\}$$

that increases and decreases monotonically for $\theta < \theta_M$ and $\theta > \theta_M$, respectively.

Proof: See the Appendix.

For example, when $G(u,\theta) = u - \theta$, we obtain $\theta_M = \bar{X} = n^{-1}\sum_{i=1}^{n} X_i$ and the function $W(\theta) = \mathrm{EL}_1(\theta)$. Now, we can obtain the following results that are analogous to the asymptotic propositions that are well addressed in the parametric literatures (e.g., Carlin and Louis, 2000; DasGupta, 2008).

Proposition 3.1

Assume $E|X_1|^4 < \infty$, $\int|\theta|\pi(\theta)d\theta < \infty$, and $\pi(\theta)$ is twice continuously differentiable in a neighborhood of $\bar{X} = n^{-1}\sum_{i=1}^{n} X_i$, then the proposed estimator (3.2) satisfies

$$\hat{\theta} = \frac{\int \theta \exp\left[-\frac{n(\bar{X}-\theta)^2}{2\sigma_n{}^2}\right]\pi(\theta)d\theta}{\int \exp\left[-\frac{n(\bar{X}-\theta)^2}{2\sigma_n{}^2}\right]\pi(\theta)d\theta} + \frac{M_n^3}{\sigma_n^2 n} + g_n,$$

where $\sigma_n^2 = n^{-1}\sum_{i=1}^{n}(X_i - \bar{X})^2$, $M_n^3 = n^{-1}\sum_{i=1}^{n}(X_i - \bar{X})^3$, $g_n = O_p(n^{-3/2+\varepsilon})$ for all $\varepsilon > 0$, as $n \to \infty$.

Proof: See the Appendix.

Corollary 3.1

Let $\pi(\theta) = (2\pi\sigma_\pi^2)^{-1/2}\exp[-(\theta-\mu_\pi)^2/2\sigma_\pi^2]$, where μ_π and σ_π^2 are known hyperparameters, and the conditions of Proposition 3.1 hold. Then the posterior expectation at (3.2) can be approximated as

$$\hat{\theta} = \tilde{\theta} + \frac{M_n^3}{\sigma_n^2 n} + O_p\left(n^{-3/2+\varepsilon}\right),$$

where $$\tilde{\theta} = \frac{(\mu_\pi\sigma_n^2 + \bar{X}\sigma_\pi^2 n)}{(n\sigma_\pi^2 + \sigma_n^2)} = \frac{\left(\sigma_\pi^2\right)^{-1}\mu_\pi}{\left(\sigma_\pi^2\right)^{-1} + n\left(\sigma_n^2\right)^{-1}} + \frac{n\left(\sigma_n^2\right)^{-1}\bar{X}}{\left(\sigma_\pi^2\right)^{-1} + n\left(\sigma_n^2\right)^{-1}}.$$

Proof: See the Appendix.

The estimator $\tilde{\theta}$ is equivalent to the form of the parametric posterior expectation derived under the Normal/Normal model (e.g., Carlin and Louis, 2000). The integral mentioned in Proposition 3.1 can be sometimes obtained analytically depending upon the form of $\pi(\theta)$. However, following the process of the asymptotic evaluation of the parametric posterior expectations we can easily show the following results.

Corollary 3.2

Under the conditions of Proposition 3.1, let $\pi(\theta)$ be a prior function with $|d^3 \log(\pi(\theta))/d\theta^3| < \infty$, for all θ. Then we have

$$\hat{\theta} = \frac{n\bar{X} + \sigma_n^2\{\log \pi(\bar{X})\}' - \sigma_n^2\{\log \pi(\bar{X})\}''\bar{X}}{n - \sigma_n^2\{\log \pi(\bar{X})\}''} + \frac{M_n^3}{\sigma_n^2 n} + O_p(n^{-3/2+\varepsilon}), \varepsilon > 0, \text{ as } n \to \infty.$$

Proof: See the Appendix.

Now, we consider the normal prior, $\pi(\theta)$, when μ_π and σ_π^2 are unknown. Following the empirical Bayes concepts (e.g., Carlin and Louis, 2000) the unknown hyperparameters can be estimated by, e.g., maximizing the respective marginal distributions. This method can be applied to the nonparametric posterior expectation yielding double empirical posterior estimation. In this case, we define

$$\hat{\theta}_E = \frac{\int \theta \exp[\log \mathrm{EL}_1(\theta)] \exp[-(\theta - \hat{\mu}_\pi)^2/2\hat{\sigma}_\pi^2] d\theta}{\int \exp[\log \mathrm{EL}_1(\theta)] \exp[-(\theta - \hat{\mu}_\pi)^2/2\hat{\sigma}_\pi^2] d\theta}, \tag{3.3}$$

where $(\hat{\mu}_\pi, \hat{\sigma}_\pi^2) = \arg\max_{\mu,\sigma} [(2\pi\sigma^2)^{-1/2} \int_{-\infty}^{\infty} \exp\{\log \mathrm{EL}_1(\theta)\} \exp\{-(\theta-\mu)^2/2\sigma^2\} d\theta]$.
The next result implies a simple asymptotic form of $\hat{\theta}_E$.

Corollary 3.3

Assume $E|X_1|^4 < \infty$, then the posterior expectation $\hat{\theta}_E$ satisfies

$$\hat{\theta}_E = \frac{\hat{\mu}_\pi \sigma^2 + \bar{X}\hat{\sigma}_\pi^2 n}{n\hat{\sigma}_\pi^2 + \sigma^2} + \frac{M_n^3}{\sigma_n^2 n} + O_p\left(n^{-3/2+\varepsilon}\right)$$

$$= \frac{\left(\hat{\sigma}_\pi^2\right)^{-1} \mu_\pi}{\left(\hat{\sigma}_\pi^2\right)^{-1} + n\left(\hat{\sigma}_n^2\right)^{-1}} + \frac{n\left(\hat{\sigma}_n^2\right)^{-1} \bar{X}}{\left(\hat{\sigma}_\pi^2\right)^{-1} + n\left(\hat{\sigma}_n^2\right)^{-1}} + \frac{M_n^3}{\sigma_n^2 n} + O_p\left(n^{-3/2+\varepsilon}\right),$$

where $\hat{\mu}_\pi = \bar{X}, \hat{\sigma}_\pi^2 - \max\{0, \sigma_n^2 - \sigma^2\} \to 0, \sigma^2 = \mathrm{Var}(X_1), \varepsilon > 0$ as $n \to \infty$.

The proof of Corollary 3.3 is technical and follows directly from the proof scheme of Proposition 3.1. Thus the proof is omitted.

Remark 3.1: Note that, according to the Central Limit Theorem it follows that $\sqrt{n}(\bar{X}-\theta)\sim N(0,\sigma^2)$, as $n\to\infty$. Then under the conditions of Proposition 3.1 the nonparametric posterior expectations $\hat{\theta}$ and $\hat{\theta}_E$ have the following asymptotic distributions, respectively, given as $\sqrt{n}\left((\hat{\theta}-M_n^3(\sigma_\pi^2 n)^{-1})(\sigma_n^2+\sigma_\pi^2 n)(\sigma_\pi^2 n)^{-1}-\mu_\pi\sigma_n^2(\sigma_\pi^2 n)^{-1}-\theta\right)\sim N(0,\sigma^2)$ and $\sqrt{n}\left((\hat{\theta}_E-M_n^3(\sigma_n^2 n)^{-1})(\sigma_n^2+\hat{\sigma}_\pi^2 n)(\hat{\sigma}_\pi^2 n)^{-1}-\hat{\mu}_\pi\sigma_n^2(\hat{\sigma}_\pi^2 n)^{-1}-\theta\right)\sim N(0,\sigma^2)$.

To extend the above results to more general situations, we assume that $D(\theta)$ defines a function of θ and we denote. The nonparametric posterior expectation of $D(\theta)$ to be

$$\hat{D}=\int D(\theta)e^{\mathrm{EL}_1(\theta)}\pi(\theta)d\theta\left(\int e^{\mathrm{EL}_1(\theta)}\pi(\theta)d\theta\right)^{-1}.$$

Proposition 3.2

Under the conditions that $D(\theta)>0$, $\int|D(\theta)|\pi(\theta)d\theta<\infty$, $|[\log D(\theta)]'''|<\infty$, and $|\log(\pi(\theta))'''|<\infty$, for all θ, it can be shown that the nonparametric posterior expectation of $D(\theta)$, satisfies, for all $\varepsilon>0$,

$$\hat{D}=\int D(\theta)e^{-\frac{1}{2n}\frac{\left(\sum X_i-n\theta\right)^2}{\sigma_n^2}}\pi(\theta)d\theta\left(\int e^{-\frac{1}{2n}\frac{\left(\sum X_i-n\theta\right)^2}{\sigma_n^2}}\pi(\theta)d\theta\right)^{-1}+\frac{D'(\bar{X})M_n^3}{\sigma_n^2 n}+O_p\left(n^{-3/2+\varepsilon}\right),$$

where $\sigma_n^2=n^{-1}\sum_{i=1}^n(X_i-\bar{X})^2$, $M_n^3=n^{-1}\sum_{i=1}^n(X_i-\bar{X})^3$ as $n\to\infty$.

The proof of this proposition is similar to that of Proposition 3.1.

Now, in a similar manner to Tierney et al. (1989) under the assumptions stated above we apply the proof strategies used for Proposition 3.1 and Corollary 3.2 to show that the posterior expectation of $D(\theta)$ can be approximated by

$$\begin{aligned}\hat{D}=D(\bar{X})&\left(\frac{n-\sigma_n^2\{\log\pi(\bar{X})\}''}{n-\sigma_n^2\{\log D(\bar{X})\}''-\sigma_n^2\{\log\pi(\bar{X})\}''}\right)^{1/2}\\
&\times\exp\left\{\left(\frac{n\bar{X}+\sigma_n^2\{\log D(\bar{X})\}-\sigma_n^2\{\log D(\bar{X})\}''\bar{X}+\sigma_n^2\{\log\pi(\bar{X})\}'-\sigma_n^2\{\log\pi(\bar{X})\}''\bar{X}}{n-\sigma_n^2\log D''(\bar{X})-\sigma_n^2\log\pi''(\bar{X})}\right)^2\right.\\
&\left.-\left(\frac{n\bar{X}+\sigma_n^2\{\log\pi(\bar{X})\}'-\sigma_n^2\{\log\pi(\bar{X})\}''\bar{X}}{n-\sigma_n^2\{\log\pi(\bar{X})\}''}\right)^2-\{\log D(\bar{X})\}'\bar{X}+\frac{\{\log D(\bar{X})\}''\bar{X}^2}{2}\right\}\\
&+\frac{D'(\bar{X})M_n^3}{\sigma_n^2 n}+O_p(n^{-3/2+\varepsilon}).\end{aligned}$$

3.2.2 Nonparametric Posterior Expectations of General Functionals

In order to consider more general cases and to extend the results found in the previous section, we begin with the definition of the EL function presented in the form

$$\mathrm{EL}_2(\theta) = \max\left\{ \prod_{i=1}^{n} p_i : 0 < p_i < 1, \sum_{i=1}^{n} p_i = 1, \sum_{i=1}^{n} p_i \; G(X_i, \theta) = 0 \right\},$$

where we assume for simplicity that $\partial G(u,\theta)/\partial\theta > 0$ or $\partial G(u,\theta)/\partial\theta < 0$, for all u, and $E|G(X_1,\theta)|^4 < \infty$. In this framework the posterior expectation takes the form

$$\hat{\theta} = \frac{\int_{X_{(1)}}^{X_{(n)}} \theta e^{\log \mathrm{EL}_2(\theta)} \pi(\theta) d\theta}{\int_{X_{(1)}}^{X_{(n)}} e^{\log \mathrm{EL}_2(\theta)} \pi(\theta) d\theta} = \frac{\int_{X_{(1)}}^{X_{(n)}} \theta e^{\log \mathrm{ELR}_2(\theta)} \pi(\theta) d\theta}{\int_{X_{(1)}}^{X_{(n)}} e^{\log \mathrm{ELR}_2(\theta)} \pi(\theta) d\theta}, \quad \mathrm{ELR}_2(\theta) = n^n \; \mathrm{EL}_2(\theta). \quad (3.4)$$

According to Lemma 3.1, $\mathrm{EL}_2(\theta)$ increases and decreases monotonically for $\theta < \theta_M$ and $\theta > \theta_M$, respectively, where θ_M is a root of

$$\frac{1}{n}\sum_{i=1}^{n} G(X_i, \theta_M) = 0.$$

Then, employing the same technique used in the proof of Proposition 3.1, we can derive the following result:

Proposition 3.3

If $\int |\theta| \pi(\theta) d\theta < \infty$, and $\pi(\theta)$ is twice continuously differentiable in a neighborhood of θ_M, then the estimator defined at (3.4) has the asymptotic form

$$\hat{\theta} = \left[\int \theta \exp\left\{ -\frac{\left[\sum_{i=1}^{n} G(X_i,\theta) \right]^2}{2\sigma_{Gn}^2 n} \right\} \pi(\theta) d\theta \right] \left[\int \exp\left\{ -\frac{\left[\sum_{i=1}^{n} G(X_i,\theta) \right]^2}{2\sigma_{Gn}^2 n} \right\} \pi(\theta) d\theta \right]^{-1}$$

$$+ \frac{M_{Gn}^3}{\sigma_{Gn}^2 n} + g_n,$$

where $\sigma_{Gn}^2 = n^{-1}\sum_{i=1}^{n} G(X_i,\theta)^2$, $M_{Gn}^3 = n^{-1}\sum_{i=1}^{n} G(X_i,\theta)^3$, $g_n = O_p(n^{-3/2+\varepsilon})$.

Moreover, if $\pi(\theta)$ is a prior distribution function with $|\log(\pi(\theta))'''| < \infty$ and $|\partial^2 G(X_i,\theta)/\partial\theta^2| < \infty$, for all θ, we have that

$$\hat{\theta} = \left[\left\{\sum_{i=1}^{n} \partial G(X_i,\theta_M)/\partial\theta_M\right\}^2 - \{\log \pi(\theta_M)\}''\sum_{i=1}^{n} G(X_i,\theta_M)^2\right]^{-1} \left[\theta_M \left\{\sum_{i=1}^{n} \frac{\partial G(X_i,\theta_M)}{\partial\theta_M}\right\}^2\right.$$

$$+ \{\log \pi(\theta_M)\}'\sum_{i=1}^{n} G(X_i,\theta_M)^2$$

$$\left. - \sum_{i=1}^{n} G(X_i,\theta_M)\sum_{i=1}^{n} \frac{\partial G(X_i,\theta_M)}{\partial\theta_M} - \{\log \pi(\theta_M)\}''\sum_{i=1}^{n} G(X_i,\theta_M)^2\theta_M\right]$$

$$+ \frac{M_{Gn}^3}{\sigma_{Gn}^2 n} + O_p(n^{-3/2+\varepsilon}), \text{ for all } \varepsilon > 0, \text{ as } n \to \infty.$$

The proof of this proposition is similar to that of Proposition 3.1 and Corollary 3.2.

Remark 3.2: The nonparametric posterior expectation of $D(\theta)$ defined earlier and given in the more general form as

$$\hat{D} = \frac{\int_{X_{(1)}}^{X_{(n)}} D(\theta)e^{\log \mathrm{EL}_2(\theta)}\pi(\theta)d\theta}{\int_{X_{(1)}}^{X_{(n)}} e^{\log \mathrm{EL}_2(\theta)}\pi(\theta)d\theta}$$

can be analyzed in a similar manner to that used in Propositions 3.2 and 3.3.

Generally, we can define the EL function as

$$\mathrm{EL}_3(\theta_1,\theta_2,\ldots,\theta_K)$$

$$= \max\left\{\prod_{i=1}^{n} p_i : 0 < p_i < 1, \sum_{i=1}^{n} p_i = 1, \sum_{i=1}^{n} p_i\ G_k(X_i,\theta_k) = 0, k = 1,\ldots,K\right\}$$

to propose the estimation

$$\hat{D}_G = \frac{\underbrace{\iint\cdots\int}_{k-\text{times}} D(\theta_1,\ldots,\theta_k)e^{\log \mathrm{ELR}_3(\theta_1,\ldots,\theta_k)}\pi(\theta_1,\ldots,\theta_k)d\theta_1\ldots d\theta_k}{\underbrace{\iint\cdots\int}_{k-\text{times}} e^{\log \mathrm{ELR}_3(\theta_1,\ldots,\theta_k)}\pi(\theta_1,\ldots,\theta_k)d\theta_1\ldots d\theta_k}, \quad \mathrm{ELR}_3 = n^n\mathrm{EL}_3.$$

Without loss of generality and for ease of presentation, we consider $K = 2$, $G_k(X_i,\theta_k) = X_i^k - \theta_k, k = 1,2$ and

$$\hat{D}_G = \frac{\int_{X_{(1)}}^{X_{(n)}}\int_{V_1}^{V_2} D(\theta_1,\theta_2)e^{\log \mathrm{ELR}_3(\theta_1,\theta_2)}\pi(\theta_1,\theta_2)d\theta_1 d\theta_2}{\int_{X_{(1)}}^{X_{(n)}}\int_{V_1}^{V_2} e^{\log \mathrm{ELR}_3(\theta_1,\theta_2)}\pi(\theta_1,\theta_2)d\theta_1 d\theta_2}, \; V_1 = \min_i X_i^2,\, V_2 = \max_i X_i^2.$$

If we assume that $\iint |D(\theta_1,\theta_2)|\pi(\theta_1,\theta_2)d\theta_1 d\theta_2 < \infty$ exists, D and π are twice continuously differentiable in neighborhoods of $(\overline{X}, \overline{X^2})$, then the following proposition yields the relevant asymptotic result, where $\overline{X^2} = \sum_{i=1}^{n} X_i^2/n$.

Proposition 3.4

Assume $E|X_1|^4 < \infty$, then the asymptotic approximation to the proposed posterior expectation of $D(\theta_1,\theta_2)$ is given by

$$\hat{D}_G = \frac{\iint D(\theta_1,\theta_2) e^{-\frac{0.5n(\theta_1-\bar{X})^2}{\sigma_n^2-(\sigma_{XX^2n})^2/\sigma_{X^2n}^2} - \frac{0.5n\left(\theta_2-\overline{X^2}\right)^2}{\sigma_{X^2n}^2-(\sigma_{XX^2n})^2/\sigma_n^2} + \frac{n(\theta_1-\bar{X})\left(\theta_2-\overline{X^2}\right)}{\sigma_{X^2n}^2\,\sigma_n^2/\sigma_{XX^2n}-\sigma_{XX^2n}}} \pi(\theta_1,\theta_2)d\theta_1 d\theta_2}{\iint e^{-\frac{0.5n(\theta_1-\bar{X})^2}{\sigma_n^2-(\sigma_{XX^2n})^2/\sigma_{X^2n}^2} - \frac{0.5n\left(\theta_2-\overline{X^2}\right)^2}{\sigma_{X^2n}^2-(\sigma_{XX^2n})^2/\sigma_n^2} + \frac{n(\theta_1-\bar{X})\left(\theta_2-\overline{X^2}\right)}{\sigma_{X^2n}^2\,\sigma_n^2/\sigma_{XX^2n}-\sigma_{XX^2n}}} \pi(\theta_1,\theta_2)d\theta_1 d\theta_2}$$

$$+\frac{J_n}{n} + O_p(n^{-3/2+\varepsilon}), \quad J_n = O_p(1),$$

for all $\varepsilon > 0$, as $n \to \infty$, where

$$\overline{X^2} = n^{-1}\sum_{i=1}^{n} X_i^2, \; \sigma_{X^2n}^2 = \frac{1}{n}\sum_{i=1}^{n}\left(X_i^2 - \overline{X^2}\right)^2,$$

$$\sigma_{XX^2n} = \frac{1}{n}\sum_{i=1}^{n}(X_i - \bar{X})\left(X_i^2 - \overline{X^2}\right),$$

and the term J_n has a complicated form depicted in Equation (A.3.14) of the Appendix.

Proof: See the Appendix.

3.2.3 Nonparametric Analog of James–Stein Estimation

Let us begin by outlining the classic James–Stein estimation process assuming the observations $X_1,\ldots,X_n$ are independent and identically distributed as multivariate normal with corresponding mean vector $\boldsymbol{\theta} = (\theta_1,\theta_2,\ldots,\theta_K)$ and covariance matrix $\boldsymbol{\Sigma}$, that is, $X_i = (X_{i1}, X_{i2},\ldots,X_{iK})^T \sim N((\theta_1,\theta_2,\ldots,\theta_K)^T, \Sigma)$, $i = 1,2,\ldots,n$. In this case, Stein (1956) proved that for $K \geq 3$, the MLE of $\boldsymbol{\theta}$ is inadmissible, that is, there exists another estimator with MSE that is less than or equal to that of the MLE. Through the analysis of the quadratic loss function, one such dominating estimator was derived by James and Stein (1961). Efron and Morris (1972) showed that the James–Stein estimator belongs to a class of the PEB point estimators related to the Gaussian/Gaussian model.

In Section 3.2, we showed that when $K = 1$ and the prior function is a normal density function the proposed nonparametric posterior expectation is asymptotically equivalent to the parametric posterior expectation derived under assumptions of the Gaussian/Gaussian model. In this section, we assume $X_1,...,X_n$ are independent random vectors, $X_i=(X_{i1},X_{i2},...,X_{iK})^T$, with an unknown distribution, and $E|X_{ij}|^4<\infty$, $j=1,...,K$, $i=1,...,n$. Under these set of assumptions we propose a nonparametric estimate of the mean $(\theta_1,\theta_2,...,\theta_K)^T$ using the double empirical posterior estimation, in the form of

$$\hat{\theta}_{Ej}=\frac{\int \theta\exp\{\log \mathrm{EL}_{4j}(\theta)\}\exp(-\theta^2/2\tilde{\sigma}_\pi^2)d\theta}{\int \exp\{\log \mathrm{EL}_{4j}(\theta)\}\exp(-\theta^2/2\tilde{\sigma}_\pi^2)d\theta}, \tag{3.5}$$

with

$$\tilde{\sigma}_\pi^2=\arg\max_{\sigma^2}\sum_{j=1}^{K}\log\left[(2\pi\sigma^2)^{-1/2}\int\exp\{\log \mathrm{EL}_{4j}(\theta)\}\exp(-\theta^2/2\sigma^2)d\theta\right],$$

where $\mathrm{EL}_{4j}(\theta_j)=\max\left\{\prod_{i=1}^n p_{ij}:0<p_{ij}<1,\sum_{i=1}^n p_{ij}=1,\sum_{i=1}^n p_{ij}\ X_{ij}=\theta_j\right\}, j=1,2,\ldots,K$. In the following proposition we will show the proposed distribution-free estimation is asymptotically equivalent to the parametric version of the James–Stein estimator.

Proposition 3.5

For all $\varepsilon>0$ and as $n\to\infty$ the double empirical posterior estimator (3.5) *has the following asymptotic form:*

$$\hat{\theta}_{Ej}=\left\{1-\frac{(K-2)/n}{\bar{X}^T S^{-1}\bar{X}}\right\}\bar{X}_j+\frac{1}{n}\sum_{r=1}^{K}\frac{\sum_{i=1}^{n}\left(X_{ir}-\bar{X}_r\right)^3}{\sum_{i=1}^{n}\left(X_{ir}-\bar{X}_r\right)^2}+O_p(n^{-3/2+\varepsilon}), j=1,...,K,$$

where $\bar{X}=(\bar{X}_1,...,\bar{X}_K)^T$, $\bar{X}_j=n^{-1}\sum_{i=1}^n X_{ij}$ and S is the sample estimator of Σ.

The proof of Proposition 3.5 is technical and follows directly from the steps used to prove Propositions 3.1 and 3.4, respectively. Thus the proof is omitted.

3.2.4 Performance of the Empirical Likelihood Bayesian Estimators

Vexler et al. (2014b) compared the nonparametric posterior expectation (3.2), its asymptotic forms stated in Proposition 3.1 and Corollary 3.1, the classical nonparametric estimator $\bar{X}$, and the corresponding MLEs of $\theta=EX_1$ through an extensive Monte Carlo study based on normally and lognormally distributed underlying data and various prior distributions depicting a degree of confidence of the prior information. It is shown that, with the normally distributed data, the variance of the EL-based estimator $\hat{\theta}$ has smaller variance than that of $\bar{X}$ indicating an increased efficiency of $\hat{\theta}$.

With the lognormally distributed data, $\hat{\theta}$ shows impressive reduction of variances compared with both $\bar{X}$ and the MLE. The approximated forms of $\hat{\theta}$ in Proposition 3.1 and Corollary 3.1 show similar performance to $\hat{\theta}$ with fairly small sample sizes, e.g., $n = 20$. It is also shown that the EL-based estimator has a high efficiency in the case of skewed data. It has been discussed in the literature that the traditional estimation of the mean of a lognormal distribution is inaccurate due to the nonquadratic and asymmetric shape of the likelihood profile (e.g., Wu et al., 2003). In this case the estimator $\hat{\theta}$ can serve as valid alternatives to the traditional techniques. Also, the performance of the approximations shown in Proposition 3.1 and Corollary 3.1 is observed to be similar to $\hat{\theta}$ across a wide range of scenarios. Vexler et al. (2014b) showed that the double empirical Bayesian estimator $\hat{\theta}_E$ given by (3.3) and the corresponding asymptotic form from Corollary 3.3 are comparable to $\bar{X}$, the MLE, when data are normally distributed. When data have a lognormal distribution, $\hat{\theta}_E$ demonstrates an improvement efficiency as compared with the classical nonparametric estimator $\bar{X}$. With sample sizes ranging from small to large, the proposed nonparametric James–Stein estimator consistently outperforms the classical nonparametric estimator, $\bar{X}$, in the multivariate setting.

3.3 Confidence Interval Estimation with Adjustment for Skewed Data

The Bayesian display of the upper and lower bounds of a credible set (Szabó et al., 2015), which contains a large fraction of the posterior mass (typically 95%) related to a functional parameter, is an analog of a frequentist confidence interval and commonly termed in the literature as a credible set or simply *confidence interval* (e.g., Carlin and Louis, 2000, p. 35). Due to its efficiency and natural interpretation, the Bayesian approach for confidence interval estimation is widely used in statistical practice. There is a rich statistical literature regarding the theoretical and applied aspects of the Bayesian CI estimation (e.g., Broemeling, 2007; Carlin and Louis, 2000; Gelman et al., 2013).

To outline this technique, we assume that the dataset X consists of n independent and identically distributed observations $X = (X_1, \ldots, X_n)$ from density function $f(x|\theta)$ with an unknown parameter θ of interest. For simplicity, suppose that θ is scalar. In the Bayesian framework we define the prior distribution $\pi(\theta)$ representing the prior information for θ. Using the likelihood function $\prod_{i=1}^{n} f(X_i|\theta)$ and Bayes' theorem, the posterior density function of θ can be presented as

$$h(\theta|X) = \prod_{i=1}^{n} f(X_i \mid \theta)\pi(\theta) \Big/ \int \prod_{i=1}^{n} f(X_i|\theta)\pi(\theta)\, d\theta. \qquad (3.6)$$

Assume that $h(\theta|X)$ is unimodal. The $(1-\alpha)100\%$ Bayesian CI estimate for θ can be presented as an interval $[q_L, q_U]$ such as the posterior probability $\Pr(q_L < \theta < q_U) = 1-\alpha$ at a fixed significant level α. To calculate the interval $[q_L, q_U]$, one can employ the following two strategies: (1) The CI bounds q_L and q_U are computed as roots of the equations

$$\frac{\alpha}{2} = \int_{-\infty}^{q_L} h(\theta|X)d\theta \quad \text{and} \quad \frac{\alpha}{2} = \int_{q_U}^{\infty} h(\theta|X)d\theta.$$

This implies the Bayesian ET CI estimation and (2) we can derive values of the CI bounds q_L and q_U as roots of the equations

$$h(q_L|X) = h(q_U|X) \quad \text{and} \quad \int_{q_L}^{q_U} h(\theta|X)d\theta = 1-\alpha.$$

This implies the Bayesian HPD CI estimation.

Method (1) is computationally simple and oftentimes used in practice. The practical implementation of Method (2) usually requires using complicated computation schemes based on Markov Chain Monte Carlo techniques (e.g., Chen and Shao, 1999). It is known that Method (2) provides shorter length CIs than that of Method (1) (e.g., Vexler and Hutson, 2018). In order to apply the earlier methods in practice, the form of density function $f(x|\theta)$ used in (3.6) needs to be specified. Daniels and Hogan (2008) showed significant issues relative to verifying the parametric assumptions for various cases as to when the Bayesian CI estimation can be applied efficiently. Zhou and Reiter (2010) demonstrated that when parametric assumptions are not met exactly, the posterior estimators are generally biased. The statistical literature has displayed many examples when parametric forms of data distributions are not available and there are vital concerns relative to using the Bayesian parametric CI approach. We employ EL functions to replace the corresponding unknown parametric likelihood functions in the posterior probability construction. We also derive higher order asymptotic approximations related to the EL CI estimation similar to that mentioned in Section 3.2.

3.3.1 Data-Driven Equal-Tailed CI Estimation

Without loss of generality, we begin by considering a scenario where the parameter of interest θ corresponds to the mean. With respect to the mean θ of a random sample $X_1, X_2, ..., X_n$, the log EL function has the form

$$l(\theta) = \max_{0<p_1...p_n<1} \left\{ \sum_{i=1}^{n} \log p_i : \sum_{i=1}^{n} p_i = 1, \sum_{i=1}^{n} p_i X_i = \theta \right\},$$

where the probability weights $p_i \in (0,1)$, for $i = 1,...,n$. Note that without further restrictions on the mean EX_1, the log EL function is $\sum_{i=1}^{n}\log(1/n)$. The posterior density function, $h_E(\theta|X)$, based on the EL function can be written as

$$h_E(\theta|X) = \frac{e^{lr(\theta)}\pi(\theta)}{\int_{X_{(1)}}^{X_{(n)}} e^{lr(\theta)}\pi(\theta)d\theta}, \tag{3.7}$$

where $lr(\theta) = \log\left(\exp(l(\theta))n^n\right)$ is the log ELR and the statistics $X_{(1)}$, $X_{(n)}$ are the minimal and maximum order statistics based on random sample $X_1, X_2,..., X_n$. The EL-based ET CI estimation requires one to find the interval $[q_L, q_U]$ that satisfies the following equations:

$$\frac{\alpha}{2} = \int_{X_{(1)}}^{q_L} h_E(\theta|X)d\theta \text{ and } \frac{\alpha}{2} = \int_{q_U}^{X_{(n)}} h_E(\theta|X)d\theta. \tag{3.8}$$

We remark that an R function *uniroot* (R Development Core Team, 2014) can be easily applied to find numerical solutions for q_L and q_U under constraints (3.8). Now, we have the following asymptotic results similar to those mentioned in Section 3.2.

Proposition 3.6

Assume $E|X_1|^4 < \infty$, *and* $\pi(\theta)$ *is twice continuously differentiable in a neighborhood of* $\bar{X} = n^{-1}\sum_{i=1}^{n}X_i$, *then the estimates* q_L *and* q_U *in* (3.8), *as the sample size* $n \to \infty$, *satisfy the equations:*

$$\frac{\alpha}{2} = \frac{\int_{X_{(1)}}^{q_L} \exp\left[-\frac{n}{2\sigma_n^2}(\theta - \bar{X})^2\right]\pi(\theta)d\theta}{\int_{X_{(1)}}^{X_{(n)}} \exp\left[-\frac{n}{2\sigma_n^2}(\theta - \bar{X})^2\right]\pi(\theta)d\theta} + M_n^3 C_n + O_p(n^{-1+\varepsilon}), \tag{3.9}$$

$$1 - \frac{\alpha}{2} = \frac{\int_{X_{(1)}}^{q_U} \exp\left[-\frac{n}{2\sigma_n^2}(\theta - \bar{X})^2\right]\pi(\theta)d\theta}{\int_{X_{(1)}}^{X_{(n)}} \exp\left[-\frac{n}{2\sigma_n^2}(\theta - \bar{X})^2\right]\pi(\theta)d\theta} + M_n^3 C_n + O_p(n^{-1+\varepsilon}), \tag{3.10}$$

where $\bar{X} = \sum_{i=1}^{n}X_i/n$, $\sigma_n^2 = n^{-1}\sum_{i=1}^{n}(X_i - \bar{X})^2$, $M_n^3 = n^{-1}\sum_{i=1}^{n}(X_i - \bar{X})^3$, $C_n = 2n^{-0.5}(1 + z_{1-\alpha/2}^2/2)\varphi\left(z_{1-\alpha/2}\right)/3\sigma_n^3$, and $\varphi(\cdot)$ denotes the standard normal density function.

Proof: See the Appendix.

This proposition simplifies the calculations of q_L and q_U. The second terms in (3.9) and (3.10) involve the third moment estimate, M_n^3. Chen (1995) applied a M_n^3-type correction to improve the t-test statistic for the mean because the short right tail in the sampling distribution of t-test leads to a loss of power for tests of the population mean. This correction was shown to be a very efficient one for t-test applications based on skewed data. Proposition 3.6 shows that the proposed CI estimators automatically adjust the CI estimation with respect to skewness of the data using Chen's M_n^3-type correction.

A wide range of Bayesian statistical models are based on the assumption that the prior information can be modeled via normal (Gaussian) distributions. In this case we have the following results:

Lemma 3.2

Assume that $\pi(\theta)$ is a normal density function with mean μ and variance σ^2. Then (3.9) and (3.10) imply

$$\frac{\alpha}{2} = \Phi\left(u_L\right) + M_n^3 C_n + O_p(n^{-1+\varepsilon}),$$

$$1 - \frac{\alpha}{2} = \Phi\left(u_U\right) + M_n^3 C_n + O_p(n^{-1+\varepsilon}),$$

where $\Phi(\cdot)$ is a cumulative distribution of the standard normal random variable and

$$u_L = \left(q_L - \frac{\sigma_n^2\mu + n\sigma^2\bar{X}}{\sigma_n^2 + n\sigma^2}\right)\left(\frac{\sigma_n^2\sigma^2}{\sigma_n^2 + n\sigma^2}\right)^{-0.5}, \quad u_U = \left(q_u - \frac{\sigma_n^2\mu + n\sigma^2\bar{X}}{\sigma_n^2 + n\sigma^2}\right)\left(\frac{\sigma_n^2\sigma^2}{\sigma_n^2 + n\sigma^2}\right)^{-0.5}.$$

Proof: See the Appendix.

Proposition 3.7

Under assumptions of Proposition 3.6 and Lemma 3.2, we have

$$q_L = \frac{\sigma_n^2\mu + n\sigma^2\bar{X}}{\sigma_n^2 + n\sigma^2} - z_{1-\alpha/2}\sqrt{\frac{\sigma_n^2\sigma^2}{\sigma_n^2 + n\sigma^2}} + \frac{M_n^3}{3n\sigma_n^2}\left(2 + z_{1-\alpha/2}^2\right) + o_p\left(n^{-1}\right), \quad (3.11)$$

$$q_U = \frac{\sigma_n^2\mu + n\sigma^2\bar{X}}{\sigma_n^2 + n\sigma^2} + z_{1-\alpha/2}\sqrt{\frac{\sigma_n^2\sigma^2}{\sigma_n^2 + n\sigma^2}} + \frac{M_n^3}{3n\sigma_n^2}\left(2 + z_{1-\alpha/2}^2\right) + o_p\left(n^{-1}\right). \quad (3.12)$$

Proof: See the Appendix.

Regarding this result, one can remark that the first two asymptotic components of the estimator q_L and q_U are equivalent to those derived by using the Normal/Normal model in the context of the classical Bayesian CI mean estimation (e.g., Carlin and Louis, 2000). In order to compare the asymptotic CI bounds (3.11) and (3.12) with the classical mean confidence interval estimator $\left[\bar{X} \pm z_{1-\alpha/2}\sqrt{\sigma_n^2/n}\right]$, Equations (3.11) and (3.12) can be *informally* rewritten providing the interval

$$\left[\bar{X} \pm z_{1-\alpha/2}\sqrt{\sigma_n^2/n} + M_n^3(4+2z_{1-\alpha/2}^2)/(6n\sigma_n^2) + o_p(n^{-1})\right]$$

when the prior hyperparameter σ^2 increases to infinity providing the case with very vague prior information. This formula is also similar to that derived by Hall (1983) to construct the skewness-corrected confidence interval estimation in the form

$$\left[\bar{X} \pm z_{1-\alpha/2}\sqrt{\sigma_n^2/n} + M_n^3(1+2z_{1-\alpha/2}^2)/(6n\sigma_n^2) + o_p(n^{-1})\right].$$

The M_n^3-skewness correction terms involved in both the proposed CI estimator and Hall's confidence interval estimator improve the accuracy of the procedures with an adjustment for skewed data.

To prove the consistency of the proposed approach in the probabilistic manner, we present the following proposition:

Proposition 3.8

Under assumptions of Proposition 3.6, the CI bounds q_L and q_U from (3.8) *satisfy*

$$\Pr(q_L < \theta < q_U) = 1 - \alpha + O_p(n^{-0.5}).$$

The proof of Proposition 3.8 is omitted as it directly follows from the application of Slutsky's theorem and an Edgeworth expansion technique.

3.3.2 Data-Driven Highest Posterior Density CI Estimation

In the context of the data-driven HPD CI estimation, we compute the bounds for the CI interval $[\tilde{q}_L, \tilde{q}_U]$ as the roots of the equations

$$1-\alpha = \int_{\tilde{q}_L}^{\tilde{q}_U} h_E(\theta \mid X)d\theta \text{ and } h_E(\tilde{q}_L \mid X) = h_E(\tilde{q}_U \mid X). \tag{3.13}$$

We remark that an R function `optim` (R Development Core Team, 2014) can be easily used to find numerical solutions for $\tilde{q}_L$ and $\tilde{q}_U$ under the constraints at (3.13). We have the following asymptotic result for the HPD CI estimation.

Proposition 3.9

Under the assumptions of Proposition 3.6, the estimates $\tilde{q}_L$ and $\tilde{q}_U$ in (3.13) satisfy the equations

$$\exp\left[-n(\tilde{q}_L-\bar{X})^2/2\sigma_n^2+nM_n^3(\tilde{q}_L-\bar{X})^3/3(\sigma_n^2)^3+O_p(n)(\tilde{q}_L-\bar{X})^4\right]\pi(\tilde{q}_L)$$
$$=\exp\left[-n(\tilde{q}_U-\bar{X})^2/2\sigma_n^2+nM_n^3(\tilde{q}_U-\bar{X})^3/3(\sigma_n^2)^3+O_p(n)(\tilde{q}_U-\bar{X})^4\right]\pi(\tilde{q}_U),$$

$$\int_{\tilde{q}_L}^{\tilde{q}_U}\exp\left[-\frac{n}{2\sigma_n^2}(\theta-\bar{X})^2\right]\pi(\theta)d\theta\Big/\int_{X_{(1)}}^{X_{(n)}}\exp\left[-\frac{n}{2\sigma_n^2}(\theta-\bar{X})^2\right]\pi(\theta)d\theta$$
$$=1-\alpha+O_p(n^{-1+\varepsilon}).$$

We note that the proof of Proposition 3.9 is omitted as the proof scheme is similar to those used in Propositions 3.6 and 3.7.

The result of Proposition 3.9 can be simplified, given that $\pi(\theta)$ is a normal density function with mean μ and variance σ^2. Lemma 3.3 and Proposition 3.10 represent the results.

Lemma 3.3

Under assumptions of Lemma 3.2, $\tilde{q}_L$ and $\tilde{q}_U$ can be approximated as the roots of the equations

$$-n(\tilde{q}_L-\bar{X})^2/2\sigma_n^2+nM_n^3(\tilde{q}_L-\bar{X})^3/3(\sigma_n^2)^3-(\tilde{q}_L-\mu)^2/2\sigma_n^2+O_p(n)(\tilde{q}_L-\bar{X})^4$$
$$=-n(\tilde{q}_U-\bar{X})^2/2\sigma_n^2+nM_n^3(\tilde{q}_U-\bar{X})^3/3(\sigma_n^2)^3-(\tilde{q}_U-\mu)^2/2\sigma_n^2+O_p(n)(\tilde{q}_U-\bar{X})^4,$$

$$\Phi(u_U)-\Phi(u_L)=1-\alpha+O_p(n^{-1+\varepsilon}).$$

Proposition 3.10

Under the assumptions of Proposition 3.6 and Lemma 3.2, the asymptotic expansions for the bounds of the HPD CI, $[\tilde{q}_L,\tilde{q}_U]$, are

$$\tilde{q}_L = \bar{X} - z_{1-\alpha/2}\sqrt{\frac{\sigma_n^2\sigma^2}{\sigma_n^2 + n\sigma^2}} + \left[\frac{M_n^3 z_{1-\alpha/2}^2}{3n\sigma_n^2} - \frac{\sigma_n^2}{n\sigma^2}(\bar{X} - \mu)\right] + o_p(n^{-1}),$$

$$\tilde{q}_U = \bar{X} + z_{1-\alpha/2}\sqrt{\frac{\sigma_n^2\sigma^2}{\sigma_n^2 + n\sigma^2}} + \left[\frac{M_n^3 z_{1-\alpha/2}^2}{3n\sigma_n^2} - \frac{\sigma_n^2}{n\sigma^2}(\bar{X} - \mu)\right] + o_p(n^{-1}).$$

For the consistency of the proposed HPD approach we present the next Proposition.

Proposition 3.11

Under the assumptions of Proposition 3.8, the CI bounds $\tilde{q}_L$ and $\tilde{q}_U$ in Equation (3.13) satisfy

$$\Pr(\tilde{q}_L < \theta < \tilde{q}_U) = 1 - \alpha + O_p(n^{-0.5}).$$

3.3.3 General Cases for CI Estimation

In order to extend the results in the previous sections, we can define the log EL function as

$$l_G(\theta) = \max_{0<p_1,\ldots,p_n<1}\left\{\sum_{i=1}^n \log p_i : \sum_{i=1}^n p_i = 1, \sum_{i=1}^n p_i G(X_i,\theta) = 0\right\},$$

where the probability weights $p_i \in (0,1)$, for $i = 1,\ldots,n$. We assume that $\partial G(u,\theta)/\partial\theta > 0$ or $\partial G(u,\theta)/\partial\theta < 0$, for all u. Define θ_M as a solution of the equation $n^{-1}\sum_{i=1}^n G(X_i,\theta) = 0$. In the case of $G(X_i,\theta) = X_i - \theta$, the parameter θ is the mean of data as previously considered. We construct the nonparametric posterior density function as

$$h_{EG}(\theta|X) = \frac{e^{lr_G(\theta)}\pi(\theta)}{\int_{X_{(1)}}^{X_{(n)}} e^{lr_G(\theta)}\pi(\theta)d\theta},$$

where $lr_G(\theta) = \log\left(\exp\left(l_G(\theta)\right)n^n\right)$ is the log ELR. The posterior density function $h_{EG}(\theta \mid X)$ can be applied to denote the data-driven CI estimation via two strategies, the Bayesian ET and HPD CI estimations. Toward this end, one can use Equations (3.8) and (3.13) by applying the function $h_{EG}(\theta \mid X)$ instead of $h_E(\theta \mid X)$.

In a similar manner to the data-driven ET CI estimation, we have the following asymptotic propositions:

Proposition 3.12

Assume $E|G(X_1,\theta)|^4<\infty$, *and* $\pi(\theta)$ *is twice continuously differentiable in a neighborhood of* θ_M, *then the lower and upper CI bounds* Q_L *and* Q_U *satisfy the equations*

$$\frac{\alpha}{2}=\frac{\int_{X_{(1)}}^{Q_L}\exp\left[-\frac{n}{2\sigma_{Gn}^2}(\theta-\theta_M)^2\right]\pi(\theta)d\theta}{\int_{X_{(1)}}^{X_{(n)}}\exp\left[-\frac{n}{2\sigma_{Gn}^2}(\theta-\theta_M)^2\right]\pi(\theta)d\theta}+M_{Gn}^3C_{Gn}+O_p(n^{-1+\varepsilon}),$$

$$1-\frac{\alpha}{2}=\frac{\int_{X_{(1)}}^{Q_U}\exp\left[-\frac{n}{2\sigma_{Gn}^2}(\theta-\theta_M)^2\right]\pi(\theta)d\theta}{\int_{X_{(1)}}^{X_{(n)}}\exp\left[-\frac{n}{2\sigma_{Gn}^2}(\theta-\theta_M)^2\right]\pi(\theta)d\theta}+M_{Gn}^3C_{Gn}+O_p(n^{-1+\varepsilon}),$$

where $\sigma_{Gn}^2=n^{-1}\sum_{i=1}^n G(X_i,\theta)^2$, $M_{Gn}^3=n^{-1}\sum_{i=1}^n G(X_i,\theta)^3$, and $C_{Gn}=2n^{-0.5}(1+z_{1-\alpha/2}^2/2)\varphi(z_{1-\alpha/2})/3\sigma_{Gn}^3$.

The next proposition provides the asymptotic evaluations of the HPD CI estimation with the bounds $\left[\hat{Q}_L,\hat{Q}_U\right]$.

Proposition 3.13

Under the assumptions of Proposition 3.12, the lower and upper HPD CI bounds $\hat{Q}_L$ and $\hat{Q}_U$, asymptotically satisfy the equations

$$\exp\left[-n(\hat{Q}_L-\bar{X})^2/2\sigma_{Gn}^2+nM_n^3(\hat{Q}_L-\bar{X})^3/3(\sigma_{Gn}^2)^3+O_p(n)(\hat{Q}_L-\bar{X})^4\right]\pi(\hat{Q}_L)$$
$$=\exp\left[-n(\hat{Q}_U-\bar{X})^2/2\sigma_{Gn}^2+nM_n^3(\hat{Q}_U-\bar{X})^3/3(\sigma_{Gn}^2)^3+O_p(n)(\hat{Q}_U-\bar{X})^4\right]\pi(\hat{Q}_U),$$

$$\int_{\hat{Q}_L}^{\hat{Q}_U}\exp\left[-\frac{n}{2\sigma_{Gn}^2}(\theta-\theta_M)^2\right]\pi(\theta)d\theta\Big/\int_{X_{(1)}}^{X_{(n)}}\exp\left[-\frac{n}{2\sigma_{Gn}^2}(\theta-\theta_M)^2\right]\pi(\theta)d\theta$$
$$=1+O_p(n^{-1+\varepsilon}).$$

We note that one can easily derive asymptotic expression for the CI bounds in general case by directly using the proof strategies of Propositions 3.7 and 3.10 when the prior distribution is in a Gaussian form. The following proposition confirms that the proposed nonparametric procedures are consistent.

Proposition 3.14

Under assumptions of Proposition 3.12, we have

$$\Pr(Q_L < \theta < Q_U) = 1 - \alpha + O_p(n^{-0.5}) \quad \text{and} \quad \Pr(\hat{Q}_L < \theta < \hat{Q}_U) = 1 - \alpha + O_p(n^{-0.5}).$$

3.3.4 Performance of the Empirical Likelihood Bayesian CIs

The performances of the EL Bayesian CIs are evaluated based on the various scenarios and sample sizes using an extensive Monte Carlo (MC) study. The prior is set up as the normal distribution with different variances reflecting relative confidence on the prior information regarding the parameter $\theta = EX$ (a larger variance indicates a less confidence on the prior information). With the lognormal data and the correct normal prior, the coverage rates of both ET and HPD CIs incorporating the EL are close to the target confidence level, whereas the lengths of the CIs are shorter than the classical CI $\left[\bar{X} \pm C_{1-\alpha/2}\sqrt{\sigma_n^2/n}\right]$, where $C_{1-\alpha/2}$ is the normal quantile corresponding to the probability $1-\alpha/2$ and the sample variance σ_n^2. When an incorrect prior is used by using incorrect mean in the normal prior, the EL Bayesian CIs maintain similar coverage rates with a little increase in interval lengths as compared to the classical method. For the cases of baseline data from normal distributions with the correctly specified priors, the performance of the proposed methods is comparable to the classical method. In these cases the classical CI method is a product of the parametric maximum likelihood technique and then can be expected to be very efficient. In comparison with other confidence interval construction methods, the EL Bayesian CIs outperform the classical EL confidence intervals or the CI based on inverse Edgeworth expansion (Hall, 1983). In a setting of known normal prior and normal data, the EL Bayesian CIs show a similar performance to the parametric Bayesian CIs.

3.3.5 Strategy to Analyze Real Data

In the real data analysis, reasonable prior distributions are required. Oftentimes, such information is available from previous studies. For example, consider a sample from epidemiological studies about atherosclerotic coronary heart disease (Schisterman et al., 2001, see Chapter 1 for explanation) that have been carried forth for the purpose of examining the association between biomarkers and myocardial infarction (MI) disease. We consider

TABLE 3.1

The 95% CI estimators of the mean of the glucose biomarker

	Equal-Tailed CI	HPD CI	Classical CI
Case group	[106.17, 116.85]	[105.87, 116.46]	[105.26, 115.55]
Control group	[99.78, 105.98]	[99.61, 105.76]	[99.28, 105.28]

glucose level (a total of 386 measurements) that is often used as a discriminant factor between individuals with and without MI disease (e.g., Schisterman et al., 2001). Half of them were collected on cases who survived on MI and the other half on controls who had no previous MI. In order to implement the proposed method, results of the population-based study described in Schisterman et al. (2001) were employed to provide the prior information of the parameter, the population mean of the glucose level. Based on the research of Schisterman et al. (2001), it is reasonable to assume that $N(105.04, 33.38^2)$ and $N(161.85, 68.04^2)$ are the prior distributions for the mean of glucose in the control and the case groups, respectively. Table 3.1 presents the results of the proposed 95% CI estimation of the mean of the glucose biomarker.

Based on the Shapiro–Wilk test for normality we reject the normality assumption for the glucose data for both the case and control groups (p-values < 0.05) due to the right-skewed distributions. The nonoverlapping CIs provided by the proposed method for the case and control groups suggest there is a significant difference in means of glucose levels between the two groups. By contrast, the 95% classical CIs for the case and control groups overlap and do not provide this conclusion. A relevant R code for the data analysis is provided in the Appendix.

3.4 Some Warnings

Fang and Mukerjee (2006) and Chang and Mukerjee (2008) proposed a general class of empirical-type likelihoods via the asymptotic form

$$L(\theta) \propto \exp(-y^2/2)$$
$$\left[1+\frac{1}{3}n^{-1/2}g_3y^3+n^{-1}\left\{\frac{1}{4}(g_4-2g_3^2-2)y^4+\frac{1}{18}g_3^2y^6\right\}+o_p(n^{-1})\right], \tag{3.14}$$

where $y=(n/m_2)^{1/2}(\theta-\bar{X})$, $\bar{X}=n^{-1}\sum_{i=1}^{n}X_i$, $m_s=n^{-1}\sum_{i=1}^{n}(X_i-\bar{X})^s$, $s=2,3,\ldots$, $g_3=m_3/m_2^{3/2}$, and $g_4=m_4/m_2^2$. Then the authors applied this asymptotic proposition to obtain and examine the approximately correct posterior density function $\pi^*(y|X)$ based on the general empirical-type likelihood form resulting in

$$\pi^*(y|X) = (2\pi)^{-1/2}\exp(-y^2/2)\Big[1+n^{-1/2}(R_1y+R_3y^3)+n^{-1}\left\{R_2(y^2-1)\right.$$
$$\left.+R_4(y^4-3)\right\}+R_6(y^6-15)+o_p(n^{-1})\Big], \tag{3.15}$$

where R_i, $i=1,\ldots,6$, denote functions of g_j, $j=3,4$, $\pi'(\bar{X})$, and $\pi''(\bar{X})$. Unfortunately, in general, this direction is not completely appropriate in terms of constructing and evaluating Bayesian-type statistical schemes, including, e.g., BFs and posterior expectations. The following arguments should be taken into accounts. In the EL framework the asymptotic notation given in (3.14) is valid only when $\theta = \theta_T + O_p(n^{-1/2})$, where θ_T is the true value of parameter θ (Lazar and Mykland, 1998). For example, in the simple case of the EL mentioned above, we have $\theta_T = EX_1$. The posterior distribution should be considered to have support over a large range of θ values. In order to derive the corresponding marginal distributions, one needs to integrate $\exp\{l(\theta)\}\pi(\theta)$ over $\theta\in(-\infty,\infty)$, where

$$l(\theta) = \max_{0<p_1,\ldots,p_n<1}\left\{\sum_{i=1}^n \log p_i : \sum_{i=1}^n p_i = 1, \sum_{i=1}^n p_iX_i = \theta\right\}.$$

The remainder term in (3.14) will not vanish to zero, as the order of this term depends on $y=(n/m_2)^{1/2}(\theta-\bar{X})$, where $\theta-\bar{X}$ does not converge to zero when θ is not relatively close to θ_T. Similarly, when θ is not in the neighborhood of θ_T, e.g., the component, $n^{-1/2}g_3y^3/3$, of (3.14) is unbounded as $n\to\infty$ and the remainder term might be the dominant term in (3.14). In several scenarios, corresponding to the Bayesian principle, we can be interested to consider the posterior density function, where θ is not relatively close to $\bar{X}$, e.g., according to prior information. Note that EL-type procedures are commonly not defined for relatively large or small values of their parameters depending on the existence conditions used to obtain the probability weights (p_i's, $i=1,\ldots,n$). For example, in the case mentioned above, the EL is defined as $\exp\{l(\theta)\}=\prod_{i=1}^n p_i$ only when $\theta\in(\min(X_1,\ldots,X_n),\max(X_1,\ldots,X_n))$.

In order to correct this problem, one can show a similarity between behaviors of parametric likelihoods and their nonparametric counterparts subjected to a set of theoretical assumptions (Vexler et al., 2014b, 2016). The end results of Fang and Mukerjee (2006) may be technically correct as the authors applied the general asymptotic form with a known limiting distribution. These asymptotic forms can be easily modified to be associated with many statistical objects, including parametric Bayesian forms (Tierney and Kadane, 1986). The use of Equations (3.14) and (3.15) to develop and evaluate Bayesian procedures may lead investigators to neglect appropriate assumptions on the prior $\pi(\theta)$ and data distributions. We also remark that the probability weights in the EL definition can be defined to satisfy the constraint $\sum_{i=1}^n p_iG(X_i,\theta)=0$

and it is clear that the function G should be restricted to satisfy several conditions while considering Bayesian-type inference based on the corresponding EL. Alternatively, the Bayesian integral form

$$\int_{q_L}^{q_U} \exp\{l(\theta)\}\pi(\theta)d\theta\left[\int_{X_{(1)}}^{X_{(n)}} \exp\{l(\theta)\}\pi(\theta)d\theta\right]^{-1} = 1-\alpha$$

can be directly used to obtain the $100(1-\alpha)\%$ credible set $[q_L, q_U]$ (Vexler et al., 2016). To this end, Laplace's method used in the parametric Bayesian analysis by Tierney and Kadane (1986) should be extended and adapted to the nonparametric setting (Vexler et al., 2014b, 2016).

Note that the practical performance of the credible set scheme proposed by Fang and Mukerjee (2006) strongly depends on convergence rates of higher order moment estimators. In contrast to that, the natural definition of the Bayesian scheme based on the EL does not consist of high-order moment estimators.

We would like to remark the arguments mentioned above yield a concern regarding the general form of empirical-type likelihoods derived via asymptotic explanations similar to (3.14).

3.5 An Example of the Use of Empirical Likelihood-Based Bayes Factors in the Bayesian Manner

Define, e.g., q to be a quintile that satisfies $F(q) = 0.1$, where F is a distribution function of independent and identically distributed data points $X_1,\dots,X_n$. Assume, in the Bayesian framework (when parameters of data distributions are treated as random variables), we would like to compare the model $M_0 : q \sim \pi_0 = Unif[0,1]$ with the model $M_1 : q \sim \pi_1 = Unif[1,1.5]$.

Consider a scenario, when we presume that observations $X_1,\dots,X_n$ are exponentially distributed with the density function $f(x \mid \lambda_q)$, where the parameter λ_q satisfies $\int_0^q f(u \mid \lambda_q)du = 0.1$. Then, the parametric BF is

$$BF = \frac{\int_1^{1.5} \prod_{i=1}^{n} f(X_i \mid \lambda_q)dq}{\int_0^{1} \prod_{i=1}^{n} f(X_i \mid \lambda_q)dq}.$$

Alternatively, assuming the distribution function F is unknown, one can use the empirical likelihood based Bayes Factor defined as

$$ELBF = \frac{\int_1^{1.5} \left\{\frac{0.1}{nF_n(q)}\right\}^{nF_n(q)} \left\{\frac{1-0.1}{n(1-F_n(q))}\right\}^{n(1-F_n(q))} dq}{\int_0^1 \left\{\frac{0.1}{nF_n(q)}\right\}^{nF_n(q)} \left\{\frac{1-0.1}{n(1-F_n(q))}\right\}^{n(1-F_n(q))} dq}, \quad F_n(u) = \frac{1}{n}\sum_{i=1}^{n} I(X_i \le u).$$

In this construction, we use the EL in the form $EL = \prod_{i=1}^{n} p_i$, where in order to find values of $p_1, \ldots, p_n$ that maximize EL given the constraints $\sum_{i=1}^{n} p_i = 1$ and $\sum_{i=1}^{n} p_i I(X_i \le q) = 0.1$, we can use the Lagrange function

$$\Lambda = \sum_{i=1}^{n} \log(p_i) + \lambda_1 \left(1 - \sum_{i=1}^{n} p_i\right) + \lambda_2 \left(0.1 - \sum_{i=1}^{n} p_i I(X_i \le q)\right),$$

where λ_1 and λ_2 are the Lagrange multipliers. Simple considerations of $\partial\Lambda / \partial p_i = 0, i = 1, .., n$, show that

$$p_i = \left(n + \lambda_2 \left(I(X_i \le q) - 0.1\right)\right)^{-1},$$

where λ_2 is the root of the equation

$$\sum_{i=1}^{n} p_i I(X_i \le q) = \sum_{i=1}^{n} \left(n + \lambda_2 \left(I(X_i \le q) - 0.1\right)\right)^{-1} I(X_i \le q) = 0.1$$

that can be simplified as $\sum_{i=1}^{n} (n + 0.9\lambda_2)^{-1} I(X_i \le q) = 0.1$. Thus, we have $\lambda_2 = (0.1(1-0.1))^{-1} n(F_n(q) - 0.1)$. Now

$$p_i = \left(n - \frac{nF_n(q) - 0.1n}{(1-0.1)} + \frac{nF_n(q) - 0.1n}{0.1(1-0.1)} I(X_i \le q)\right)^{-1}.$$

Let $X_{(1)}, \ldots, X_{(n)}$ be the order statistics based on $X_1, .., X_n$. Suppose k_0 is the index such that $X_{(k_0)} \le q$ and $X_{(k_0+1)} > q$. Note that $k_0 = nF_n(q)$. Define

$$p_{[i]} = \left(n - \frac{nF_n(q) - 0.1n}{(1-0.1)} + \frac{nF_n(q) - 0.1n}{0.1(1-0.1)} I(X_{(i)} \le q)\right)^{-1}$$

$$= \frac{0.1}{nF_n(q)} I(i \le k_0) + \frac{1-0.1}{n(1-F_n(q))} I(i > k_0).$$

Then

$$EL = \prod_{i=1}^{n} p_i = \prod_{i=1}^{n} p_{[i]} = \prod_{i=1}^{k_0} \frac{0.1}{nF_n(q)} \prod_{i=k_0+1}^{n} \frac{1-0.1}{n(1-F_n(q))} \text{ with } k_0 = nF_n(q).$$

This implies the form of *ELBF*. (*ELBF*-type statistics were evaluated and applied in Vexler at al., 2017; Yu et al, 2011, 2014b.)

Since a problem of misclassification can be in effect, we suppose that, in practice, observed data points $X_1,...,X_n \sim Gamma(\gamma_q, 0.1)$, where $\gamma_q : F(q) = 0.1$. Commonly, BF values are used following the table (e.g., Kass and Raftery, 1995):

BF Value	Strength of Evidence
$< 10^0$	negative (*supports* M_0)
10^0 to $10^{1/2}$	barely worth mentioning
$10^{1/2}$ to 10^1	substantial
10^1 to $10^{3/2}$	strong
$10^{3/2}$ to 10^2	very strong

We generated 25,000 times the scenario mentioned above under the model M_0 with $n = 25$, and compared the parametric Bayes factor and *ELBF*. To this end the following R code was used.

```
alpha<-0.1
n<-25
MC<-25000 #Number of the MC repetitions
BF<-array()
ELBF<-array()
for(mc in 1:MC)
{
a0<-0
b0<-1
a1<-b0
b1<-b0+0.5
q<-runif(1,a0,b0) #under model M0
#q<-runif(1,a1,b1) #under model M1

QQ<-function(u) pexp(q,u)-alpha
lambda<-uniroot(QQ,c(0,1000000))$root
#xt<-rexp(n,lambda) #expected data point to be observed
#x<-xt

gam2<-0.1
GG<-function(u) pgamma(q,u,gam2)-alpha
GGV<-Vectorize(GG)
gam1<-uniroot(GGV,c(0,100000))$root
pgamma(q,gam1,gam2)
x<-rgamma(n,gam1,gam2) #Observed data points

Inegr<-function(uu){
fix<-uu
QQ1<-function(u) pexp(fix,u)-alpha
QQ1V<-Vectorize(QQ1)
```

```
lambda1<-uniroot(QQ1V,c(0,100000000))$root
S<-sum(log(dexp(x,lambda1)))
return(exp(S))
}
Intr<-Vextorize(Inegr)
Num<-integrate(Intr,a1,b1)[[1]]
Den<-integrate(Intr,a0,b0,stop.on.error = FALSE)[[1]]

BF[mc]<-Num/Den #BF

EDF<-function(u) {
y<-1*(x<=u)
return(mean(y))
}

EDFV<-Vectorize(EDF)
EL<-function(u) ((alpha/(n*EDFV(u)))^(n*EDFV(u)))*((1-alpha)/
(n*(1-EDFV(u))))^(n*(1-EDFV(u)))
ELV<-Vectorize(EL)
NumEL<-integrate(ELV,a1,b1)[[1]]
DenEL<-integrate(ELV,a0,b0)[[1]]
ELBF[mc]<-NumEL/DenEL #ELBF

print(c(mc,BF[mc],ELBF[mc]))
print(c(length(BF[BF<1]),length(ELBF[ELBF<1])))
print(c(length(BF[(BF>=1)&(BF<10^0.5)]),length(ELBF[(ELBF>=1)&
(ELBF<10^0.5)])))
print(c(length(BF[(BF>=10^0.5)&(BF<10^1)]),length(ELBF[(ELBF>=
10^0.5)&(ELBF<10^1)])))
print(c(length(BF[(BF>=10^1)&(BF<10^1.5)]),length(ELBF[(ELBF>=
10^1)&(ELBF<10^1.5)])))
#See also https://en.wikipedia.org/wiki/Bayes_factor
#par(mfrow=c(2,1))
#hist(BF,xlim=c(0,50))
#hist(ELBF,xlim=c(0,50))
}
```

The results are:

Strength of Evidence	**Parametric BF**	**ELBF**
negative (*supports* M_0)	18514 times (74.1%)	22579 times (90.3%)
barely worth mentioning	3787 (15.1%)	2077 (8.3%)
substantial	1925 (7.7%)	344 (1.4%)
strong and very strong	774 (3.1%)	0 (0%)

Thus, it is clear that the empirical likelihood based method provides more frequently correct results demonstrating the robustness of *ELBF* comparing with the parametric BF.

3.6 Concluding Remarks

We demonstrated how to incorporate the EL in the Bayesian framework by showing a novel approach for developing the nonparametric Bayesian posterior expectation and the nonparametric Bayesian CI estimation. The asymptotic approximations to the new distribution-free posterior expectations are developed and shown to be quite accurate, even in the finite sample setting. The asymptotic forms are similar to those derived in the well-known parametric Bayesian and frequentist statistical literature. In the case when the prior distribution function depends on unknown hyperparameters we proposed a nonparametric version of the empirical Bayesian method. This yielded double empirical Bayesian estimators. In the multivariate setting, with prior functions defined to be normal distributions with unknown hyperparameters, the double empirical Bayesian estimation yields a nonparametric version of the well-known James–Stein estimator. The Monte Carlo study in the multivariate setting confirmed that the proposed nonparametric James–Stein estimator has smaller variances than the classical nonparametric estimator $\bar{X}$ for data generated from *MVN* and *MVLogNorm* distributions. The asymptotic propositions showed that the proposed method can improve the CI estimation with an adjustment for skewed data. The Bayesin CI estimation is more accurate relative to the coverage probability (CP) aspect than that of the classical CI estimation and has shorter length of CI estimation.

Appendix

R Codes to Obtain Confidence Intervals in Section 3.3.

In the following codes, we assume that the baseline data distribution is *Lognormal*$(0, 1)$ (and centered to make mean 0), and the prior distribution is normal with mean zero and variance 1.

```
library(emplik)                                          #library in R
n<-50; alpha<-0.05              #sample size and significance level
x<-rlnorm(n,0,1)-exp(0.5)  #random numbers for a sample of size n
```

The following code creates function (`integ`) for $e^{lr(\theta)}\pi(\theta)$ in Equation (3.7).

```
integ<-function(u){exp((el.test(x,u)$'-2LLR')*(-0.5))*dnorm(u,0,1)}
```

The following code calculates the denominator in Equation (3.7).

```
c<-min(x); a<-mean(x)-n^(-0.5+1/6); b<-mean(x)+n^(-0.5+1/6);
d<-max(x)
dem2<-integrate(Vectorize(integ),c,2*a,stop.on.error=FALSE)$value+
integrate(Vectorize(integ),2*a,a,stop.on.error=FALSE)$value+
integrate(Vectorize(integ),a,mean(x),
stop.on.error=FALSE)$value+
integrate(Vectorize(integ),mean(x),b,
stop.on.error=FALSE)$value+
integrate(Vectorize(integ),b,2*b,stop.on.error=FALSE)$value+
integrate(Vectorize(integ),2*b,d,stop.on.error=FALSE)$value
```

The following are the functions to calculate the confidence interval (3.8).

```
f1<-function(q){
((integrate(Vectorize(integ),lower=c,upper=a/2,
stop.on.error=FALSE)$value+
integrate(Vectorize(integ),lower=a/2,upper=a,
stop.on.error=FALSE)$value+
integrate(Vectorize(integ),lower=a,upper=q,
stop.on.error=FALSE)$value)/
dem2-alpha/2)}
f2<-function(q){
((integrate(Vectorize(integ),lower=q,upper=b,
stop.on.error=FALSE)$value+
integrate(Vectorize(integ),lower=b,upper=2*b,
stop.on.error=FALSE)$value+
integrate(Vectorize(integ),lower=2*b,upper=d,
stop.on.error=FALSE)$value)/
dem2-alpha/2)}
```

The following code provides the confidence interval (3.8).

```
c11<-uniroot(f1,c(c,d))$root
c12<-uniroot(f2,c(c,d))$root
print(c(c11,c12))
```

The following codes are to obtain the HPD confidence interval (3.13).

```
integ1<-Vectorize(integ)
f2<-function(u){
integrate(integ1,lower=u[1],upper=u[2],
stop.on.error=FALSE)$value/dem2 }
Model1 <-function(u){ F1<-(integ1(u[1])-integ1(u[2]))
F2<-(f2(u)-1+alpha);FF<- (F1^2+F2^2);return(FF)}
solu3<-optim(c(c11,c12),f=Model1)$par #Data-driven HPD CI
print(solu3)
```

Proof of Lemma 3.1

It is clear that the argument θ_M, a root of $n^{-1}\sum_{i=1}^{n}G(X_i,\theta_M)=0$, maximizes the function $W(\theta)$, as in this case $W(\theta_M)=n^{-n}$ with $p_i=n^{-1}$, $i=1,\dots,n$, that maximize $\prod_{i=1}^{n}p_i$ given the sole constraint $\sum_{i=1}^{n}p_i=1$, $0\le p_i\le 1, i=1,\dots,n$.
Using the Lagrange method, one can represent $W(\theta)$ as

$$W(\theta)=\prod_{i=1}^{n}p_i,\quad 0<p_i=\frac{1}{n+\lambda G(X_i,\theta)}<1,\ i=1,\dots,n,$$

where the Lagrange multiplier λ is a root of the equation $\sum G(X_i,\theta)\left(n+\lambda G(X_i,\theta)\right)^{-1}=0$ (e.g., Owen, 2001). This then yields the following expression:

$$\frac{d\log\left(W(\theta)\right)}{d\theta}=-\lambda\sum_{i=1}^{n}\frac{\partial G(X_i,\theta)/\partial\theta}{n+\lambda G(X_i,\theta)}-\sum_{i=1}^{n}\frac{G(X_i,\theta)}{n+\lambda G(X_i,\theta)}\frac{\partial\lambda}{\partial\theta}=-\lambda\sum_{i=1}^{n}\frac{\partial G(X_i,\theta)/\partial\theta}{n+\lambda G(X_i,\theta)},\tag{A.3.1}$$

where without loss of generality we assume $\partial G(X_i,\theta)/\partial\theta>0, i=1,\dots,n$.

Now define the function $L(\lambda)=\sum_{i=1}^{n}G(X_i,\theta)\left(n+\lambda G(X_i,\theta)\right)^{-1}$. As $dL(\lambda)/d\lambda<0$ the function $L(\lambda)$ decreases with respect to λ and has just one root relative to solving $L(\lambda)=0$. Consider the scenario with $\theta>\theta_M$. In this case when $\lambda_0=0$ we can conclude that

$$L(\lambda_0)=\sum_{i=1}^{n}G(X_i,\theta)(n)^{-1}\ge\sum_{i=1}^{n}G(X_i,\theta_M)(n)^{-1}=0,$$

as $G(X_i,\theta)$ increases with respect to θ ($\partial G(X_i,\theta)/\partial\theta>0$).

The function $L(\lambda)$ decreases. This implies that the root of $L(\lambda)=0$ should be located on the right side from $\lambda_0=0$ and then this root is positive. For a graphical representation of this case, see Figure A.3.1a. Thus, by virtue of Equation (A.3.1), we prove that the function $W(\theta)$ decreases, when $\theta>\theta_M$.

Taking the same approach, one can show that the root of $L(\lambda)=0$ should be to the left of $\lambda_0=0$, when $\theta<\theta_M$. For a graphical representation of this case, see Figure A.3.1b. This result combined with Equation (A.3.1) completes the proof of Lemma 3.1.

Proof of Proposition 3.1

To prove the proposition, we first show that

$$\int_{X_{(1)}}^{X_{(n)}}\theta^{\upsilon}e^{\log \mathrm{ELR}_1(\theta)}\pi(\theta)d\theta\cong\int_{\bar{X}-\varphi_n n^{-1/2}}^{\bar{X}+\varphi_n n^{-1/2}}\theta^{\upsilon}e^{\log \mathrm{ELR}_1(\theta)}\pi(\theta)d\theta,\ \upsilon=0,1,$$

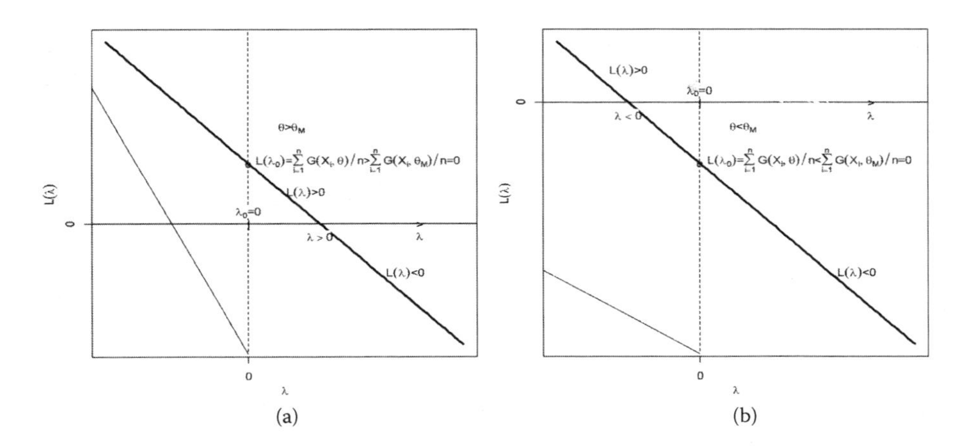

FIGURE A.3.1
The schematic behaviors of $L(\lambda)$ plotted against λ (the axis of abscissa), when (a) $\theta > \theta_M$ and (b) $\theta < \theta_M$, respectively.

where a positive sequence $\varphi_n n^{-1/2} \to 0, \varphi_n \to \infty$, as $n \to \infty$. This approximation allows us to analyze the numerator ($\upsilon = 1$) and the denominator ($\upsilon = 0$) defined at (3.2). Let us rewrite the function $\mathrm{EL}_1(\theta)$ in the form of $\log \mathrm{EL}_1(\theta) = \sum_{i=1}^{n} \log p_i$, where p_i can be defined by maximizing the Lagrangian

$$\Lambda = \sum_{i=1}^{n} \log p_i + \lambda_1\left(1 - \sum_{i=1}^{n} p_i\right) + \lambda_2\left(\theta - \sum_{i=1}^{n} p_i X_i\right),$$

where λ_1 and λ_2 are Lagrange multipliers. Thus one can show that $p_i = (n + \lambda(X_i - \theta))^{-1}$, where λ is a root of the equation $\sum_{i=1}^{n}(X_i - \theta)/[n + \lambda(X_i - \theta)] = 0$.

Now we define the function

$$L(\lambda) = \sum_{i=1}^{n}(X_i - \theta)/[n + \lambda(X_i - \theta)]. \quad \text{(A.3.2)}$$

According to Lemma 3.1, when $\theta < \bar{X}$ then the function $\log \mathrm{ELR}_1(\theta)$ is strictly increasing and when $\theta > \bar{X}$ then the function $\log \mathrm{ELR}_1(\theta)$ is strictly decreasing. This implies that the function $\log \mathrm{ELR}_1(\theta)$ is maximized at the point $\theta = \bar{X}$. Now, denote $a = \bar{X} - \varphi_n n^{-1/2}$ and $b = \bar{X} + \varphi_n n^{-1/2}$, where $\varphi_n = n^{1/6-\beta}$ and $\beta \in (0, 1/6)$. Then it follows that

$$\int_{X_{(1)}}^{X_{(n)}} e^{\log \mathrm{ELR}_1(\theta)} \pi(\theta) d\theta = \int_{X_{(1)}}^{a} e^{\log \mathrm{ELR}_1(\theta)} \pi(\theta) d\theta + \int_{a}^{b} e^{\log \mathrm{ELR}_1(\theta)} \pi(\theta) d\theta + \int_{b}^{X_{(n)}} e^{\log \mathrm{ELR}_1(\theta)} \pi(\theta) d\theta.$$

By virtue of the previous considerations we can bound the remainder term

$$\int_{X_{(1)}}^{a} e^{\log \mathrm{ELR}_1(\theta)} \pi(\theta) d\theta \le e^{\log \mathrm{ELR}_1(a)} \int_{X_{(1)}}^{X_{(n)}} \pi(\theta) d\theta \le e^{\log \mathrm{ELR}_1(a)}.$$

In order to arrive at an expression for the value of $\log \mathrm{ELR}_1(a)$, taking into account the definition of ELR_1 in (3.2), we evaluate (A.3.2) at $\theta = a$ such that

$$\begin{aligned} L(\lambda) &= \sum_{i=1}^{n} \frac{(X_i - \bar{X} + \varphi_n n^{-1/2})}{n + \lambda(X_i - \bar{X} + \varphi_n n^{-1/2})} \\ &= \frac{1}{n} \sum_{i=1}^{n} \frac{(X_i - \bar{X} + \varphi_n n^{-1/2})\left[(1 + \lambda n^{-1}(X_i - \bar{X} + \varphi_n n^{-1/2}) - \lambda n^{-1}(X_i - \bar{X} + \varphi_n n^{-1/2})\right]}{1 + \lambda n^{-1}(X_i - \bar{X} + \varphi_n n^{-1/2})} \\ &= \frac{1}{n}\left[\sum_{i=1}^{n}(X_i - \bar{X} + \varphi_n n^{-1/2}) - \lambda n^{-1} \sum_{i=1}^{n} \frac{(X_i - \bar{X} + \varphi_n n^{-1/2})^2}{1 + \lambda n^{-1}(X_i - \bar{X} + \varphi_n n^{-1/2})}\right]. \end{aligned} \quad \text{(A.3.3)}$$

Defining $\lambda_c = n^{2/3} \tau_n^{-1}$, where $\tau_n = n^{\gamma}$, $0 < \gamma < \beta < 1/6$, and substituting it into Equation (A.3.3) yields

$$\sqrt{n} L(\lambda_c) = \varphi_n - \sqrt{n} \frac{n^{2/3-1}}{\tau_n} \frac{1}{n} \sum_{i=1}^{n} \frac{(X_i - \bar{X} + \varphi_n n^{-1/2})^2}{1 + n^{-1/3} \tau_n^{-1}(X_i - \bar{X} + \varphi_n n^{-1/2})},$$

Since

$$\frac{X_i - \bar{X}}{n^{1/3} \tau_n} = O_p(1)$$

(e.g., Owen, 1988), we have

$$\sqrt{n} L(\lambda_c) = \varphi_n - \frac{n^{1/6}}{\tau_n} \frac{1}{n} \sum_{i=1}^{n} \frac{(X_i - \bar{X} + \varphi_n n^{-1/2})^2}{1 + O_p(1)}.$$

Now, it follows that $\sqrt{n} L(\lambda_c) \to -\infty$, as $n \to \infty$. In a similar manner, $\sqrt{n} L(-\lambda_c) \to \infty$, as $n \to \infty$. Thus, the solution, λ_0, of equation $\sqrt{n} L(\lambda_0) = 0$ belongs to the interval $(-\lambda_c, \lambda_c)$, that is, $\lambda_0 = O_p(n^{2/3} \tau_n^{-1})$.

Let us now derive the approximate value corresponding to λ_0 as $n \to \infty$. Since $L(\lambda_0) = 0$,

$$\sum_{i=1}^{n}(X_i - \bar{X} + \varphi_n n^{-1/2})\frac{1}{1+\lambda_0 n^{-1}(X_i - \bar{X} + \varphi_n n^{-1/2})} = 0 \quad \text{(A.3.4)}$$

Applying a Taylor series expansion to (A.3.4) we then obtain

$$\sum_{i=1}^{n}(X_i - \bar{X} + \varphi_n n^{-1/2})[1 - \lambda_0 n^{-1}(X_i - \bar{X} + \varphi_n n^{-1/2}) + \frac{\lambda_0^2 n^{-2}(X_i - \bar{X} + \varphi_n n^{-1/2})^2}{(1+\omega_i)^2}] = 0, \quad \text{(A.3.5)}$$

where $0 < \omega_i < \lambda_0 n^{-1}(X_i - \bar{X} + \varphi_n n^{-1/2})$. Since $\lambda_0 = O(n^{2/3}\tau_n^{-1})$, we can re-express (A.3.5) as

$$\sum_{i=1}^{n}(X_i - \bar{X} + \frac{\varphi_n}{n^{1/2}}) - \frac{\lambda}{n}\sum_{i=1}^{n}(X_i - \bar{X} + \frac{\varphi_n}{n^{1/2}})^2 + \frac{O(n^{1/3})}{\tau_n^2}\frac{1}{n}\sum_{i=1}^{n}(X_i - \bar{X} + \frac{\varphi_n}{n^{1/2}})^3 = 0. \quad \text{(A.3.6)}$$

Then it follows that the approximate solution based on solving (A.3.6) is given by

$$\lambda_0 = \frac{\varphi_n n^{1/2}}{n^{-1}\sum_{i=1}^{n}(X_i - \bar{X} + \varphi_n n^{-1/2})^2} + \frac{O(n^{1/3})}{\tau_n^2}. \quad \text{(A.3.7)}$$

Applying a Taylor series expansion to $\log \mathrm{ELR}_1(\theta)$ by (3.2) with $\theta = a$ yields the following expression:

$$\begin{aligned}\log \mathrm{ELR}_1(a) &= -\sum_{i=1}^{n}\log\,[1 + \frac{\lambda_0}{n}(X_i - \bar{X} + \varphi_n n^{-1/2})] \\ &= -\sum_{i=1}^{n}\frac{\lambda_0}{n}(X_i - \bar{X} + \varphi_n n^{-1/2}) \\ &\quad + \frac{1}{2}\sum_{i=1}^{n}\frac{\lambda_0^2}{n^2}(X_i - \bar{X} + \varphi_n n^{-1/2})^2 - \frac{1}{3}\sum_{i=1}^{n}\frac{\lambda_0^3}{n^3}\frac{(X_i - \bar{X} + \varphi_n n^{-1/2})^3}{(1+\omega_i^*)^3},\end{aligned}$$

where $0 < \omega_i^* < \lambda_0 n^{-1}(X_i - \bar{X} + \varphi_n n^{-1/2})$. By virtue of (A.3.7) and the fact that $\lambda_0 = O(n^{2/3}/\tau_n)$ we then have

$$\log \mathrm{ELR}_1(a) = -\frac{\lambda}{n}\varphi_n n^{1/2} + \frac{1}{2}\sum_{i=1}^{n}\frac{\lambda^2}{n^2}(X_i - \bar{X} + \varphi_n n^{-1/2})^2 - O(n^{-3\gamma})$$

$$= -\frac{\varphi_n^{\,2} n}{n n^{-1}\sum_{i=1}^{n}(X_i - \bar{X} + \varphi_n n^{-1/2})^2} - \frac{O(n^{4/3})}{\tau_n^2 n^2}\varphi_n n^{1/2}$$

$$+\frac{1}{2}\left[\frac{\varphi_n^{\,2} n}{\left[n^{-1}\sum_{i=1}^{n}(X_i - \bar{X} + \varphi_n n^{-1/2})^2\right]^2} + 2\frac{O(n^{4/3})}{\tau_n^{\,2} n}\frac{\varphi_n n^{1/2}}{n^{-1}\sum_{i=1}^{n}(X_i - \bar{X} + \varphi_n n^{-1/2})^2}\right.$$

$$\left. + \frac{O(n^{8/3})}{\tau_n^4 n^2}\right]\frac{1}{n^2}\sum_{i=1}^{n}(X_i - \bar{X} + \varphi_n n^{-1/2})^2 - O(n^{-3\gamma})$$

$$= -\frac{1}{2}\frac{\varphi_n^{\,2}}{n^{-1}\sum_{i=1}^{n}(X_i - \bar{X} + \varphi_n n^{-1/2})^2} - O(n^{\frac{4}{3}-2-2\gamma+\frac{1}{6}-\beta+\frac{1}{2}})$$

$$+ O(n^{\frac{4}{3}-1-2\gamma+\frac{1}{6}-\beta+\frac{1}{2}-1}) + O(n^{\frac{8}{3}-2-4\gamma-1}) - O(n^{-3\gamma})$$

$$= -\frac{1}{2}\frac{\varphi_n^{\,2}}{n^{-1}\sum_{i=1}^{n}(X_i - \bar{X} + \varphi_n n^{-1/2})^2} - O(n^{-3\gamma}) \to -\infty \text{ as } n \to \infty,$$

where $\varphi_n^{\,2} = n^{1/3-2\beta} \to \infty$ and $0 < \gamma < \beta < 1/6$. Thus, we arrive at the result that

$$\int_{X_{(1)}}^{a} \exp\left(\log \mathrm{ELR}_1(\theta)\right)\pi(\theta)d\theta \le \exp\left(\log \mathrm{ELR}_1(a)\right)$$

$$= O\left(\exp\left(-wn^{1/3-2\beta}\right)\right) \to 0 \text{ as } n \to \infty,$$

where w is a positive constant. It follows similarly that $\int_b^{X_{(n)}} \exp(\log \mathrm{ELR}_1(\theta))\pi(\theta)d\theta \le \exp(\log \mathrm{ELR}_1(b)) = O\left(\exp\left(-w_1 n^{1/3-2\beta}\right)\right) \to 0$ as well as

$$\int_{X_{(1)}}^{a} \theta e^{\log \mathrm{ELR}_1(\theta)} \pi(\theta) d\theta \le O\left(e^{-w_2 n^{1/3-2\beta}}\right) \to 0,$$

$$\int_{b}^{X_{(n)}} \theta e^{\log \mathrm{ELR}_1(\theta)} \pi(\theta) d\theta \le O\left(e^{-w_3 n^{1/3-2\beta}}\right) \to 0,$$

where w_1, w_2, and w_3 are positive constants and $n \to \infty$.

Now we consider the main term $\int_a^b e^{\log \mathrm{ELR}_1(\theta)} \pi(\theta) d\theta$ of the marginal distribution defined at (3.2). This integral consists of $\log \mathrm{ELR}_1(\theta)$ that, by virtue of the Taylor theorem and (A.3.1), is

$$\log \mathrm{ELR}_1(\theta) = \log \mathrm{ELR}_1(\bar{X}) + (\theta - \bar{X})\lambda(\bar{X}) + \frac{1}{2}(\theta - \bar{X})^2 \left(\left. \frac{d\lambda(u)}{du} \right|_{u=\bar{X}} \right)$$
$$+ \frac{1}{6}(\theta - \bar{X})^3 \left(\left. \frac{d^2\lambda(u)}{du^2} \right|_{u=\bar{X}} \right) + \frac{1}{24}(\theta - \bar{X})^4 \left(\left. \frac{d^3\lambda(u)}{du^3} \right|_{u=\theta+\varpi(\bar{X}-\theta)} \right), \ \varpi \in (0,1). \tag{A.3.8}$$

Since the function $\lambda(u)$ is defined by $\sum (X_i - u)/[n + \lambda(u)(X_i - u)] = 0$, one can show that

$$\frac{d\lambda(\theta)}{d\theta} = -\frac{n\sum_{i=1}^{n} p_i^2}{\sum_{i=1}^{n} (X_i - \theta)^2 p_i^2},$$

$$\frac{d^2\lambda(\theta)}{d\theta^2} = \frac{2(d\lambda(\theta)/d\theta)^2 \sum_{i=1}^{n} (X_i - \theta)^3 p_i^3 + 4n(d\lambda(\theta)/d\theta) \sum_{i=1}^{n} (X_i - \theta) p_i^3 - 2n\lambda(\theta) \sum_{i=1}^{n} p_i^3}{\sum_{i=1}^{n} (X_i - \theta)^2 p_i^2},$$

$$\frac{d^3\lambda(\theta)}{d\theta^3} = \left[\sum_{i=1}^{n} (X_i - \theta)^2 p_i^2 \right]^{-1} \left[6 \frac{d\lambda(\theta)}{d\theta} \frac{d^2\lambda(\theta)}{d\theta^2} \sum_{i=1}^{n} (X_i - \theta)^3 p_i^3 \right.$$
$$+ 6n \frac{d^2\lambda(\theta)}{d\theta^2} \sum_{i=1}^{n} (X_i - \theta) p_i^3 - 6 \left(\frac{d\lambda(\theta)}{d\theta} \right)^3 \sum_{i=1}^{n} (X_i - \theta)^4 p_i^4$$
$$- 18n \left(\frac{d\lambda(\theta)}{d\theta} \right)^2 \sum_{i=1}^{n} (X_i - \theta)^2 p_i^4$$
$$\left. + 12n \left(\frac{d\lambda(\theta)}{d\theta} \right) \sum_{i=1}^{n} p_i^3 - \left(18n^2 \left(\frac{d\lambda(\theta)}{d\theta} \right) + 6n(\lambda(\theta))^2 \right) \sum_{i=1}^{n} p_i^4 \right],$$

where $p_i = \left(n + \lambda(\theta)(X_i - \theta)\right)^{-1}$. Noting that the argument $\bar{X}$ maximizes the function $\log \mathrm{ELR}_1(\theta)$, $\log \mathrm{ELR}_1(\bar{X}) = 0$, and $\lambda(\bar{X}) = 0$, we have

$$\left.\frac{d\lambda(\theta)}{d\theta}\right|_{\theta=\bar{X}} = -\frac{n}{\frac{1}{n}\sum_{i=1}^{n}(X_i - \bar{X})^2} = -\frac{n}{\sigma_n^2}, \quad \left.\frac{d^2\lambda(\theta)}{d\theta^2}\right|_{\theta=\bar{X}} = \frac{2n\sum_{i=1}^{n}(X_i - \bar{X})^3/n}{\left(\frac{1}{n}\sum_{i=1}^{n}(X_i - \bar{X})^2\right)^3} = \frac{2nM_n^3}{(\sigma_n^2)^3}$$

as well as $d^3\lambda(\theta)/d\theta^3 = O(n)$, for $\theta \in (a,b)$, since, in this case, by using the same techniques applied to the previous proofs and using results found in Owen (1988) and Lazar and Mykland (1998) one can derive the following expressions:

$$\lambda = \frac{\sum_{i=1}^{n}(X_i - \theta)}{\frac{1}{n}\sum_{i=1}^{n}(X_i - \theta)^2} + \frac{O(n^{1/3})}{\tau_n^2} = O\left(n^{2/3-\beta}\right), \quad \frac{\lambda(\theta)}{n}(X_i - \theta) = O(1),$$

$$p_i = \frac{1}{n}\left(1 + \frac{\lambda(\theta)}{n}(X_i - \theta)\right)^{-1} = O(n^{-1}), \text{ when } \left|\bar{X} - \theta\right| \le \varphi_n n^{-1/2} = n^{-1/3-\beta}, 0 < \beta < 1/6.$$

The above asymptotic results, (A.3.8), and a Taylor expansion imply

$$\begin{aligned}
&\int_a^b e^{\log \mathrm{ELR}_1(\theta)}\pi(\theta)d\theta \\
&= \int_a^b \exp\left(-\frac{n}{2\sigma_n^2}(\theta - \bar{X})^2 + \frac{nM_n^3}{3(\sigma_n^2)^3}(\theta - \bar{X})^3 + O(n)(\theta - \bar{X})^4\right)\pi(\theta)d\theta \\
&= \int \exp\left(-\frac{n}{2\sigma_n^2}(\theta - \bar{X})^2\right)\pi(\theta)d\theta + \frac{nM_n^3}{3(\sigma_n^2)^3}\int(\theta - \bar{X})^3 \exp\left(-\frac{n}{2\sigma_n^2}(\theta - \bar{X})^2\right)\pi(\theta)d\theta \\
&\quad + O(n)\int_a^b (\theta - \bar{X})^4 \exp\left(-\frac{n}{2\sigma_n^2}(\theta - \bar{X})^2\right)\pi(\theta)d\theta.
\end{aligned} \tag{A.3.9}$$

It follows similarly that

$$\int_a^b (\theta - \bar{X})e^{\log \mathrm{ELR}_1(\theta)}\pi(\theta)d\theta = \int (\theta - \bar{X})\exp\left(-\frac{n}{2\sigma_n^2}(\theta - \bar{X})^2\right)\pi(\theta)d\theta$$

$$+\frac{nM_n^3}{3(\sigma_n^2)^3}\int (\theta - \bar{X})^4 \exp\left(-\frac{n}{2\sigma_n^2}(\theta - \bar{X})^2\right)\pi(\theta)d\theta \tag{A.3.10}$$

$$+O(n)\int_a^b (\theta - \bar{X})^5 \exp\left(-\frac{n}{2\sigma_n^2}(\theta - \bar{X})^2\right)\pi(\theta)d\theta.$$

By virtue of the definition (3.2), the nonparametric posterior expectation $\hat{\theta}$ can be represented in the form of

$$\hat{\theta} = \frac{\int \theta \exp\left(-\frac{n}{2\sigma_n^2}(\theta - \bar{X})^2\right)\pi(\theta)d\theta}{\int \exp\left(-\frac{n}{2\sigma_n^2}(\theta - \bar{X})^2\right)\pi(\theta)d\theta} + Q_n,$$

where

$$Q_n \equiv \frac{\int_a^b \theta e^{\log \mathrm{ELR}_1(\theta)}\pi(\theta)d\theta \int e^{-\frac{n}{2\sigma_n^2}(\theta-\bar{X})^2}\pi(\theta)d\theta - \int \theta e^{-\frac{n}{2\sigma_n^2}(\theta-\bar{X})^2}\pi(\theta)d\theta \int_a^b e^{\log \mathrm{ELR}_1(\theta)}\pi(\theta)d\theta}{\int e^{-\frac{n}{\sigma_n^2}(\theta-\bar{X})^2}\pi(\theta)d\theta \int_a^b e^{\log \mathrm{ELR}_1(\theta)}\pi(\theta)d\theta}$$

$$= \frac{\int_a^b (\theta - \bar{X})e^{\log \mathrm{ELR}_1(\theta)}\pi(\theta)d\theta \int e^{-\frac{n}{2\sigma_n^2}(\theta-\bar{X})^2}\pi(\theta)d\theta - \int (\theta - \bar{X})e^{-\frac{n}{2\sigma_n^2}(\theta-\bar{X})^2}\pi(\theta)d\theta \int_a^b e^{\log \mathrm{ELR}_1(\theta)}\pi(\theta)d\theta}{\int e^{-\frac{n}{2\sigma_n^2}(\theta-\bar{X})^2}\pi(\theta)d\theta \int_a^b e^{\log \mathrm{ELR}_1(\theta)}\pi(\theta)d\theta}.$$

It is clear that, taking into account the results (A.3.9) and (A.3.10), the facts

$$\pi(\theta) = \pi(\bar{X}) + (\theta - \bar{X})\pi'(\bar{X}) + 0.5(\theta - \bar{X})^2\pi''(\bar{X} + q(\theta - \bar{X})), q \in (0,1),$$

$\int (\theta - \bar{X})e^{-\frac{n}{2\sigma_n^2}(\theta-\bar{X})^2} d\theta = 0$, and $b - a = n^{1/6-\beta}/\sqrt{n}$, we obtain

$$Q_n = \left[\frac{nM_n^3}{3(\sigma_n^2)^3} \int (\theta - \bar{X})^4 e^{-\frac{n}{2\sigma_n^2}(\theta-\bar{X})^2} \pi(\theta)d\theta \int e^{-\frac{n}{2\sigma_n^2}(\theta-\bar{X})^2} \pi(\theta)d\theta \right.$$

$$+O(n)\int_a^b (\theta - \bar{X})^5 e^{-\frac{n}{2\sigma_n^2}(\theta-\bar{X})^2} \pi(\theta)d\theta \int e^{-\frac{n}{2\sigma_n^2}(\theta-\bar{X})^2} \pi(\theta)d\theta$$

$$-\frac{nM_n^3}{3(\sigma_n^2)^3} \int (\theta - \bar{X})^4 e^{-\frac{n}{2\sigma_n^2}(\theta-\bar{X})^2} \pi(\theta)d\theta \int (\theta - \bar{X}) e^{-\frac{n}{2\sigma_n^2}(\theta-\bar{X})^2} \pi(\theta)d\theta$$

$$\left. -O(n)\int_a^b (\theta - \bar{X})^4 e^{-\frac{n}{2\sigma_n^2}(\theta-\bar{X})^2} \pi(\theta)d\theta \int (\theta - \bar{X}) e^{-\frac{n}{2\sigma_n^2}(\theta-\bar{X})^2} \pi(\theta)d\theta \right] \times$$

$$\left[\left(\int e^{-\frac{n}{2\sigma_n^2}(\theta-\bar{X})^2} \pi(\theta)d\theta \right)^2 \right.$$

$$+\frac{nM_n^3}{3(\sigma_n^2)^3} \int (\theta - \bar{X})^3 e^{-\frac{n}{2\sigma_n^2}(\theta-\bar{X})^2} \pi(\theta)d\theta \int e^{-\frac{n}{2\sigma_n^2}(\theta-\bar{X})^2} \pi(\theta)d\theta$$

$$\left. + O(n)\int_a^b (\theta - \bar{X})^4 e^{-\frac{n}{2\sigma_n^2}(\theta-\bar{X})^2} \pi(\theta)d\theta \int e^{-\frac{n}{2\sigma_n^2}(\theta-\bar{X})^2} \pi(\theta)d\theta \right]^{-1}$$

$$= \left[\frac{nM_n^3}{3(\sigma_n^2)^3} \int (\theta - \bar{X})^4 e^{-\frac{n}{2\sigma_n^2}(\theta-\bar{X})^2} d\theta \int e^{-\frac{n}{2\sigma_n^2}(\theta-\bar{X})^2} d\theta \right.$$

$$\left. +O(n)\int_a^b (\theta - \bar{X})^5 e^{-\frac{n}{2\sigma_n^2}(\theta-\bar{X})^2} d\theta \int e^{-\frac{n}{2\sigma_n^2}(\theta-\bar{X})^2} d\theta \right] \times$$

$$\left[\int e^{-\frac{n}{2\sigma_n^2}(\theta-\bar{X})^2} d\theta \right]^{-2} + O(n^{-1/2-6\beta}).$$

Computing the integrals written above, we deduce that

$$\hat{\theta} = \frac{\int \theta \exp\left(-\frac{n}{2\sigma_n^2}(\theta - \bar{X})^2 \right) \pi(\theta)d\theta}{\int \exp\left(-\frac{n}{2\sigma_n^2}(\theta - \bar{X})^2 \right) \pi(\theta)d\theta}$$

$$+ \frac{\frac{2nM_n^3}{3(\sigma_n^2)^3} \frac{4!(\pi)^{1/2}(2\sigma_n^2)^{5/2}}{2!n^{5/2}2^5} \frac{(2\pi\sigma_n^2)^{1/2}}{n^{1/2}} + O\left(n(n^{1/6-\beta-1/2})^6\right) \frac{(2\pi\sigma_n^2)^{1/2}}{n^{1/2}}}{\frac{(2\pi\sigma_n^2)}{n}}$$

$$+O(n^{-1/2-6\beta}).$$

Making use of $\beta = 1/6 - \varepsilon/6, \varepsilon > 0$ we complete the proof of Proposition 3.1.

Proof of Corollary 3.1

Corollary 3.1 can be proven by applying directly the result of Proposition 3.1.

Proof of Corollary 3.2

To prove this corollary, we can use the result

$$\hat{\theta} = \frac{\int_a^b \theta \exp[-\frac{1}{2n}\frac{(\sum X_i - n\theta)^2}{\sigma_n{}^2}]\pi(\theta)d\theta}{\int_a^b \exp[-\frac{1}{2n}\frac{(\sum X_i - n\theta)^2}{\sigma_n{}^2}]\pi(\theta)d\theta} + \frac{M_n^3}{\sigma_n^2 n} + O_p\left(n^{-3/2+\varepsilon}\right),$$

where $a = \bar{X} - \varphi_n n^{-1/2}$, $b = \bar{X} + \varphi_n n^{-1/2}$, $\varphi_n = n^{1/6-\beta}$, $0 < \gamma < \beta < 1/6$, and $\beta = 1/6 - \varepsilon/6,\ \varepsilon > 0$.

This approximation was obtained previously via the process related to the proof of Proposition 3.1. Applying the Taylor expansion $\pi(\theta) = \pi(\bar{X}) + (\theta - \bar{X})\pi'(\bar{X}) + (\theta - \bar{X})^2\pi''(\bar{X})/2 + (\theta - \bar{X})^3\pi'''(\tilde{X})/6,\ \tilde{X} \in (\theta, \bar{X})$ to the asymptotic form of $\hat{\theta}$ and in a similar manner of the Laplace method (e.g., Bleistein and Handelsman, 1975, p. 180), we complete the proof.

Proof of Proposition 3.4

We begin with the asymptotic analysis related to the numerator of the definition of the nonparametric posterior expectation $\hat{D}_G$. To approximate the double integral $\iint D(\theta_1, \theta_2)e^{\log \mathrm{ELR}_3(\theta_1,\theta_2)}\pi(\theta_1, \theta_2)d\theta_1 d\theta_2$, we first show that the main term of the integral is

$$\int_a^b \int_{a_1}^{b_1} D(\theta_1, \theta_2)e^{\log \mathrm{ELR}_3(\theta_1,\theta_2)}\pi(\theta_1, \theta_2)d\theta_1 d\theta_2,$$

where $a = \bar{X} - \varphi_n n^{-1/2}, b = \bar{X} + \varphi_n n^{-1/2}, a_1 = \overline{X^2} - \varphi_n n^{-1/2}, b_1 = \overline{X^2} + \varphi_n n^{-1/2}, \varphi_n = n^{1/6-\beta}$, $0 < \beta < 1/6$ and $\overline{X^2} = \sum_{i=1}^n X_i^2/n$. Since

$$\int_{X_{(1)}}^a \int_{X_{(1)}^2}^{X_{(n)}^2} D(\theta_1, \theta_2)e^{\log \mathrm{ELR}_3(\theta_1,\theta_2)}\pi(\theta_1, \theta_2)d\theta_1 d\theta_2$$

$$\leq \int_{X_{(1)}}^a \int_{X_{(1)}^2}^{X_{(n)}^2} D(\theta_1, \theta_2)\pi(\theta_1, \theta_2)d\theta_2 e^{\log \mathrm{ELR}_1(\theta_1)}d\theta_1, X_{(1)}^2 = \min(X_i^2), X_{(n)}^2 = \max(X_i^2),$$

in a similar manner to the proof of Proposition 3.1, we conclude

$$\int_{X_{(1)}}^{a}\int_{X_{(1)}^2}^{X_{(n)}^2} D(\theta_1,\theta_2)\pi(\theta_1,\theta_2)d\theta_2 e^{\log \mathrm{ELR}_1(\theta_1)}d\theta_1$$
$$\le \int_{X_{(1)}}^{a}\int_{X_{(1)}^2}^{X_{(n)}^2} D(\theta_1,\theta_2)\pi(\theta_1,\theta_2)d\theta_2 d\theta_1 e^{\log \mathrm{ELR}_1(a)}$$
$$= O(e^{-wn^{1/3-2\beta}}) \to 0,$$

where w is a positive constant and $n \to \infty$.

Likewise, we have

$$\int_{b}^{X_{(n)}}\int_{X_{(1)}^2}^{X_{(n)}^2} D(\theta_1,\theta_2)e^{\log \mathrm{ELR}_3(\theta_1,\theta_2)}\pi(\theta_1,\theta_2)d\theta_1 d\theta_2 = O(e^{-wn^{1/3-2\beta}}) \to 0, \text{ as } n \to \infty.$$

Now, we define $\mathrm{ELR}_5(\theta) = n^n \max_{0<p_1,\ldots,p_n<1}\{\prod_{i=1}^n p_i : \sum_{i=1}^n p_i = 1, \sum_{i=1}^n p_i X_i^2 = \theta\}$. It is clear that $\mathrm{ELR}_5(\theta) \ge \mathrm{ELR}_3(\theta_1,\theta)$, for all (θ_1,θ), and hence

$$\int_{a}^{b}\int_{X_{(1)}^2}^{a_1} D(\theta_1,\theta_2)e^{\log \mathrm{ELR}_3(\theta_1,\theta_2)}\pi(\theta_1,\theta_2)d\theta_1 d\theta_2$$
$$\le \int_{a}^{b}\int_{X_{(1)}^2}^{a_1} D(\theta_1,\theta_2)\pi(\theta_1,\theta_2)d\theta_1 e^{\log \mathrm{ELR}_5(\theta_2)}d\theta_2$$
$$\le \int_{a}^{b}\int_{X_{(1)}^2}^{a_1} D(\theta_1,\theta_2)\pi(\theta_1,\theta_2)d\theta_1 d\theta_2 e^{\log \mathrm{ELR}_5(a_1)} = O(e^{-wn^{1/3-2\beta}}) \to 0,$$

and $\int_{a}^{b}\int_{b_1}^{X_{(n)}^2} D(\theta_1,\theta_2)e^{\log \mathrm{ELR}_3(\theta_1,\theta_2)}\pi(\theta_1,\theta_2)d\theta_1 d\theta_2 \to 0,\ n \to \infty.$

In order to apply almost directly the proof scheme of Proposition 3.1, we note that

$$\log \mathrm{ELR}_3(\theta_1,\theta_2) = -\sum_{i=1}^{n}\log\left\{1+\frac{\lambda_1}{n}(X_i-\theta_1)+\frac{\lambda_2}{n}(X_i^2-\theta_2)\right\},$$

where the Lagrange multipliers λ_1 and λ_2 satisfy

$$L_1(\theta_1,\theta_2) \equiv \sum_{i=1}^{n}\frac{X_i-\theta_1}{n+\lambda_1(X_i-\theta_1)+\lambda_2(X_i^2-\theta_2)} = 0 \text{ and}$$
$$L_2(\theta_1,\theta_2) \equiv \sum_{i=1}^{n}\frac{X_i^2-\theta_2}{n+\lambda_1(X_i-\theta_1)+\lambda_2(X_i^2-\theta_2)} = 0. \tag{A.3.11}$$

Since (A.3.11), one can show that

$$\frac{\partial \log \mathrm{ELR}_3(\theta_1,\theta_2)}{\partial \theta_1} = \lambda_1(\theta_1,\theta_2) \text{ and } \frac{\partial \log \mathrm{ELR}_3(\theta_1,\theta_2)}{\partial \theta_2} = \lambda_2(\theta_1,\theta_2). \quad \text{(A.3.12)}$$

Then the facts $\lambda_1(\bar{X},\overline{X^2})=0, \lambda_2(\bar{X},\overline{X^2})=0$, and a Taylor expansion argument yield

$$\begin{aligned}\log \mathrm{ELR}_3(\theta_1,\theta_2) &= \frac{1}{2}(\theta_1-\bar{X})^2 \left.\frac{\partial\lambda_1}{\partial\theta_1}\right|_{\substack{\theta_1=\bar{X}\\ \theta_2=\overline{X^2}}} + (\theta_1-\bar{X})(\theta_2-\overline{X^2})\left.\frac{\partial\lambda_1}{\partial\theta_2}\right|_{\substack{\theta_1=\bar{X}\\ \theta_2=\overline{X^2}}} \\ &+ \frac{1}{2}(\theta_2-\overline{X^2})^2 \left.\frac{\partial\lambda_2}{\partial\theta_2}\right|_{\substack{\theta_1=\bar{X}\\ \theta_2=\overline{X^2}}} + \frac{1}{3!}\left[(\theta_1-\bar{X})^3 \left.\frac{\partial^2\lambda_1}{\partial\theta_1^2}\right|_{\substack{\theta_1=\bar{X}\\ \theta_2=\overline{X^2}}}\right. \\ &+ 3(\theta_1-\bar{X})^2(\theta_2-\overline{X^2})\left.\frac{\partial^2\lambda_1}{\partial\theta_1\partial\theta_2}\right|_{\substack{\theta_1=\bar{X}\\ \theta_2=\overline{X^2}}} \\ &+ 3(\theta_1-\bar{X})(\theta_2-\overline{X^2})^2\left.\frac{\partial^2\lambda_2}{\partial\theta_1\partial\theta_2}\right|_{\substack{\theta_1=\bar{X}\\ \theta_2=\overline{X^2}}} \\ &\left. + (\theta_2-\overline{X^2})^3\left.\frac{\partial^2\lambda_2}{\partial\theta_2^2}\right|_{\substack{\theta_1=\bar{X}\\ \theta_2=\overline{X^2}}}\right] + O(n^{-1/3-4\beta}),\end{aligned}$$

when $\theta_1 \in (a,b), \theta_2 \in (a_1,b_1), 0<\beta<1/6$ and where

$$\left.\frac{\partial\lambda_1}{\partial\theta_1}\right|_{\substack{\theta_1=\bar{X}\\ \theta_2=\overline{X^2}}} = -\frac{n}{\sigma_n^2-(\sigma_{XX^2n})^2/\sigma_{X^2n}^2}, \quad \left.\frac{\partial\lambda_2}{\partial\theta_2}\right|_{\substack{\theta_1=\bar{X}\\ \theta_2=\overline{X^2}}} = -\frac{n}{\sigma_{X^2n}^2-(\sigma_{XX^2n})^2/\sigma_n^2}, \quad \text{(A.3.13)}$$

$$\left.\frac{\partial\lambda_1}{\partial\theta_2}\right|_{\substack{\theta_1=\bar{X}\\ \theta_2=\overline{X^2}}} = \left.\frac{\partial\lambda_2}{\partial\theta_1}\right|_{\substack{\theta_1=\bar{X}\\ \theta_2=\overline{X^2}}} = \frac{n}{\sigma_{X^2n}^2\sigma_n^2/\sigma_{XX^2n}-\sigma_{XX^2n}},$$

$$\left.\frac{\partial^2\lambda_1}{\partial\theta_k^2}\right|_{\substack{\theta_1=\bar{X}\\ \theta_2=\overline{X^2}}} = 2n^{-2}\left[\sigma_{XX^2n}\sum_{i=1}^{n}(X_i^2-\overline{X^2})\psi_{ki}-\sigma_{X^2n}^2\sum_{i=1}^{n}\left(X_i-\bar{X}\right)\psi_{ki}\right]\times \left[(\sigma_{XX^2n})^2-\sigma_{X^2n}^2\sigma_n^2\right]^{-1},$$

$$\left.\frac{\partial^2\lambda_2}{\partial\theta_k^2}\right|_{\substack{\theta_1=\bar{X}\\ \theta_2=\overline{X^2}}} = 2n^{-2}\left[\sigma_n^2\sum_{i=1}^{n}(X_i^2-\overline{X^2})\psi_{ki}-\sigma_{XX^2n}\sum_{i=1}^{n}(X_i-\bar{X})\psi_{ki}\right]\times \left[\sigma_{X^2n}^2\sigma_n^2-(\sigma_{XX^2n})^2\right]^{-1},$$

$$\frac{\partial^2\lambda_1}{\partial\theta_1\partial\theta_2} = \frac{\partial^2\lambda_2}{\partial\theta_1^2} \text{ and } \frac{\partial^2\lambda_1}{\partial\theta_1\partial\theta_2} = \frac{\partial^2\lambda_2}{\partial\theta_1^2}$$

that can be obtained by using (A.3.11) and (A.3.12) with the definitions

$$\psi_{ki} = \left(\left.\frac{\partial \lambda_1}{\partial \theta_k}\right|_{\substack{\theta_1=\bar{X} \\ \theta_2=\overline{X^2}}} (X_i - \bar{X}) + \left.\frac{\partial \lambda_2}{\partial \theta_k}\right|_{\substack{\theta_1=\bar{X} \\ \theta_2=\overline{X^2}}} (X_i^2 - \overline{X^2}) \right)^2, \; k = 1, 2,$$

$$\sigma^2_{X^2 n} = \frac{1}{n}\sum_{i=1}^{n}\left(X_i^2 - \overline{X^2}\right)^2,$$

$$\sigma_{XX^2 n} = \frac{1}{n}\sum_{i=1}^{n}\left(X_i - \bar{X}\right)\left(X_i^2 - \overline{X^2}\right).$$

The validity of the Proposition 3.4 follows by arguments similar to those of the proof of Proposition 3.1 (see the proof scheme from (A.3.8) to the end of the Proposition 3.1's proof) where the Taylor expansion for

$$D(\theta_1, \theta_2) = D(\bar{X}, \overline{X^2}) + (\theta_1 - \bar{X}) \left.\frac{\partial D(\theta_1, \theta_2)}{\partial \theta_1}\right|_{\substack{\theta_1=\bar{X} \\ \theta_2=\overline{X^2}}} + (\theta_2 - \overline{X^2}) \left.\frac{\partial D(\theta_1, \theta_2)}{\partial \theta_2}\right|_{\substack{\theta_1=\bar{X} \\ \theta_2=\overline{X^2}}} + \ldots$$

is applied evaluating a Q_n-type remainder term (see the remainder term Q_n and its analysis in the proof of Proposition 3.1). In this case, we present the remainder term, J_n, which appears in the expansion of Proposition 3.4, in the integral form

$$J_n = \left\{ \iint \left[(\theta_1 - \bar{X}) \left.\frac{\partial D(t_1, t_2)}{\partial t_1}\right|_{\substack{t_1=\bar{X} \\ t_2=\overline{X^2}}} + (\theta_2 - \overline{X^2}) \left.\frac{\partial D(t_1, t_2)}{\partial t_2}\right|_{\substack{t_1=\bar{X} \\ t_2=\overline{X^2}}} \right] \frac{1}{6} \left[(\theta_1 - \bar{X})^3 \left.\frac{\partial^2 \lambda_1}{\partial t_1^2}\right|_{\substack{t_1=\bar{X} \\ t_2=\overline{X^2}}} \right.\right.$$

$$+ 3\left(\theta_1 - \bar{X}\right)^2 \left(\theta_2 - \overline{X^2}\right) \left.\frac{\partial^2 \lambda_1}{\partial t_1 \partial t_2}\right|_{\substack{t_1=\bar{X} \\ t_2=\overline{X^2}}}$$

$$\left. + 3\left(\theta_1 - \bar{X}\right)\left(\theta_2 - \overline{X^2}\right)^2 \left.\frac{\partial^2 \lambda_2}{\partial t_1 \partial t_2}\right|_{\substack{t_1=\bar{X} \\ t_2=\overline{X^2}}} + \left(\theta_2 - \overline{X^2}\right)^3 \left.\frac{\partial^2 \lambda_2}{\partial t_2^2}\right|_{\substack{t_1=\bar{X} \\ t_2=\overline{X^2}}} \right]$$

$$\left. \times e^{-\frac{0.5n(\theta_1 - \bar{X})^2}{\sigma_n^2 - ()\left(\sigma_{XX^2 n}\right)^2 / \sigma^2_{X^2 n}} - \frac{0.5n(\theta_2 - \overline{X^2})^2}{\sigma^2_{X^2 n} - \left(\sigma_{XX^2 n}\right)^2 / \sigma_n^2} + \frac{n(\theta_1 - \bar{X})(\theta_2 - \overline{X^2})}{\sigma^2_{X^2 n}\, \sigma_n^2 / \sigma_{XX^2 n} - \sigma_{XX^2 n}}} \pi(\theta_1, \theta_2)\, d\theta_1 d\theta_2 \right\}$$

$$\times \left\{ \iint e^{-\frac{0.5n(\theta_1 - \bar{X})^2}{\sigma_n^2 - \left(\sigma_{XX^2 n}\right)^2 / \sigma^2_{X^2 n}} - \frac{0.5n(\theta_2 - \overline{X^2})^2}{\sigma^2_{X^2 n} - \left(\sigma_{XX^2 n}\right)^2 / \sigma_n^2} + \frac{n(\theta_1 - \bar{X})(\theta_2 - \overline{X^2})}{\sigma^2_{X^2 n}\, \sigma_n^2 / \sigma_{XX^2 n} - \sigma_{XX^2 n}}} \pi(\theta_1, \theta_2)\, d\theta_1 d\theta_2 \right\}^{-1}, \quad \text{(A.3.14)}$$

where the corresponding derivatives of λ_1 and λ_2 are defined in (A.3.13).

Proof of Proposition 3.6

The proof of Proposition 3.6 is based on the fact that function $lr(\theta)$ is highly peaked about its maximum $\bar{X} = \sum_{i=1}^{n} X_i/n$. We will use that $lr(\theta)$ can be well approximated by the function $-n(\theta - \bar{X})^2/2\sigma_n^2$, when values of θ are close to $\bar{X}$. Toward this end, we first show that

$$\int_{X_{(1)}}^{X_{(n)}} e^{lr(\theta)}\pi(\theta)d\theta = \int_{\bar{X}-\varphi_n n^{-1/2}}^{\bar{X}+\varphi_n n^{-1/2}} e^{lr(\theta)}\pi(\theta)d\theta + O\left(\exp\left(-c\varphi_n^2\right)\right),$$

where $c > 0$ is a constant, a positive sequence $\varphi_n = O(n^{\varepsilon}) \to \infty$, for some $\varepsilon > 0$, $\varphi_n n^{-0.5} \to 0$, and $\int_{\bar{X}-\varphi_n n^{-1/2}}^{\bar{X}+\varphi_n n^{-1/2}} e^{lr(\theta)}\pi(\theta)d\theta = O(n^{-1/2})$, as $n \to \infty$. This approximation allows us to analyze the numerator and denominator in (3.8). Denote the log EL function $l(\theta) = \sum_{i=1}^{n} \log p_i$, where p_i's maximize the Lagrangian

$$\Delta = \sum_{i=1}^{n} \log(p_i) + \lambda_1(1 - \sum_{i=1}^{n} p_i) + \lambda_2(\theta - \sum_{i=1}^{n} p_i X_i),$$

with λ_1 and λ_2 that are the Lagrange multipliers. One can show that $p_i = (n + \lambda(X_i - \theta))^{-1}$, where λ is a root of the equation $\sum_{i=1}^{n}(X_i - \theta)/(n + \lambda(X_i - \theta)) = 0$.

By virtue of Lemma 3.1, when $\theta < \bar{X}$, $lr(\theta)$ increases and when $\theta > \bar{X}$, $lr(\theta)$ decreases. This implies that the log ELR function $lr(\theta)$ defined in (3.7) has the maximum at $\theta = \bar{X}$. Denote $a = \bar{X} - \varphi_n n^{-0.5}$ and $b = \bar{X} + \varphi_n n^{-0.5}$ where $\varphi_n = n^{1/6-\beta}$ and $\beta \in (0, 1/6)$. Then it turns out that

$$\int_{X_{(1)}}^{X_{(n)}} e^{lr(\theta)}\pi(\theta)d\theta = \int_{X_{(1)}}^{a} e^{lr(\theta)}\pi(\theta)d\theta + \int_{a}^{b} e^{lr(\theta)}\pi(\theta)d\theta + \int_{b}^{X_{(n)}} e^{lr(\theta)}\pi(\theta)d\theta,$$

$$\text{and } \int_{X_{(1)}}^{q_L} e^{lr(\theta)}\pi(\theta)d\theta = \int_{X_{(1)}}^{a} e^{lr(\theta)}\pi(\theta)d\theta + \int_{a}^{q_L} e^{lr(\theta)}\pi(\theta)d\theta.$$

By the virtue of the previous considerations we can bound the remainder term

$$\int_{X_{(1)}}^{a} e^{lr(\theta)}\pi(\theta)d\theta \le e^{lr(a)} \int_{X_{(1)}}^{X_{(n)}} \pi(\theta)d\theta \le e^{lr(a)}.$$

In order to evaluate $lr(a)$, we define the function

$$L(\lambda) = \sum_{i=1}^{n} (X_i - \theta)/(n + \lambda(X_i - \theta)). \tag{A.3.15}$$

We rewrite (A.3.15) at $\theta = a$ such that

$$L(\lambda) = \sum\nolimits_{i=1}^{n} (X_i - \bar{X} + \varphi_n n^{-0.5}) / (n + \lambda(X_i - \bar{X} + \varphi_n n^{-0.5}))$$

$$= \frac{1}{n} \sum_{i=1}^{n} \frac{(X_i - \bar{X} + \varphi_n n^{-0.5}) \left[\left(1 + \lambda n^{-1}(X_i - \bar{X} + \varphi_n n^{-0.5})\right) - \lambda n^{-1}(X_i - \bar{X} + \varphi_n n^{-0.5}) \right]}{1 + \lambda n^{-1}(X_i - \bar{X} + \varphi_n n^{-0.5})}$$

$$= \frac{1}{n} \left[\sum_{i=1}^{n} (X_i - \bar{X} + \varphi_n n^{-0.5}) - \lambda n^{-1} \sum_{i=1}^{n} \frac{(X_i - \bar{X} + \varphi_n n^{-0.5})^2}{1 + \lambda n^{-1}(X_i - \bar{X} + \varphi_n n^{-0.5})} \right]. \tag{A.3.16}$$

Defining $\lambda_c = n^{2/3}\tau_n^{-1}$, where $\tau_n = n^{\gamma}$, $0 < \gamma < \beta < 1/6$, and plugging it into Equation (A.3.16) we have

$$\sqrt{n}L(\lambda_c) = \varphi_n - \sqrt{n}\frac{n^{2/3-1}}{\tau_n}\frac{1}{n}\sum_{i=1}^{n} \frac{(X_i - \bar{X} + \varphi_n n^{-0.5})^2}{1 + n^{-1/3}\tau_n^{-1}(X_i - \bar{X} + \varphi_n n^{-0.5})},$$

Since $\frac{X_i - \bar{X}}{n^{1/3}\tau_n} = O_p(1)$ (e.g., Owen, 1988), we have

$$\sqrt{n}L(\lambda_c) = \varphi_n - \frac{n^{1/6}}{\tau_n}\frac{1}{n}\sum_{i=1}^{n} \frac{(X_i - \bar{X} + \varphi_n n^{-0.5})^2}{1 + O_p(1)}.$$

Thus $\sqrt{n}L(\lambda_c) \to -\infty$, as $n \to \infty$. In a similar manner, $\sqrt{n}L(-\lambda_c) \to \infty$, as $n \to \infty$. And then the solution, λ_0, of equation $\sqrt{n}L(\lambda_0) = 0$ belongs to the interval $[-\lambda_c, \lambda_c]$, that is, $\lambda_0 = O_p\left(n^{2/3}\tau_n^{-1}\right)$.

Let us now derive the approximate value of λ_0 as $n \to \infty$. Since $L(\lambda_0) = 0$,

$$\sum\nolimits_{i=1}^{n} \frac{(X_i - \bar{X} + \varphi_n n^{-0.5})}{1 + \lambda_0 n^{-1}(X_i - \bar{X} + \varphi_n n^{-0.5})} = 0. \tag{A.3.17}$$

Applying a Taylor series expansion to (A.3.17) considering $\lambda_0 n^{-1}(X_i - \bar{X} + \varphi_n n^{-0.5})$ around zero we obtain

$$\sum_{i=1}^{n} \left(X_i - \bar{X} + \phi_n n^{-0.5}\right) \left[1 - \lambda_0 n^{-1}\left(X_i - \bar{X} + \phi_n n^{-0.5}\right) + \frac{\lambda_0^{\,2} n^{-2}\left(X_i - \bar{X} + \phi_n n^{-0.5}\right)^2}{\left(1 + \omega_i\right)^3} \right] = 0. \tag{A.3.18}$$

where $0 < \omega_i < \lambda_0 n^{-1}(X_i - \bar{X} + \varphi_n n^{-0.5})$. As $\lambda_0 = O_p\left(n^{2/3}\tau_n^{-1}\right)$, we can rewrite Equation (A.3.18) in the form

$$\sum_{i=1}^{n}\left(X_i - \bar{X} + \frac{\varphi_n}{n^{1/2}}\right) - \frac{\lambda}{n}\sum_{i=1}^{n}\left(X_i - \bar{X} + \frac{\varphi_n}{n^{1/2}}\right)^2 + \frac{O(n^{1/3})}{\tau_n^2}\frac{1}{n}\sum_{i=1}^{n}\left(X_i - \bar{X} + \frac{\varphi_n}{n^{1/2}}\right)^3 = 0. \tag{A.3.19}$$

Then solving (A.3.19) gives the approximate solution by

$$\lambda_0 = \frac{\varphi_n n^{1/2}}{n^{-1}\sum_{i=1}^{n}(X_i - \bar{X} + \varphi_n n^{-1/2})^2} + \frac{O(n^{1/3})}{\tau_n^2}. \tag{A.3.20}$$

Applying a Taylor series expansion to $lr(a)$ considering $\lambda_0 n^{-1}(X_i - \bar{X} + \varphi_n n^{-0.5})$ around zero yields

$$\begin{aligned} lr(a) &= -\sum_{i=1}^{n}\log\left[1+\frac{\lambda_0}{n}(X_i - \bar{X} + \varphi_n n^{-0.5})\right] \\ &= -\sum_{i=1}^{n}\frac{\lambda_0}{n}(X_i - \bar{X} + \varphi_n n^{-0.5}) + \frac{1}{2}\sum_{i=1}^{n}\frac{\lambda_0{}^2}{n^2}(X_i - \bar{X} + \varphi_n n^{-0.5})^2 \\ &\quad -\frac{1}{3}\sum_{i=1}^{n}\frac{\lambda_0{}^3}{n^3}\frac{(X_i - \bar{X} + \varphi_n n^{-0.5})^3}{(1+\omega_i^*)^3}, \end{aligned}$$

where $0 < \omega_i^* < \lambda_0 n^{-1}(X_i - \bar{X} + \varphi_n n^{-0.5})$. By virtue of (A.3.20) and the fact that $\lambda_0 = O(n^{2/3}/\tau_n)$ we have

$$lr(a) = -\frac{\lambda_0}{n}\varphi_n n^{1/2} + \frac{1}{2}\sum_{i=1}^{n}\frac{\lambda_0{}^2}{n^2}(X_i - \bar{X} + \varphi_n n^{-0.5})^2 - O(n^{-3\gamma})$$

$$= \frac{-\varphi_n{}^2 n}{nn^{-1}\sum_{i=1}^{n}(X_i - \bar{X} + \varphi_n n^{-0.5})^2} - \frac{O(n^{4/3})}{\tau_n^2 n^2}\varphi_n n^{1/2} + \frac{1}{2}\left[\frac{\varphi_n{}^2 n}{\left[n^{-1}\sum_{i=1}^{n}(X_i - \bar{X} + \varphi_n n^{-0.5})^2\right]^2}\right.$$

$$\left. + 2\frac{O(n^{4/3})}{\tau_n^2 n}\frac{\varphi_n{}^2 n^{1/2}}{n^{-1}\sum_{i=1}^{n}(X_i - \bar{X} + \varphi_n n^{-0.5})^2} + \frac{O(n^{8/3})}{\tau_n^4 n^2}\right] \times$$

$$\frac{1}{n^2}\sum_{i=1}^{n}(X_i - \bar{X} + \varphi_n n^{-0.5})^2 - O(n^{-3\gamma})$$

$$= -\frac{1}{2}\frac{\varphi_n{}^2}{n^{-1}\sum_{i=1}^{n}(X_i - \bar{X} + \varphi_n n^{-0.5})^2} - O(n^{-3\gamma}) \to -\infty, \text{ as } n \to \infty,$$

where ${\varphi_n}^2 = n^{1/3-2\beta} \to \infty$ and $0 < \gamma < \beta < 1/6$. Thus we conclude that

$$\int_{X_{(1)}}^{a} \exp(lr(\theta))\pi(\theta)d\theta \le \exp(lr(a)) = O\left(\exp\left(-wn^{1/3-2\beta}\right)\right) \to 0, \text{ as } n \to \infty,$$

where w is a positive constant.

Now define $b = \bar{X} + \varphi_n n^{-1/2}$ and in a similar manner to the proof scheme above we have

$$\int_{b}^{X_{(n)}} e^{lr(\theta)}\pi(\theta)d\theta \le \exp(lr(b)) = O\left(\exp\left(-w_1\varphi_n^2\right)\right) \to 0,$$

where w_1 is a positive constant and $n \to \infty$. Thus we show that

$$\int_{X_{(1)}}^{X_{(n)}} e^{lr(\theta)}\pi(\theta)d\theta \cong \int_{\bar{X}-\varphi_n n^{-1/2}}^{\bar{X}+\varphi_n n^{-1/2}} e^{lr(\theta)}\pi(\theta)d\theta.$$

Similarly we have that

$$\int_{X_{(1)}}^{q_L} e^{lr(\theta)}\pi(\theta)d\theta \cong \int_{\bar{X}-\phi_n n^{-1/2}}^{q_L} e^{lr(\theta)}\pi(\theta)d\theta.$$

Now we consider the main term $\int_a^b e^{lr(\theta)}\pi(\theta)d\theta$ of the marginal distribution defined in (3.7). This integral consists of the log ELR function $lr(\theta)$ and we expand $lr(\theta)$ at $\theta = \bar{X}$ using Taylor theorem,

$$\begin{aligned} lr(\theta) = {} & lr(\bar{X}) + (\theta - \bar{X})\lambda(\bar{X}) + \frac{1}{2}(\theta - \bar{X})^2\left(\left.{d\lambda(u)}\middle/{du}\right|_{u=\bar{X}}\right) \\ & + \frac{1}{6}(\theta - \bar{X})^3\left(\left.{d^2\lambda(u)}\middle/{du^2}\right|_{u=\bar{X}}\right) \\ & + \frac{1}{24}(\theta - \bar{X})^4\left(\left.{d^3\lambda(u)}\middle/{du^3}\right|_{u=\theta+\varpi(\bar{X}-\theta)}\right), \varpi \in [0,1]. \end{aligned} \tag{A.3.21}$$

By virtue of Proposition 10.2.1 in Vexler et al. (2014a), we have

$$\left.\frac{d\lambda(u)}{du}\right|_{u=\bar{X}} = -\frac{n}{n^{-1}\sum_{i=1}^{n}(X_i - \bar{X})^2} = -\frac{n}{\sigma_n^2}, \left.\frac{d^2\lambda(u)}{du^2}\right|_{u=\bar{X}} = -\frac{2n\sum_{i=1}^{n}(X_i - \bar{X})^3/n}{\left[n^{-1}\sum_{i=1}^{n}(X_i - \bar{X})^2\right]^3} = \frac{2nM_n^3}{(\sigma_n^2)^3},$$

and $d^3\lambda(\theta)/d\theta^3 = O_p(n)$, for $\theta \in [a,b]$. The argument $\bar{X}$ maximizes the function $l(\theta) = \sum_{i=1}^{n} \log p_i$, $l(\bar{X}) = n\log(1/n)$ and then $lr(\bar{X}) = 0$ as well as $\lambda(\bar{X}) = 0$.

Using the aforementioned results, Equation (A.3.21) and a Taylor expansion for $nM_n^3(\theta - \bar{X})^3/3(\sigma_n^2)^3$ and $O_p(n)(\theta - \bar{X})^4$ around zero, we have

$$\int_a^b e^{lr(\theta)}\pi(\theta)\,d\theta = \int_a^b \exp\left[-\frac{n}{2\sigma_n^2}(\theta-\overline{X})^2 + \frac{nM_n^3}{3(\sigma_n^2)^3}(\theta-\overline{X})^3 + O_p(n)(\theta-\overline{X})^4\right]\pi(\theta)d\theta$$
$$= \int \exp\left[-\frac{n}{2\sigma_n^2}(\theta-\overline{X})^2\right]\pi(\theta)d\theta$$
$$+\frac{nM_n^3}{3(\sigma_n^2)^3}\int(\theta-\overline{X})^3\exp\left[-\frac{n}{2\sigma_n^2}(\theta-\overline{X})^2\right]\pi(\theta)d\theta$$
$$+O_p(n)\int(\theta-\overline{X})^4\exp\left[-\frac{n}{2\sigma_n^2}(\theta-\overline{X})^2\right]\pi(\theta)d\theta. \tag{A.3.22}$$

Now by virtue of the definition (3.8), the formula $\alpha/2 = \int_{X_{(1)}}^{q_L} h_E(\theta \mid X)d\theta$ can be rewritten as

$$\frac{\alpha}{2} = \frac{\int^{q_L}\exp\left[-\frac{n}{2\sigma_n^2}(\theta-\overline{X})^2\right]\pi(\theta)d\theta}{\int\exp\left[-\frac{n}{2\sigma_n^2}(\theta-\overline{X})^2\right]\pi(\theta)d\theta} + R_n,$$

where

$$R_n = \left\{\int_a^{q_L} e^{lr(\theta)}\pi(\theta)\,d\theta\int\exp\left[-\frac{n}{2\sigma_n^2}(\theta-\overline{X})^2\right]\pi(\theta)d\theta\right.$$
$$\left.-\int^{q_L}\exp\left[-\frac{n}{2\sigma_n^2}(\theta-\overline{X})^2\right]\pi(\theta)d\theta\int_a^b e^{lr(\theta)}\pi(\theta)\,d\theta\right\}$$
$$\left\{\int_a^b e^{lr(\theta)}\pi(\theta)\,d\theta\int\exp\left[-\frac{n}{2\sigma_n^2}(\theta-\overline{X})^2\right]\pi(\theta)d\theta\right\}^{-1}.$$

It is clear that one can use (A.3.22) and the facts:

(1) $\pi(\theta) = \pi(\overline{X}) + (\theta-\overline{X})\pi'(\overline{X}) + 1/2(\theta-\overline{X})^2\pi''(\overline{X}+q(\theta-\overline{X})),\ q\in[0,1]$;
(2) $b-a = n^{1/6-\beta}/n^{1/2}$;
(3) $\int(\theta-\overline{X})\exp\left[-\frac{n}{2\sigma_n^2}(\theta-\overline{X})^2\right]d\theta = 0$

to represent the remainder term R_n in the form

$$R_n = M_n^3 C_n + O_p(n^{-1+\varepsilon}),$$

where $C_n = 2n^{-0.5}(1+z_{1-\alpha/2}^2/2)\varphi(z_{1-\alpha/2})/3\sigma_n^3$ and $\varepsilon>0$.

Combing the above asymptotic approximations, we have

$$\frac{\alpha}{2} = \frac{\int_{X_{(1)}}^{q_L}\exp\left[-\frac{n}{2\sigma_n^2}(\theta-\overline{X})^2\right]\pi(\theta)d\theta}{\int_{X_{(1)}}^{X_{(n)}}\exp\left[-\frac{n}{2\sigma_n^2}(\theta-\overline{X})^2\right]\pi(\theta)d\theta} + M_n^3C_n + O_p(n^{-1+\varepsilon}). \tag{A.3.23}$$

Similarly one can show that

$$1-\frac{\alpha}{2}=\frac{\int_{X_{(1)}}^{q_U}\exp\left[-\frac{n}{2\sigma_n^2}(\theta-\overline{X})^2\right]\pi(\theta)d\theta}{\int_{X_{(1)}}^{X_{(n)}}\exp\left[-\frac{n}{2\sigma_n^2}(\theta-\overline{X})^2\right]\pi(\theta)d\theta}+M_n^3C_n+O_p(n^{-1+\varepsilon}).$$

The proof of Proposition 3.6 is complete.

Proof of Lemma 3.2

The proof of Lemma 3.2 is just a straightforward rearrangement of the equations in Proposition 3.6. It shows a similar structure as compared to the classic Bayesian Normal/Normal model. For details, see Carlin and Louis (2000).

Proof of Proposition 3.7

We assume that $\pi(\theta)$ is a normal density function with mean μ and variance σ^2. We first derive a Lemma that is useful for this proof.

Lemma 3.4

$|u_L - z_{\alpha/2}| = O(n^{-0.5+\varepsilon})$ where u_L is defined in Proposition 3.7.

Proof: First note the order of a component in remainder term R_n, used in the notations above (A.3.23) $M_n^3C_n = O_p(n^{-0.5+\varepsilon})$.

Equation (A.3.23) with the aforementioned fact imply

$$\frac{\alpha}{2}=\Phi(u_L)+O_p(n^{-0.5+\varepsilon}),$$

where $\Phi(\cdot)$ is a cumulative distribution function of the standard normal random variable.

Now we rearrange Equation (A.3.20) as

$$\Phi(u_L)-\Phi(z_{1-\alpha/2})=O_p(n^{-0.5+\varepsilon}),$$

where $z_{1-\alpha/2}$ is defined as $\Phi(z_{1-\alpha/2})=\alpha/2$.

We also have the inequality $\Phi(u_L)-\Phi(z_{\alpha/2})=\frac{1}{\sqrt{2\pi}}\int_{z_{1-\alpha/2}}^{u_L}\exp(-\frac{z^2}{2})dz \le \frac{|u_L - z_{\alpha/2}|}{\sqrt{2\pi}}$.

Combining Equation (A.3.21) and the above result, we have, as $n \to \infty$,

$$|u - z_{\alpha/2}| = O_p(n^{-0.5+\varepsilon}).$$

This shows the proof of Lemma 3.4.

Based on Lemma 3.2, Equation (A.3.23) becomes

$$\frac{\alpha}{2} = \Phi(u_L) + M_n^3 C_n + O_p(n^{-1+\varepsilon}). \qquad \text{(A.3.24)}$$

Now we expand function $\Phi(u_L)$ using the Taylor theorem with respect to u_L around $u_L = z_{1-\alpha/2}$, we have

$$\Phi(u_L) = \Phi(u_L)_{u_L = z_{1-\alpha/2}} + \Phi(u_L)'_{u_L = z_{1-\alpha/2}}(u_L - z_{\alpha/2}) + O_p(n^{-1+\varepsilon}). \qquad \text{(A.3.25)}$$

Combining Equations (A.3.24) and (A.3.25), we obtain

$$\frac{\alpha}{2} = \Phi(u)_{u=z_{\alpha/2}} + \Phi(u)'_{u=z_{\alpha/2}}(u - z_{\alpha/2}) + M_n^3 C_n + O_p(n^{-1+\varepsilon}).$$

Then, we have the expression for q_L as

$$q_L = \frac{\sigma_n^2 \mu + n\sigma^2 \overline{X}}{\sigma_n^2 + n\sigma^2} - z_{1-\alpha/2}\sqrt{\frac{\sigma_n^2 \sigma^2}{\sigma_n^2 + n\sigma^2}} + \frac{M_n^3}{3n\sigma_n^2}(2 + z_{1-\alpha/2}^2) + o_p(n^{-1}).$$

In a similar manner, one can show that the expression for q_U is

$$q_U = \frac{\sigma_n^2 \mu + n\sigma^2 \overline{X}}{\sigma_n^2 + n\sigma^2} + z_{1-\alpha/2}\sqrt{\frac{\sigma_n^2 \sigma^2}{\sigma_n^2 + n\sigma^2}} + \frac{M_n^3}{3n\sigma_n^2}(2 + z_{1-\alpha/2}^2) + o_p(n^{-1}).$$

The proof of Proposition 3.7 is complete.

Proofs of Propositions 3.8 through 3.14

The proof of Proposition 3.8 is omitted, since it directly follows from the application of Slutsky's theorem and an Edgeworth expansion technique. One can use the proof schemes of Propositions 3.6 and 3.7 to show Propositions 3.9 through 3.14 in a similar manner.

4

Empirical Likelihood for Probability Weighted Moments

4.1 Introduction

Greenwood et al. (1979) introduced probability weighted moments (PWMs) as a generalization of the conventional moments of a probability distribution. PWMs are widely used for modeling extremes of natural phenomena. For example, applications of statistical methods based on PWMs are of considerable importance in hydrology, as the concept of the PWMs is very efficient for estimating statistical characteristics of the tails of distribution functions pertaining to features such as 50, 100, and 1,000 year floods. Commonly, PWM-based techniques provide favorable estimation properties when using samples with relatively small sizes and are computationally straightforward to calculate (Hosking et al., 1985b; Katz et al., 2002). Researchers have proposed using PWM-based methods to quantify the uncertainty related to annual maxima of daily stream flows of rivers (Flood Studies Report, 1975; Hosking et al., 1985a; Wallis and Wood, 1985).

Hosking et al. (1985b) studied PWMs in the form of $\beta_r = E\left[X(F(X))^r\right]$, the expectation of $X(F(X))^r$, where X is a random variable with distribution function F and r is an integer. The authors applied the method of PWMs to estimate characteristics of the generalized extreme value distribution, which is related to the limiting distribution of the maximum of a series of independent and identically distributed (i.i.d) observations. Several important properties of data distributions can be estimated and summarized in functional forms depending on β_r's. For example, certain linear combinations of β_r's can be interpreted as measures of the scale and shape of a probability distribution, e.g., multiples of $2\beta_1 - \beta_0$ can be used as assessments of scale parameters of a distribution function (e.g., Hosking et al., 1985b), and $6\beta_2 - 6\beta_1 + \beta_0$ denotes a skewness characteristic of a distribution function (Stedinger, 1983). More generalized linear combinations of the PWMs can be constructed by employing orthogonal polynomials in a manner of specific PWMs called L-moments (Hosking, 1990).

Following the approach of Hosking et al. (1985b), we focus on the PWMs in the form of β_r.

An empirical likelihood (EL)-based method can be used for inferences about β_r. In this chapter, we show how to develop the EL inference of β_r as an extension to the classical EL technique. The asymptotic distribution of the corresponding EL ratio (ELR) test under the null distribution will be derived as an appropriate nonparametric version of the Wilks theorem.

4.2 Incorporating the Empirical Likelihood for β_r

4.2.1 Estimators of the Probability Weighted Moments

Given a random sample $X_1,\ldots,X_n$ of size n from an unknown distribution function F, estimation of β_r is most conveniently based on the order statistics $X_{(1)} \le X_{(2)} \le \cdots \le X_{(n)}$. Landwehr et al. (1979) proposed the estimator of β_r as

$$\tilde{b}_r = n^{-1}\sum_{j=1}^{n} k_{j,n}X_{(j)} \text{ with } k_{j,n} = \prod_{l=1}^{r}\frac{j-l}{n-l}.$$

To construct this estimator the authors focused on the relationships between moments of order statistics and β_r. van Gelder and Pandy (2005) numerically compared the value of $k_{j,n}$ with $(j/n)^r$ to show that $k_{j,n} \approx (j/n)^r$ for all j's. Hosking et al. (1985b) estimated β_r using the form

$$b_r = n^{-1}\sum_{j=1}^{n} q_{j,n}^{r} X_{(j)},$$

where $q_{j,n}$ is a plotting position, which is a distribution-free estimate of $F(X_{(j)})$ and usually it is chosen to be $q_{j,n} = (j-a)/n$, $0 < a < 1$. Here $F(x) = P(X_1 \le x)$. Hosking et al. (1985b) employed an extensive simulation study to confirm that b_r with the choice of $a = 0.35$ was the overall best estimator of β_r among a wide set of estimators. This estimator is asymptotically equivalent to $\tilde{b}_r$, derived by Landwehr et al. (1979). More recently in section 11.4 of the book presented by David and Nagaraja (2003), the empirical estimator of β_r is shown to be

$$\bar{b}_r = n^{-1}\sum_{i=1}^{n}\left(\frac{i}{n}\right)^{r} X_{(i)}.$$

The idea of constructing $\bar{b}_r$ and b_r is directly followed by replacing the unknown distribution function F in the definition of β_r with its empirical counterpart $F_n(u) = \sum_{i=1}^{n} I\left(X_{(i)} \le u\right)/n$, where $I(\cdot)$ denotes the indicator function. We consider the following approximation scheme:

$$\beta_r = \int x\left[F(x)\right]^r dF(x) \cong \sum_{i=1}^{n} \int_{X_{(i-1)}}^{X_{(i)}} x\left[F(x)\right]^r dF(x) \cong \sum_{i=1}^{n} X_{(i)} \int_{X_{(i-1)}}^{X_{(i)}} \left[F(x)\right]^r dF(x)$$

$$\cong \sum_{i=1}^{n} X_{(i)} \left[F_n^{r+1}\left(X_{(i)}\right) - F_n^{r+1}\left(X_{(i-1)}\right)\right] \frac{1}{r+1}, \quad X_{(0)} = -\infty.$$

This simple technique implies the new formula to estimate β_r using

$$\hat{b}_r = \sum_{i=1}^{n} X_{(i)} \left\{ \left(\frac{i}{n}\right)^{r+1} - \left(\frac{i-1}{n}\right)^{r+1} \right\} \frac{1}{r+1}.$$

It turns out that asymptotically $\hat{b}_r$ behaves similar to the well-known estimator $\bar{b}_r$ (for details, see Remark A.4.1 at the end of this chapter).

Using an extensive Monte Carlo study, it is shown that the estimator $\hat{b}_r$ has smaller variances with relatively small sample sizes and various distributions compared with $\tilde{b}_r$ and $\bar{b}_r$. This fact is true for all investigated cases of r ($r = 1, 2, 3, 4$) (Vexler et al., 2017).

One can extend the estimation scheme based on $F_n(u)$ by using the general form of the empirical distribution function $\tilde{F}_n(u) = \sum_{i=1}^{n} w_i I\left(X_{(i)} \le u\right)$, where the weights w_i's, $0 < w_1, \ldots, w_n < 1$, satisfy the assumption $\sum_{i=1}^{n} w_i = 1$. This approach implies more general forms of the estimators of β_r. For example, we can rewrite the estimators $\bar{b}_r$ and $\hat{b}_r$ as

$$\bar{b}_r = \sum_{i=1}^{n} w_i \left(\sum_{j=1}^{i} w_j\right)^r X_{(i)} \text{ and } \breve{b}_r = \sum_{i=1}^{n} X_{(i)} \left\{ \left(\sum_{j=1}^{i} w_j\right)^{r+1} - \left(\sum_{j=1}^{i-1} w_j\right)^{r+1} \right\} \frac{1}{r+1}.$$

Associating the weights w_i's and the probability weights p_i's in the EL framework allows us to develop EL inference about PWMs. For clarity and simplicity of explanation, we will focus on $\hat{b}_r$-type constructions. Note that, in the context of a $\hat{b}_r$-based EL technique, we propose an exact algorithm to compute values of $p_i, i = 1, \ldots, n$, (section 4.2.3) whereas, e.g., $\bar{b}_r$-based-EL's methods require complicated schemes to estimate the corresponding probability weights. See Remark A.4.2 for details at the end of this chapter.

4.2.2 Empirical Likelihood Inference for β_r

One can define the EL function for β_r as

$$L(\beta_r) = \max_{0<p_1,\ldots,p_n<1}\left[\prod_{i=1}^{n} p_i : \sum_{i=1}^{n} p_i = 1, \sum_{i=1}^{n} X_{(i)}\left\{(S_i)^{r+1} - (S_{i-1})^{r+1}\right\}\frac{1}{r+1} = \beta_r\right],$$

where the probability weights $0 < p_1,\ldots,p_n < 1$, $S_i = \sum_{j=1}^{i} p_j$ and we let that $\sum_{i=n+1}^{n} p_i = 0$ and $S_0 = 0$.

In order to find the expressions of p_i's, $i = 1,\ldots,n$, in $L(\beta_r)$, we denote the corresponding Lagrangian function:

$$U = \sum_{i=1}^{n}\log(p_i) + \lambda_1\left(1 - \sum_{i=1}^{n} p_i\right) + \lambda_2\left(\beta_r - \sum_{i=1}^{n} X_{(i)}\left\{(S_i)^{r+1} - (S_{i-1})^{r+1}\right\}\frac{1}{r+1}\right),$$

where λ_1 and λ_2 are the Lagrange multipliers. By calculating p_k as roots of $\partial U/\partial p_k = 0$, $k = 1,\ldots,n$, one can show that

$$\frac{1}{p_k} - \lambda_1 - \lambda_2\left(X_{(k)}(S_k)^r + \sum_{i=k+1}^{n} X_{(i)}\left\{(S_i)^r - (S_{i-1})^r\right\}\right) = 0.$$

Thus, taking into account the constraint $S_n = 1$ and summing up $\sum_{k=1}^{n} p_k \partial U/\partial p_k = 0$, we have

$$n - \lambda_1 - \lambda_2 \sum_{k=1}^{n}\left(X_{(k)}(S_k)^r + \sum_{i=k+1}^{n} X_{(i)}\left\{(S_i)^r - (S_{i-1})^r\right\}\right)p_k = 0. \quad (4.1)$$

To simplify Equation (4.1), we use the following well-known result that will be oftentimes applied throughout this chapter.

Lemma 4.1

Given two sequences a_i and b_j of real numbers, $i, j = 1,\ldots,n$, we have

$$\sum_{j=1}^{n-1}\left(a_j \sum_{i=j+1}^{n} b_i\right) = \sum_{i=2}^{n}\left(b_i \sum_{j=1}^{i-1} a_j\right).$$

Applying Lemma 4.1 to a part of Equation (4.1), we obtain

$$\begin{aligned}\sum_{k=1}^{n} p_k\left(\sum_{i=k+1}^{n} X_{(i)}\left\{(S_i)^r-(S_{i-1})^r\right\}\right) &= \sum_{i=2}^{n} X_{(i)}\left\{(S_i)^r-(S_{i-1})^r\right\}\sum_{j=1}^{i-1} p_j \\ &= \sum_{i=2}^{n} X_{(i)}\left\{(S_i)^r-(S_{i-1})^r\right\} S_{i-1} \\ &= \sum_{i=2}^{n} X_{(i)}(S_i)^r(S_i-p_i)-\sum_{i=2}^{n} X_{(i)}(S_{i-1})^{r+1} \\ &= \sum_{i=2}^{n} X_{(i)}\left\{(S_i)^{r+1}-(S_{i-1})^{r+1}\right\}-\sum_{i=2}^{n} X_{(i)}(S_i)^r p_i \\ &= (r+1)\beta_r - X_{(1)}(S_1)^{r+1}-\sum_{i=2}^{n} X_{(i)}(S_i)^r p_i \\ &= (r+1)\beta_r-\sum_{i=1}^{n} X_{(i)}(S_i)^r p_i,\end{aligned} \tag{4.2}$$

where the constraint $\sum_{i=1}^{n} X_{(i)}\left\{(S_i)^{r+1}-(S_{i-1})^{r+1}\right\}/(r+1)=\beta_r$ is used. That is, Equation (4.1) can be rewritten as $n-\lambda_1-\lambda_2(r+1)\beta_r=0$. This shows that $\lambda_1=n-\lambda_2(r+1)\beta_r$ and then the equation $\partial U/\partial p_k=0$ yields the expressions for $p_1,\ldots,p_n$ in the form

$$p_k=\left[n+\lambda_2\left(J_k-(r+1)\beta_r\right)\right]^{-1},\ k=1,\ldots,n \tag{4.3}$$

where $J_k=X_{(k)}\left(S_k\right)^r+\sum_{i=k+1}^{n} X_{(i)}\left\{(S_i)^r-(S_{i-1})^r\right\}$, $S_k=1-\sum_{i=k+1}^{n} p_i$, for $k=1,\ldots,n$, and $S_0=0$. We have $S_n=1$, and λ_2 is a numerical solution of the equation

$$\sum_{i=1}^{n} X_{(i)}\left\{(S_i)^{r+1}-(S_{i-1})^{r+1}\right\}/(r+1)=\beta_r.$$

Note that values of λ_2 can be found by applying a standard numerical zero root finding algorithm, e.g., the Newton–Raphson scheme, which has been well equipped in the standard statistical software, can be readily employed for this purpose. We use the R (R Development Core Team, 2014) functions *uniroot* and *optimize* to calculate the values of λ_2 (see Section 4.3). We illustrate the computing scheme in detail in the next subsection.

In the case with $r = 0$ we have the regular expressions for $p_1, \ldots, p_n$ that are components of the classical EL methodology for the population mean estimation (Owen, 2001).

Now we define the log ELR for the parameter β_r as $\log \text{ELR}(\beta_r) = \log(L(\beta_r)/n^{-n})$. In a similar manner to the classical ELR definition, we denote $\log \text{ELR}(\beta_r) = -\infty$ if there are no such p_i's that satisfy the constraints $\sum_{i=1}^{n} p_i = 1$ and $\sum_{i=1}^{n} X_{(i)} \{(S_i)^{r+1} - (S_{i-1})^{r+1}\}/(r+1) = \beta_r$. Such cases can arise when the value of β_r is strongly not appropriate for underlying data distributions.

In the case of $r = 0$, -2 logELR(β_0) has an asymptotic χ_1^2 distribution under the null hypothesis (Owen, 1988). The next proposition extends the nonparametric version of Wilks theorem in the context of the proposed EL inference of $\beta_r = EX_1(F(X_1))^r$.

Proposition 4.1

Assume that i.i.d data points $X_1, \ldots, X_n$ are from an unknown distribution function F, where its inverse function F^{-1} is continuous almost everywhere. If $E|X_1|^3 < \infty$, then

$$-2logELR(\beta_r) \xrightarrow{d} \chi_1^2 \text{ as } n \to \infty.$$

The proof of Proposition 4.1 and other proofs are found in the Appendix at the end of this chapter. According to Proposition 4.1, one can derive the ELR test for the hypothesis that says $EX(F(X))^r = \beta_r$ for a specific value of β_r. We reject the hypothesis when $-2\log \text{ELR}(\beta_r) \geq \chi_1^2(1-\alpha)$, where $\chi_1^2(1-\alpha)$ is the $100(1-\alpha)\%$ percentile of the chi-square distribution with the degree of freedom one and α is the significance level. By virtue of the relation between the testing and confidence interval (CI) estimation, we can obtain the CI estimator of $EX(F(X))^r$ in the form of

$$\text{CI}_{1-\alpha} = \{\beta_r : -2\log \text{ELR}(\beta_r) \leq \chi_1^2(1-\alpha)\},$$

assuming that the nominal coverage probability (CP) is specified as $1-\alpha$.

4.2.3 A Scheme to Implement the Empirical Likelihood Ratio Technique

To calculate values of $L(\beta_r) = \prod_{i=1}^{n} p_i$, we consider the following algorithm. Begin with defining $p_n = 1/[n + \lambda_2(X_{(n)} - (r+1)\beta_r)]$ and $S_{n-1} = 1 - p_n$ as a function of λ_2. Recursively given a value of λ_2 we have $p_{n-1} = 1/[n + \lambda_2\{X_{(n-1)}(S_{n-1})^r + X_{(n)}(1-(S_{n-1})^r) - (r+1)\beta_r\}]$ and $S_{n-2} = 1 - p_n - p_{n-1}$.

Sequentially one can obtain values of $p_1,\ldots,p_n$ depending on λ_2. The appropriate λ_2 can be calculated by a zero root finding algorithm, e.g., the Newton–Raphson technique, which is employed to solve the equation $\sum_{i=1}^{n} X_{(i)}\{(S_i)^{r+1}-(S_{i-1})^{r+1}\}/(r+1)-\beta_r=0$ with respect to λ_2. Since $\sum_{k=1}^{n} p_k=1$, we rewrite the previous equation in the form of $C(\lambda_2)=0$, where the functions $C(\lambda_2)=\sum_{k=1}^{n} p_k\left(J_k-(1+r)\beta_r\right)$ and J_k is denoted in (4.3). Note that, in the case of $r=0$, this equation is widely used in the standard EL methodology to find values of p_i's. By plugging the appropriate value for λ_2 to the expressions of p_i's, we obtain a value of $-2\log \text{ELR}(\beta_r)$. (See also relevant R-codes in the Appendix.)

4.2.4 An Application to the Gini Index

For an application, we develop an EL-based test for the Gini index. The Gini index is a widely used measure for assessing distributional inequality. Let X and Y be two independent random variables from the same distribution $F(x)=\Pr(X\le x)$. The Gini mean difference was first defined by Gini (1912) as a distributional scale measure $D=E\,|\,X-Y\,|$ and the Gini index can be regarded as the normalized Gini's mean difference $G=D/(2\mu)$, where $\mu=\int x dF(x)$ is the population mean. The Gini index can also be expressed as the area between the 45-degree line and the Lorenz curve. The Lorenz curve, proposed by Lorenz (1905), is a commonly used measure of distributional inequality, and the 45-degree line represents perfect equality.

The Gini index, G, is given as

$$G=\frac{E|X-Y|}{2EX}=\frac{1}{\beta_0}\int_0^{\infty}(2F(x)-1)x\,dF(x)=\frac{2\beta_1-\beta_0}{\beta_0},$$

where β_1 and β_0 are the PWMs defined in Section 4.1 and X, Y are two independent random variables with non-negative values following the same distribution $F(x)$. Following the method proposed in Section 4.2.2, one can define the EL function with respect to β_1 and β_0 as

$$L(\beta_1,\beta_0)=\max_{0<p_1,\ldots,p_n<1}\left[\prod_{i=1}^{n} p_i : \sum_{i=1}^{n} p_i=1,\ \sum_{i=1}^{n} X_{(i)}\left\{(S_i)^2-(S_{i-1})^2\right\}/2=\beta_1,\ \sum_{i=1}^{n} X_{(i)}p_i=\beta_0\right], \tag{4.4}$$

where the probability weights $0<p_1,\ldots,p_n<1$, $S_i=\sum_{j=1}^{i} p_j$ and $S_0=0$. In a similar manner to the computing scheme in Section 4.2.3, one can derive the expressions of p_k's, $k=1,\ldots,n$, in $L(\beta_1,\beta_0)$ by solving the corresponding Lagrangian function as

$$p_k = \left[n + \lambda_1\left(J_k - 2\beta_1\right) + \lambda_2\left(X_{(k)} - \beta_0\right)\right]^{-1},$$

where $J_k = X_{(k)}S_k + \sum_{i=k+1}^{n} X_{(i)}p_k$ and $S_k = 1 - \sum_{i=k+1}^{n} p_i$, for $k=1,\ldots,n$. We let $S_0 = 0$. In this case, $S_n = 1$, λ_1 and λ_2 are numerical solutions of the equations

$$\sum_{i=1}^{n} X_{(i)}\left\{\left(S_i\right)^2 - \left(S_{i-1}\right)^2\right\}/2 = \beta_1 \text{ and } \sum_{i=1}^{n} X_{(i)}p_i = \beta_0.$$

Note that values of λ_1 and λ_2 can be found by applying one of the numerical zero root finding algorithms (Section 4.3 and the Appendix).

Since $\beta_0 = 2\beta_1/(1+G)$, we can rewrite the EL function in the form $L_G(G,\beta_1) = L(\beta_1,\ 2\beta_1/(1+G))$. Following the Qin and Lawless (1994) inference method pertaining to G, we propose the maximum ELR $= \max_{\beta_1} L_G(G,\beta_1)/n^{-n}$. The next proposition defines the asymptotic distribution of the maximum ELR statistic.

Proposition 4.2

Under the assumptions of Proposition 4.1, we have

$$-2\log\left(\max_{\beta_1} L_G\left(G,\beta_1\right)/n^{-n}\right) \xrightarrow{d} \chi_1^2,\ as\ n \to \infty,$$

when $E\left|X_2 - X_1\right|/EX_1$ *is known to be equal to 2G.*

The proof of Proposition 4.2 is directly based on a technical combination of the proof scheme of Proposition 4.1 and the results of Qin and Lawless (1994), and thus the proof is omitted.

According to Proposition 4.2, one can derive the ELR test for the hypothesis $E\left|X-Y\right|/(2EX) = G$. We reject the null hypothesis when $-2\log \text{ELR}(G,\ \beta_1^M) \geq \chi_1^2\left(1-\alpha\right)$ where β_1^M is the value of β_1 that maximizes $L_G(G,\beta_1)$, $\chi_1^2\left(1-\alpha\right)$ is the $100(1-\alpha)\%$ percentile of the chi-square distribution with the degree of freedom one, and α is the significance level. By virtue of the relation between the testing and CI estimation, we can obtain the CI estimator of G in the form of

$$\text{CI}_{1-\alpha} = \left\{G : -2\log \text{ELR}\left(G,\beta_1^M\right) \leq \chi_1^2(1-\alpha)\right\},$$

assuming that the nominal CP is specified as $1-\alpha$. A Monte Carlo (MC) study to compare the method in Proposition 4.2 with the EL method of testing the Gini index provided by Qin et al. (2010) shows that the Type I error (TIE) control related to the proposed method is significantly more accurate than that of the method by Qin et al. (2010) (Vexler et al., 2017). We note that the method of Qin et al. (2010) suggests using the empirical distribution function $F_n(x)=\sum_{i=1}^{n} I(X_i < x)/n$ while normalizing the Gini index in the EL manner.

4.3 Performance Comparisons

In this section, we discuss results of a Monte Carlo (MC) study related to comparisons of properties of the following tests: (1) the proposed EL ratio test (say, PWM EL); (2) the classical EL ratio test; and (3) a test based on asymptotic properties of the estimator $\bar{b}_r$. In order to apply the classical EL technique, we pretend that data in the form of $Z_i = X_i\left(F(X_i)\right)^r, i=1,\ldots,n$, can be observed in order to consider the classical EL ratio test for β_1 and β_2 based on $Z_1,\ldots,Z_n$. In this context, we hypothetically assume the underlying data distribution is known. In practice, this EL method cannot be performed in the nonparametric setting. According to David and Nagaraja (2003), the estimator $\bar{b}_r$ has an asymptotic normal distribution. This implies constructing a $\bar{b}_r$-based testing procedure. By virtue of the test construction's scheme for $\bar{b}_r$, we can expect the $\bar{b}_r$-based test will provide good operating characteristics when normally distributed observations are used. In this MC experiments, the underlying data distributions were chosen to be in Normal, Exponential, Chi-square and Lognormal forms, since the statistical literature (e.g., Vexler et al. 2009) shows that EL type tests provide good properties when data are generated from a normally distributed population, and the Type I error control is not robust with respect to the scenarios based on skewed data distributions. For each baseline distribution, we repeated 50,000 samples of observations with sizes n = 20, 25, 50, 150 and 300. We set up the expected significant level of the considered tests to be $\alpha = 0.05$. In this Monte Carlo setting, we evaluated the MC Type I error rates of the tests for $H_0: E[XF^r(X)] = \beta_r$, given different sample sizes n. We observed the following results. The PWM EL test and the classical EL ratio test outperform the $\bar{b}_r$-based test in the context of the Type I error control for most of the considered scenarios. The MC Type I error rates of the PWM EL test are closer to the expected 0.05 than those of the classical EL ratio tests based on the normally distributed data with relatively small sample sizes 20, 25 and 50. The PWM EL test performs well in control of the Type I error rates for the exponential distribution based on relatively small samples with sizes 25 and 50, and has a fairly good control regarding the Type I error rates for a mildly skewed chi-square distribution, when the sample size is increased to 50. For the heavily skewed lognormal distribution, the PWM test has better Type I error rate control than the $\bar{b}_r$-based test and the classical EL test for relatively small samples sizes n = 20, 25 and r = 2.

In order to compare the MC powers of the considered tests we stated the null hypothesis to be associated with the three scenarios: (1) $\beta_1 = 0.75$ and $\beta_2 = 0.61$, (2) $\beta_1 = 0.2821$ and $\beta_2 = 0.2820$, and (3) $\beta_1 = 1.2534$ and $\beta_2 = 1.0448$. Corresponding to these scenarios, the alternative data distributions were: (a) $X \sim Exp$ (rate) with $rate$ = 0.9 ($\beta_1 = 0.83$, $\beta_2 = 0.68$); $rate$ = 0.8 ($\beta_1 = 0.94$, $\beta_2 = 0.76$); $rate$ = 0.7 ($\beta_1 = 1.07$, $\beta_2 = 0.97$); and that $rate$ = 1 is related to scenario (1); (b) $X \sim Normal(0, \sigma^2)$ with $\sigma^2 = 4$ ($\beta_1 = 0.5642$, $\beta_2 = 0.5641$); $\sigma^2 = 9$ ($\beta_1 = 0.8469$, $\beta_2 = 0.8467$); and that $\sigma^2 = 1$ corresponds to scenario (2); (c) $X \sim Lognormal(0, \sigma^2)$ with $\sigma^2 = 2.25$ ($\beta_1 = 2.6354$, $\beta_2 = 2.3589$); $\sigma^2 = 4$ ($\beta_1 = 6.8079$, $\beta_2 = 6.3972$); and that $\sigma^2 = 1$ corresponds to scenario (3). We observed the following results. When $r = 1$, the PWM EL test is more powerful than the $\bar{b}_r$-based test, and the EL test is a bit more powerful than the proposed test. Note that the EL test based on Z_i's was used for the purpose of illustrating how the PWM EL test performs by comparing with a test that uses some unobserved information as noted in the beginning of this section. For the mildly skewed exponential cases, the proposed test is the most powerful one among the considered tests for β_1. When $r = 2$, the $\bar{b}_r$-based test has the largest actual power for sample sizes n = 20, 25. As the sample size increases up to 50, the PWM EL test has the largest actual power. For the heavily skewed lognormal cases, the PWM EL test is the best of all the three test procedures for most considered cases. And the PWM EL test is significantly more powerful than the other two tests especially for relatively small sample sizes n = 20, 25 (r = 1).

The 95% CI's for β_1 and β_2 were investigated via CI mechanisms based on the considered test statistics. In the normal cases, the PWM EL test provides the actual coverage probabilities (CP) that are closer to the target 0.95 than those of the $\bar{b}_r$-based CI estimation. Specially, the PWM EL based CI estimation performs reasonably well and is more competitive than the $\bar{b}_r$-based CI estimation in cases of relatively small sample sizes n = 20, 25. Similar results hold for data generated from skewed distributions of exponential, χ_3^2 and lognormal. Note that the classical EL CI estimation is hypothetically used to compare with the proposed CI estimation. The PWM EL and the classical EL have similar results for most considered cases. In practice the EL CI estimation however cannot be used in the nonparametric setting.

Tables 4.1 and 4.2 compare the MC TIE rates of the EL procedure based on the method by Qin et al. (2010) and the PWM ELR to test $H_0: G = \theta$. In the tables, θ indicates the values of the Gini index corresponding to $Pareto(1)$, $Lognormal(0.5)$, $Exp(1)$, and χ_1^2 underlying distributions. The expected TIE rate is 0.05. Overall, the tables show that the PWM ELR is much better than the method by Qin et al. (2010).

TABLE 4.1

The Type I error control of the EL procedure based on the method of Qin et al. (2010)

Baseline Distribution		$n = 20$	50	100
Pareto(1)	$\theta = 0.05$	0.999	0.617	0.259
Lognormal(0.5)	$\theta = 0.28$	0.131	0.078	0.061
Exp(1)	$\theta = 0.50$	0.100	0.074	0.054
χ_1^2	$\theta = 0.64$	0.092	0.079	0.058

Source: Qin, Y. et al., *Econ. Model.*, 27, 1429–1435, 2010.

TABLE 4.2

The Type I error control of the PWM EL method

Baseline Distribution		$n = 20$	50	100
Pareto(1)	$G = 0.05$	0.191	0.225	0.197
Lognormal(0.5)	$G = 0.28$	0.045	0.070	0.057
Exp(1)	$G = 0.50$	0.086	0.059	0.051
χ_1^2	$G = 0.64$	0.092	0.070	0.053

The following R codes are used to obtain appropriate statistics in simulations.

1. Code to obtain the true $\beta_1 = E\left[X(F(X))^1\right]$

```
r<-1; FF<-function(u) u*(pnorm(u,0,1))^r*dnorm(u,0,1)
M1<-integrate(Vectorize(FF),-Inf,Inf)[[1]] #calculate true β1 = 0.2821
```

2. Code to obtain the classical EL test in the MC simulations

```
#This assumes that the distribution is known.
library("emplik")
n<-50                                                    #sample size
x<-rnorm(n,0,1)                              # generate random sample
xx<-x*(pnorm(x,0,1))^r                  # generate values of X(F(X))^r
el.test(xx,mu=c(M1))$'-2LLR'                  # The EL ratio statistic
[1] 0.1574862                               #This value is an example.
```

3. Code to obtain the proposed EL test

   See the Appendix.

4. Code to obtain the asymptotic normal test

```
xs<- sort(x)
ys<-xs
bhat<- n^(-1)*sum(xs*(rank(xs)/n)^r)                     # obtaining b̄r
#variance estimator (Serfling, 1980), Riemann sum is used to
#approximate the integral.
nvar<- 0
```

```
for (i in 2:n){for (j in 2:n){
deltax<- xs[i]-xs[i-1]
deltay<- ys[j]-ys[j-1]
nvar<- nvar+((i-1)/n)^r*((j-1)/n)^r*( min(i-1,j-1)/n-
(i-1)*(j-1)/n^2 )*deltax*deltay
}}
(bhat-M1)/sqrt(nvar/n)                         #test statistic
[1] 0.4225396                        #This value is an example.
```

4.4 Data Example

The example is based on data from a study that evaluated biomarkers related to the myocardial infarction (MI) focusing on the residents of Erie and Niagara counties (Schisterman et al., 2001, see Chapter 1 for the description). We consider the biomarker *Vitamin E* supplement that is often used to quantify antioxidant status of individuals (e.g., Rimm et al., 1993). A total of 2390 measurements of Vitamin E were evaluated by the study. About 547 of them were collected on cases who survived on MI and the other 1843 on controls who had no previous MI.

To illustrate and examine the proposed method based on the Vitamin E data we employ the following technique: The strategy for the case group was that a sample with size n was randomly selected from the Vitamin E data to estimate the CIs at the 95% level of the PWMs β_1, say $[a, b]$ using PWM ELR method and the $\bar{b}_r$-based CI method that uses the asymptotic normality approximation. Note that the classical ELR test cannot be used in this nonparametric setting as the distribution of the Vitamin E data is unknown. The rest of the data (547-n observations) are used to compute the β_1 using the estimator $\bar{b}_1$ (Section 4.2.1). The value of (547-n) was chosen to be relatively large so that the calculated $\bar{b}_1$ estimator is close to the theoretical value of β_1. We repeated this strategy 3,000 times observing the frequencies of the event of $\bar{b}_1 \in [a, b]$. We repeat the same process for the control group. Table 4.3 presents these results for $n = 25$ and 50. The outcomes in Table 4.3 show that the PWM ELR method provides the CP that are closer to the expected 0.95 level than those of the $\bar{b}_r$-based method.

Thus the proposed method can be recommended to construct the CI estimator of β_1. The results for 95% CI estimations of β_1 and β_2 with respect

TABLE 4.3

The coverage probabilities related to the Vitamin E evaluation. (The expected coverage probability is 0.95)

	Case Group ($N = 547$)		Control Group ($N = 1843$)	
Sample Size n	**Proposed CI**	**$\bar{b}_r$-CI**	**Proposed CI**	**$\bar{b}_r$-CI**
25	93.8%	90.3%	92.5%	89.4%
50	94.8%	91.0%	93.9%	91.4%

TABLE 4.4

The 95% CI estimation of β_1 and β_2 related to the Vitamin E biomarker with respect to the case and control groups

	Case Group (N = 547)		Control Group (N = 1843)	
	β_1	β_2	β_1	β_2
Proposed CI	(7.692, 8.345)	(5.839, 6.240)	(8.374, 8.717)	(6.227, 6.506)
$\bar{b}_r$-CI	(7.671, 8.344)	(5.696, 6.240)	(8.360, 8.770)	(6.217, 6.556)

to the Vitamin E biomarker for both the case and control groups are shown in Table 4.4. Table 4.4 shows that the proposed CI estimation is very similar to the $\bar{b}_r$-based estimation proposed by David and Nagaraja (2003), when the sample sizes are large. Both methods show evidence that the levels of β_1 and β_2 of the Vitamin E biomarker are significantly different among the case and control groups. We notice that the proposed method may have some skewness correction for the CI estimation with respect to the skewed underlying data distribution based on the advantage of the EL methodology (Vexler et al., 2009).

4.5 Concluding Remarks

In this chapter, we demonstrated a general scheme to construct EL-based procedures. The asymptotic evaluation of the PWM ELR method can be considered as an extension of the nonparametric version of the Wilks theorem. The statistical test and CI estimation of the PWMs are derived based on the asymptotic proposition. We showed that PWM ELR method can be easily applied to make inference of the Gini index. The real-life example demonstrated excellent applicability of the proposed approach.

Appendix

Remark A.4.1: The Taylor theorem shows that

$$(u-s)^{r+1} = (u)^{r+1} - s(r+1)(u)^r + 0.5s^2(r+1)r(u-\theta)^{r-1},$$

for $\theta \in (0,1)$. Then, defining $u = i/n$, $s = 1/n$, we obtain

$$\hat{b}_r = \sum_{i=1}^{n} X_{(i)} \left\{ \left(\frac{i}{n}\right)^{r+1} - \left(\frac{i-1}{n}\right)^{r+1} \right\} \frac{1}{r+1} = \frac{1}{n}\sum_{i=1}^{n} X_{(i)} \left(\frac{i}{n}\right)^{r} + \frac{r}{2n^2}\sum_{i=1}^{n} X_{(i)} \left(\frac{i}{n} - \theta_{i,n}\right)^{r-1}$$

$$= \bar{b}_r + \frac{r}{2n^2}\sum_{i=1}^{n} X_{(i)} \left(\frac{i}{n} - \theta_{i,n}\right)^{r-1}, \quad \theta_{i,n} \in (0,1).$$

Since $0 < i/n < 1$, it is clear that there exists a nonrandom constant $c_r \geq \max_{1\leq i\leq n} \left|(i/n - \theta_{i,n})^{r-1}\right|$. Thus the remainder term

$$\left|\frac{r}{2n^2}\sum_{i=1}^{n} X_{(i)}\left(\frac{i}{n} - \theta_{i,n}\right)^{r-1}\right| \leq \frac{rc_r}{2n^2}\sum_{i=1}^{n}\left|X_{(i)}\right| = \frac{rc_r}{2n^2}\sum_{i=1}^{n}\left|X_i\right|.$$

This implies, e.g., if $E\left|X_1\right|^{1+\varepsilon} < \infty$, for $\varepsilon > 0$, we have $\hat{b}_r = \bar{b}_r + O(n^{-1})$, as $n \to \infty$. Note that asymptotic properties of $\bar{b}_r$ can be found in the literature dealt with L-estimates (e.g., Serfling, 1980; David and Nagaraja, 2003).

Remark A.4.2: $\bar{b}_r$-based EL inference for β_r.

Define the EL function for β_r as

$$L(\beta_r) = \max_{0<p_1,\ldots,p_n<1}\left[\prod_{i=1}^{n} p_i : \sum_{i=1}^{n} p_i = 1, \sum_{i=1}^{n} p_i X_{(i)}\left(S_i\right)^r = \beta_r\right],$$

where the probability weights $0 < p_1,\ldots,p_n < 1$, $S_i = \sum_{j=1}^{i} p_j$.

In order to express p_i, $i = 1,\ldots,n$, we denote the corresponding Lagrangian function

$$Q = \sum_{i=1}^{n}\log(p_i) + \lambda_1\left(1 - \sum_{i=1}^{n} p_i\right) + \lambda_2\left(\beta_r - \sum_{i=1}^{n} p_i X_{(i)}\left(S_i\right)^r\right),$$

where λ_1 and λ_2 are the Lagrange multipliers. Calculating p_k as the roots of $\partial Q/\partial p_k = 0$, $k = 1,\ldots,n$, we have

$$\frac{1}{p_k} - \lambda_1 - \lambda_2\left(X_{(k)}\left(S_k\right)^r + r\sum_{i=k}^{n} p_i X_{(i)}\left(S_i\right)^{r-1}\right) = 0.$$

Thus, considering $\sum_{k=1}^{n} p_k \partial Q/\partial p_k = 0$ with $S_n = 1$, we have

$$n - \lambda_1 - \lambda_2\sum_{k=1}^{n}\left(X_{(k)}\left(S_k\right)^r + r\sum_{i=k}^{n} p_i X_{(i)}\left(S_i\right)^{r-1}\right)p_k = 0.$$

To simplify this equation, we use Lemma 4.1 presented in Section 4.2.2, obtaining that

$$r\sum_{k=1}^{n} p_k \sum_{i=k}^{n} p_i X_{(i)} \left(S_i\right)^{r-1} = r\sum_{j=1}^{n} p_j \left(S_j\right)^{r} X_{(j)} = r\beta_r,$$

where the constraint $\sum_{i=1}^{n} p_i X_{(i)}(S_i)^r = \beta_r$ is used. That is, $\sum_{k=1}^{n} p_k \partial Q/\partial p_k = 0$ can be represented in the form $n-\lambda_1-\lambda_2(r+1)\beta_r = 0$. Then $\lambda_1 = n-\lambda_2(r+1)\beta_r$ and the equation $\partial Q/\partial p_k = 0$ yield $p_k = [n+\lambda_2(D_k-(r+1)\beta_r)]^{-1}$, $k=1,\dots,n$, where $D_k = X_{(k)}(S_k)^r + r\sum_{i=k}^{n} p_i (S_i)^{r-1} X_{(i)}$ and $k=1,\dots,n$. This provides nonexplicit functions to find values of p_k, $k=1,\dots,n$, depending on λ_2 via the scheme: p_n can be derived using $p_n = [n+\lambda_2(X_{(n)}+rp_n X_{(n)}-(r+1)\beta_r)]^{-1}$, then p_{n-1} can be derived using $p_{n-1} = \left[n+\lambda_2(X_{(n-1)}(1-p_n)^r + rp_{n-1}X_{(n-1)}(1-p_n)^{r-1} + rp_n X_{(n)} - (r+1)\beta_r)\right]^{-1}$, and so on. Now, λ_2 can be computed applying the equation $\sum_{i=1}^{n} p_i [X_{(i)}(S_i)^r - \beta_r] = 0$. Note that, in general, the corresponding expression of p_k gives two root values of p_k, that we reconsider satisfying $0 < p_1,\dots,p_n < 1$ and these root values depend on λ_2. This issue may lead the direct use of the $\bar{b}_r$-based EL inference for β_r to be very complicated.

Proofs

Proof of Proposition 4.1

To outline the proof of Proposition 4.1, we use an algorithm that is similar to that applied to analyze the classical log ELR (Chapter 2). We first note that by virtue of the Taylor theorem we can expand $\log(\mathrm{ELR}(\beta_r))$ around $\hat{b}_r$ as

$$\log\left(\mathrm{ELR}(\beta_r)\right) = \log\left(\mathrm{ELR}(\hat{b}_r)\right) + (\beta_r - \hat{b}_r) \left.\frac{d\log\left(\mathrm{ELR}(\beta_r)\right)}{d\beta_r}\right|_{\beta_r=\hat{b}_r} + \frac{1}{2}(\beta_r - \hat{b}_r)^2 \left.\frac{d^2\log\left(\mathrm{ELR}(\beta_r)\right)}{d\beta_r^{\,2}}\right|_{\beta_r=\hat{b}_r} + R, \tag{A.4.0}$$

where $\hat{b}_r$ is the maximum EL estimator (MELE) of β_r having the form

$$\hat{b}_r = \sum_{i=1}^{n} X_{(i)} \left(\left(\frac{i}{n}\right)^{r+1} - \left(\frac{i-1}{n}\right)^{r+1}\right) \Big/ (r+1)$$

and

$$R = \frac{1}{6}\frac{d^3 \log\left(\text{ELR}(\beta_r)\right)}{d\beta_r^{\ 3}}\Bigg|_{\beta_r=a} (\beta_r - \hat{b}_r)^3$$

denotes the remainder term with $a = \beta_r + \varpi(\hat{b}_r - \beta_r)$ and $\varpi \in (0,1)$.

In the case where the function $\log(\text{ELR}(u))$ is considered at the argument $u = \hat{b}_r$, we obtain the maximum of this function, since, by virtue of the definition of the EL, $p_i = 1/n,\ i = 1,\dots n$, satisfy the constraints $\sum_{i=1}^{n} p_i = 1$ and $\sum_{i=1}^{n} X_{(i)}\{(S_i)^{r+1} - (S_{i-1})^{r+1}\}/(r+1) = \hat{b}_r$ as well as $p_i = 1/n,\ i = 1,\dots,n$, are arguments of $\max\left(\prod_{i=1}^{n} p_i : \sum_{i=1}^{n} p_i = 1\right)$. Thus,

$$\log\left(\text{ELR}(\hat{b}_r)\right) = \log\left(\text{EL}(\hat{b}_r)/n^{-n}\right) = 0 \text{ and } d\log\left(\text{ELR}(u)\right)/du\Big|_{u=\hat{b}_r} = 0.$$

Taking into account the results by David and Nagaraja (2003) and Serfling (1980), we have that $(\beta_r - \hat{b}_r)^2$ is asymptotically χ^2 distributed. In order to show $-2\log(\text{ELR}(\beta_r)) \sim \chi_1^2$, applying (A.4.0), we will prove that the remainder term $R \to 0$ as $n \to \infty$. To achieve the proof scheme above, the next two lemmas are presented.

Lemma 4.2

We have

$$\frac{d\log\left(\text{ELR}(\beta_r)\right)}{d\beta_r} = \lambda_2,$$

where λ_2 is the second Lagrange multiplier defined in Section 4.2.2 and $\lambda_2 = \lambda_2(\beta_r)$ is a function of β_r.

Proof of Lemma 4.2

Note that $\log(\text{ELR}(\beta_r)) = \sum_{k=1}^{n} \log p_k - \log n^{-n}$, where in accordance with the definition of ELR in Section 4.2.2 and Equation (4.3), $\text{ELR}(\beta_r) = \prod_{k=1}^{n} p_k / n^n$, $p_k = (n + \lambda_2 V_k)^{-1}$ with $V_k = X_{(k)} S_k^r + \sum_{i=k+1}^{n} X_{(i)}(S_i^r - S_{i-1}^r) - (r+1)\beta_r$, for $k = 1,\dots,n$.

Thus

$$\frac{d\log\left(\text{ELR}(\beta_r)\right)}{d\beta_r} = \sum_{k=1}^{n} \frac{1}{p_k}\frac{dp_k}{d\beta_r} = -\sum_{k=1}^{n} p_k\left(V_k \frac{d\lambda_2}{d\beta_r} + \lambda_2 \frac{dV_k}{d\beta_r}\right). \qquad \text{(A.4.1)}$$

(See the results below (4.3).)
To prove Lemma 4.2, we will show that

$$\sum_{k=1}^{n}\left(p_k V_k \frac{d\lambda_2(\beta_r)}{d\beta_r}\right)=0 \text{ and } -\sum_{k=1}^{n} p_k \frac{dV_k}{d\beta_r}=1.$$

We have

$$\sum_{k=1}^{n}\left(p_k V_k \frac{d\lambda_2(\beta_r)}{d\beta_r}\right)=\left[\sum_{k=1}^{n} p_k X_{(k)} S_k^r+\sum_{k=1}^{n} p_k\left(\sum_{i=k+1}^{n} X_{(i)}\left(S_i^r-S_{i-1}^r\right)\right)-(r+1)\beta_r\right]\frac{d\lambda_2}{d\beta_r}.$$

By virtue of Equation (4.2), one can easily show that

$$\sum_{k=1}^{n} p_k X_{(k)} S_k^r+\sum_{k=1}^{n} p_k\left(\sum_{i=k+1}^{n} X_{(i)}\left(S_i^r-S_{i-1}^r\right)\right)=(r+1)\beta_r.$$

(See the results below (4.3).)
The two equations above conclude that

$$\sum_{k=1}^{n}\left(p_k V_k \frac{d\lambda_2(\beta_r)}{d\beta_r}\right)=0.$$

The definition of V_k leads to

$$\frac{dV_k}{d\beta_r}=rX_{(k)}S_k^{r-1}\frac{dS_k}{d\beta_r}+r\sum_{i=k+1}^{n} X_{(i)}\left(S_i^{r-1}\frac{dS_i}{d\beta_r}-S_{i-1}^{r-1}\frac{dS_{i-1}}{d\beta_r}\right)-(r+1),$$

and then

$$\sum_{k=1}^{n} p_k \frac{dV_k}{d\beta_r}=r\sum_{k=1}^{n} p_k X_{(k)} S_k^{r-1}\frac{dS_k}{d\beta_r} + r\sum_{k=1}^{n} p_k \sum_{i=k+1}^{n} X_{(i)}\left(S_i^{r-1}\frac{dS_i}{d\beta_r}-S_{i-1}^{r-1}\frac{dS_{i-1}}{d\beta_r}\right)-(r+1). \tag{A.4.2}$$

Thus, we need to show that

$$\sum_{k=1}^{n} p_k X_{(k)} S_k^{r-1} \frac{dS_k}{d\beta_r} + \sum_{k=1}^{n} p_k \sum_{i=k+1}^{n} X_{(i)} \left(S_i^{r-1} \frac{dS_i}{d\beta_r} - S_{i-1}^{r-1} \frac{dS_{i-1}}{d\beta_r} \right) = 1,$$

in order to conclude that $-\sum_{k=1}^{n} p_k \left(dV_k / d\beta_r \right) = 1$. To this end, we apply Lemma 4.1 to rewrite the second term on the right side of Equation (A.4.2) in the form:

$$\begin{aligned}
\sum_{k=1}^{n} p_k \sum_{i=k+1}^{n} X_{(i)} \left(S_i^{r-1} \frac{dS_i}{d\beta_r} - S_{i-1}^{r-1} \frac{dS_{i-1}}{d\beta_r} \right) &= \sum_{i=2}^{n} X_{(i)} \left(S_i^{r-1} \frac{dS_i}{d\beta_r} - S_{i-1}^{r-1} \frac{dS_{i-1}}{d\beta_r} \right) \sum_{j=1}^{i-1} p_j \\
&= \sum_{i=2}^{n} X_{(i)} \left(S_i^{r-1} \frac{dS_i}{d\beta_r} - S_{i-1}^{r-1} \frac{dS_{i-1}}{d\beta_r} \right) S_{i-1} \\
&= \sum_{i=2}^{n} \left(X_{(i)} S_i^{r-1} \frac{dS_i}{d\beta_r} (S_i - p_i) - X_{(i)} S_{i-1}^{r-1} \frac{dS_{i-1}}{d\beta_r} \right) \\
&= \sum_{i=2}^{n} X_{(i)} S_i^{r} \frac{dS_i}{d\beta_r} - \sum_{i=2}^{n} X_{(i)} S_i^{r-1} \frac{dS_i}{d\beta_r} p_i \\
&\quad - \sum_{i=2}^{n} X_{(i)} S_i^{r} \frac{dS_{i-1}}{d\beta_r}.
\end{aligned}$$

Applying this result to Equation (A.4.2) we obtain

$$\begin{aligned}
&\sum_{k=1}^{n} p_k X_{(k)} S_k^{r-1} \frac{dS_k}{d\beta_r} + \sum_{k=1}^{n} p_k \sum_{i=k+1}^{n} X_{(i)} \left(S_i^{r-1} \frac{dS_i}{d\beta_r} - S_{i-1}^{r-1} \frac{dS_{i-1}}{d\beta_r} \right) \\
&= \sum_{k=1}^{n} p_k X_{(k)} S_k^{r-1} \frac{dS_k}{d\beta_r} + \sum_{i=2}^{n} X_{(i)} S_i^{r} \frac{dS_i}{d\beta_r} - \sum_{i=2}^{n} X_{(i)} S_i^{r-1} \frac{dS_i}{d\beta_r} p_i - \sum_{i=2}^{n} X_{(i)} S_i^{r} \frac{dS_{i-1}}{d\beta_r} \qquad \text{(A.4.3)} \\
&= \sum_{i=1}^{n} X_{(i)} \left(S_i^{r} \frac{dS_i}{d\beta_r} - S_i^{r} \frac{dS_{i-1}}{d\beta_r} \right).
\end{aligned}$$

The constraint used in the definition of the EL,

$$\beta_r = \sum_{i=1}^{n} X_{(i)} \left(\frac{S_i^{r+1}}{r+1} - \frac{S_{i-1}^{r+1}}{r+1} \right),$$

implies the equation $d\beta_r/d\beta_r = d(\sum_{i=1}^{n} X_{(i)}(S_i^{r+1} - S_{i-1}^{r+1})/(r+1))/d\beta_r$, that is,

$$\sum_{i=1}^{n} X_{(i)} \left(S_i^r \frac{dS_i}{d\beta_r} - S_i^r \frac{dS_{i-1}}{d\beta_r} \right) = 1.$$

This result and Equation (A.4.3) complete the proof of $-\sum_{k=1}^{n} p_k \left(dV_k/d\beta_r \right) = 1$. The proof of Lemma 4.2 is complete.

The next lemma is presented to evaluate $d^2 \log(\mathrm{ELR}(\beta_r))/d\beta_r^2 = d\lambda_2\left(\beta_r\right)/d\beta_r$.

Lemma 4.3

The function $\lambda_2 = \lambda_2(\beta_r)$ satisfies

$$\frac{d\lambda_2}{d\beta_r} = \frac{\sum_{k=1}^{n} p_k V_k' - \lambda_2 \sum_{k=1}^{n} p_k^2 V_k V_k'}{\sum_{k=1}^{n} p_k^2 V_k^2},$$

where V_k' denotes the derivative $dV_k/d\beta_r$.

Proof of Lemma 4.3

By virtue of definition of λ_2 in Section 4.2.2 and (4.3) with $V_k = J_k - (r+1)\beta_r$ for $k = 1,..,n$, we have

$$\sum_{k=1}^{n} \frac{V_k}{n + \lambda_2 V_k} = 0.$$

Then

$$0 = d\left(\sum_{k=1}^{n} \frac{V_k}{n + \lambda_2 V_k} \right) / d\beta_r = \sum_{k=1}^{n} \frac{V_k'\left(n + \lambda_2 V_k\right) - V_k\left(\lambda_2' V_k + \lambda_2 V_k'\right)}{\left(n + \lambda_2 V_k\right)^2}$$

$$= \sum_{k=1}^{n} \frac{V_k'\left(n + \lambda_2 V_k\right)}{\left(n + \lambda_2 V_k\right)^2} - \sum_{k=1}^{n} \frac{V_k\left(\lambda_2' V_k + \lambda_2 V_k'\right)}{\left(n + \lambda_2 V_k\right)^2} = \sum_{k=1}^{n} p_k V_k' - \lambda_2' \sum_{k=1}^{n} p_k^2 V_k^2 - \lambda_2 \sum_{k=1}^{n} p_k^2 V_k V_k'.$$

The above-mentioned equation leads to the formula of λ_2' given in Lemma 4.3. This completes the proof of Lemma 4.3.

By virtue of Lemmas 4.2 and 4.3, we can rewrite Equation (A.4.0) as

$$\log\left(\mathrm{ELR}\left(\beta_r\right)\right)=\frac{1}{2}\left(\beta_r-\hat{b}_r\right)^2\left.\frac{d\lambda_2(\beta_r)}{d\beta_r}\right|_{\beta_r=\hat{b}_r}+R, \tag{A.4.4}$$

where

$$\left(\left.\frac{d\lambda_2(\beta_r)}{d\beta_r}\right|_{\beta_r=\hat{b}_r}\right)^{-1}$$

$$=\frac{-1}{n}\sum_{k=1}^{n}\left(X_{(k)}\left(\frac{k}{n}\right)^r+\sum_{i=k+1}^{n}X_{(i)}\left(\left(\frac{i}{n}\right)^r-\left(\frac{i-1}{n}\right)^r\right)-\sum_{i=1}^{n}X_{(i)}\left(\left(\frac{i}{n}\right)^{r+1}-\left(\frac{i-1}{n}\right)^{r+1}\right)\right)^2.$$

In order to evaluate the remainder term R, we present the following lemma.

Lemma 4.4

$\lambda_2\left(\beta_r\right)=O_p\left(n^{2/3}\right)$.

Proof: In Section 4.2.2, λ_2 is defined to be a root of

$$\sum_{k=1}^{n}\frac{J_k-(r+1)\beta_r}{n+\lambda_2\left(J_k-(r+1)\beta_r\right)}=0, \tag{A.4.5}$$

where $J_k=X_{(k)}S_k^r+\sum_{i=k+1}^{n}X_{(i)}\left(S_i^r-S_{i-1}^r\right)$. Denote

$$L(\lambda_2)=\sum_{k=1}^{n}\frac{J_k-(r+1)\beta_r}{n+\lambda_2\left(J_k-(r+1)\beta_r\right)}.$$

Then we have

$$\sqrt{n}L(\lambda_2)=\frac{\sum_{k=1}^{n}\left(J_k-(r+1)\beta_r\right)}{\sqrt{n}}-\frac{\lambda_2}{\sqrt{n}}\frac{1}{n}\sum_{k=1}^{n}\frac{\left(J_k-(r+1)\beta_r\right)^2}{1+\lambda_2 n^{-1}\left(J_k-(r+1)\beta_r\right)}. \tag{A.4.6}$$

Now we employ the following facts:

$X_k=O_p(n^{1/3})$, $J_k=O_p(n^{1/3})$, $k=1,..,n$, and $\sum_{i=k}^{n}X_i p_i\le\sum_{i=1}^{n}|X_i|p_i<\infty$, considering the assumption that $E|X|^3<\infty$.

Thus we obtain that $\sqrt{n}L(\lambda) \to -\infty$ as $n \to \infty$ and $\sqrt{n}L(-\lambda) \to \infty$ as $n \to \infty$ when $\lambda = n^{2/3}$. Thus the proof of Lemma 4.4 is complete.

To evaluate $\lambda_2' = d\lambda_2(\beta_r)/d\beta_r$, we will use the following scheme. Since $p_k = (n + \lambda_2 V_k)^{-1}$ and $V_k = X_{(k)} S_k^r + \sum_{i=k+1}^n X_{(i)}(S_i^r - S_{i-1}^r) - (r+1)\beta_r$, $k = 1,\ldots,n$, applying $\lambda_2(\beta_r) = O_p(n^{2/3})$ and $X_{(k)} = O_p(n^{1/3})$ to evaluate p_k, we can conclude that $p_k = O_p(n^{-1})$. Consider $V_n' = d((X_{(n)} - (r+1)\beta_r))/d\beta_r = -(r+1)$. Then $p_n' = dp_n(\beta_r)/d\beta_r = \lambda_2' O_p(n^{-5/3})$. Since

$$V_k - V_{k+1} = \left(X_{(k)} - X_{(k+1)}\right) S_k^r = \left(X_{(k)} - X_{(k+1)}\right)\left(1 - \sum_{i=k+1}^n p_i\right),$$

the results above imply

$$V_{n-1}' = \frac{d\left(V_n + (X_{(n-1)} - X_{(n)}) S_{n-1}^r\right)}{d\beta_r} = V_n' + r(X_{(n-1)} - X_{(n)})\left(1 - p_n\right)^{r-1}\left(\sum_{i=n}^n p_i'\right)$$

$$= O_p(1) + \lambda_2' O_p\left(n^{-4/3}\right),$$

and then $p_{n-1}' = \lambda_2' O_p(n^{-5/3})$. Sequentially

$$V_{n-2}' = \frac{d\left(V_{n-1} + (X_{(n-2)} - X_{(n-1)}) S_{n-2}^r\right)}{d\beta_r} = V_{n-1}' + r(X_{(n-2)} - X_{(n-1)})\left(1 - \sum_{i=n-1}^n p_i\right)^{r-1}\left(\sum_{i=n-1}^n p_i'\right)$$

$$= O_p(1) + \lambda_2' O_p\left(n^{-4/3}\right),$$

and then $p_{n-2}' = \lambda_2' O_p(n^{-5/3})$. In this induction-type manner one can conclude that

$$V_k' = O_p(1) + \lambda_2' O_p\left(n^{-4/3}\right), \quad \text{for all } k = 1,\ldots,n.$$

Now, using Lemma 4.3, we represent $\lambda_2' = d\lambda_2(\beta_r)/d\beta_r$ in the form

$$\frac{d\lambda_2}{d\beta_r} = \frac{\sum_{k=1}^n p_k V_k' - \lambda_2 \sum_{k=1}^n p_k^2 V_k V_k'}{\sum_{k=1}^n p_k^2 V_k^2}.$$

Thus applying the above results, $\lambda_2(\beta_r) = O_p(n^{2/3})$, $p_k = O_p(n^{-1})$, and $X_{(k)} = O_p(n^{1/3})$ to the formula of $\lambda_2' = d\lambda_2(\beta_r)/d\beta_r$, we obtain that $\lambda_2' = O_p(n)$. In a similar manner, one can show that $\lambda_2'' = d\lambda_2'(\beta_r)/d\beta_r = O_p(n)$.

We use the obtained results to analyze the remainder term R in Equation (A.4.0). In this case we have

$$R = \lambda_2''(a)(\beta_r - \hat{b}_r)^3/6 = o_n(1), \text{ as } n \to \infty.$$

Taking Equation (A.4.4) into account, we will show that

$$-(\beta_r - \hat{b}_r)^2 \left.\frac{d\lambda_2(\beta_r)}{d\beta_r}\right|_{\beta_r = b_r} \xrightarrow{d} \chi_1^2.$$

To this end, we note that

$$\hat{b}_r = \sum_{i=1}^{n} X_{(i)} \left(\left(\frac{i}{n}\right)^{r+1} - \left(\frac{i-1}{n}\right)^{r+1} \right) / (r+1).$$

where $\left((i/n)^{r+1} - ((i-1)/n)^{r+1}\right)/(r+1) \cong (i/n)^r/n$ (Remark 4.1).

Thus the proposed estimator $\hat{b}_r$ is asymptotically equal to the estimator $\bar{b}_r = n^{-1}\sum_{i=1}^{n} X_{(i)}(i/n)^r$ presented in David and Nagaraja (2003, pp. 332–333). Following the book material in David and Nagaraja (2003, pp. 332–333) and Serfling (1980, p. 276), we have that the estimator $\bar{b}_r$ is asymptotically normally distributed with mean β_r and a variance that can be estimated in the following form:

$$\hat{\sigma}^2(\bar{b}_r)$$
$$= \frac{1}{n} \sum_{i=1}^{n} \sum_{j=1}^{n} \left(\frac{i-1}{n}\right)^r \left(\frac{j-1}{n}\right)^r \left(\frac{\min(i-1, j-1)}{n} - \left(\frac{i-1}{n}\right)\left(\frac{j-1}{n}\right) \right) (X_{(i)} - X_{(i-1)})(X_{(j)} - X_{(j-1)}).$$

To shorten notations, we denote $\lambda' |_{\beta_r = \hat{b}_r} = d\lambda_2(\beta_r)/d\beta_r |_{\beta_r = \hat{b}_r}$.

Lemma 4.5

Let the conditions of Proposition 4.1 be held, then

$$n\left(-1/\lambda_2'|_{\beta_r = b_r'} - \hat{\sigma}(\bar{b}_r)\right) \xrightarrow{p} 0, \text{ as } n \to \infty.$$

Proof of Lemma 4.5

Based on the formula,

$$\left(\left.\frac{d\lambda_2(\beta_r)}{d\beta_r}\right|_{\beta_r=\hat{b}_r}\right)^{-1} = \frac{-1}{n}\sum_{k=1}^{n}\left(X_{(k)}\left(\frac{k}{n}\right)^r + \sum_{i=k+1}^{n} X_{(i)}\left(\left(\frac{i}{n}\right)^r - \left(\frac{i-1}{n}\right)^r\right)\right.$$
$$\left. - \sum_{i=1}^{n} X_{(i)}\left(\left(\frac{i}{n}\right)^{r+1} - \left(\frac{i-1}{n}\right)^{r+1}\right)\right)^2,$$

and that

$$\hat{\sigma}^2(\bar{b}_r)$$
$$= \frac{1}{n}\sum_{i=1}^{n}\sum_{j=1}^{n}\left(\frac{i-1}{n}\right)^r\left(\frac{j-1}{n}\right)^r\left(\frac{\min(i-1,j-1)}{n} - \left(\frac{i-1}{n}\right)\left(\frac{j-1}{n}\right)\right)(X_{(i)} - X_{(i-1)})(X_{(j)} - X_{(j-1)}),$$

heavy algebra can be used to show that

$$-1/\lambda_2'\big|_{\beta_r=\hat{b}_r} = \sum_{k=1}^{n} C_{1k}X_{(k)}^2 + \sum_{k=1}^{n-1}\sum_{i=k+1}^{n} C_{1ki}X_{(k)}X_{(i)}, \text{ and}$$

$$\breve{\sigma}^2(\bar{b}_r) = \sum_{k=1}^{n} C_{2k}X_{(k)}^2 + \sum_{k=1}^{n-1}\sum_{i=k+1}^{n} C_{2ki}X_{(k)}X_{(i)},$$

where

$$C_{1k} = 2(k-n)\frac{1}{n}\left(\frac{k-1}{n}\right)^{1+r}\left(\frac{k}{n}\right)^r + k(n-k)\frac{1}{n^2}\left(\frac{k}{n}\right)^{2r} + (n+1-k)\frac{1}{n}\left(\frac{k-1}{n}\right)^{1+2r},$$

$$C_{1ki} = \frac{1}{n^2}\left(k(i-1-n)\left(\frac{i-1}{n}\right)^r\left(\frac{k}{n}\right)^r + k(n-i)\left(\frac{i}{n}\right)^r\left(\frac{k}{n}\right)^r + n(i-n)\left(\frac{i}{n}\right)^r\left(\frac{k-1}{n}\right)^{1+r}\right.$$
$$\left. + n(n+1-i)\left(\frac{i-1}{n}\right)^r\left(\frac{k-1}{n}\right)^{1+r}\right),$$

$$C_{2k} = 2(k-n)\frac{1}{n}\left(\frac{k-1}{n}\right)^{1+r}\left(\frac{k}{n}\right)^r + k(n-k)\frac{1}{n^2}\left(\frac{k}{n}\right)^{2r} + (n+1-k)\frac{1}{n}\left(\frac{k-1}{n}\right)^{1+2r},$$

$$C_{2ki} = \frac{1}{n^2}\left(k(i-1-n)\left(\frac{i-1}{n}\right)^r \left(\frac{k}{n}\right)^r + k(n+1-i)\left(\frac{i}{n}\right)^r \left(\frac{k}{n}\right)^r + n(i-n)\left(\frac{i}{n}\right)^r \left(\frac{k-1}{n}\right)^{1+r} \right.$$

$$\left. + n\left(n+1-i\right)\left(\frac{i-1}{n}\right)^r \left(\frac{k-1}{n}\right)^{1+r} \right).$$

Based on the above results, it can be easily seen that the two variance formulas $\hat{\sigma}^2(\bar{b}_r)$ and $-1/\lambda_2'|_{\beta_r=\hat{b}_r}$ are asymptotically equivalent. This completes the proof of Lemma 4.5.

Thus, we conclude that

$$-\left(\beta_r - \hat{b}_r\right)^2 \frac{d\lambda_2(\beta_r)}{d\beta_r}\Bigg|_{\beta_r=\hat{b}_r} \xrightarrow{d} \chi_1^2 \text{ as } n \to \infty.$$

We remark that our limited Monte Carlo study showed that the values of $-1/\lambda_2'|_{\beta_r=\hat{b}_r}$ and $\hat{\sigma}^2(\bar{b}_r)$ are very close even when the sample size n is relatively small. We do not show this numerical study in this chapter.

R Code to Obtain the PWM Empirical Likelihood Test

```
#Calculate the value of Lagrangian multiplier λ2
#The data set used here was generated by R code in Section 4.3.
ssx<-sort(x)                                          #order statistics
# compute X(i)(i/n)^r's
LLL<-array(); for(ii in 1:n) LLL[ii]<-ssx[ii]*(ii/n)^(r)
# obtain initial pi's based on X(i)(i/n)^r
P0<-el.test(LLL,mu=M1)$wts/n
P0
[1] 0.02067023 0.02074551 0.02078115 0.02083454 0.02088375 0.02086615
...omitted...
```

In the following steps, we iterate the loop 10 times to estimate "P0", which we consider to be close to true theoretical values by convergence.

```
for(kkk in 1:10){
Sw<-array()
# compute Si = Σ_{j=1}^{i} pj
Sw[1]<-P0[1]
for(ii in 2:n) {
     Sw[ii]<-sum(P0[1:ii])
     # compute X(i){(Si)^r-(S_{i-1})^r}
     LLL[ii]<-ssx[ii]*(Sw[ii]^r-Sw[(ii-1)]^r)
     }
# compute values of Jk's in (4.3)
J0<-array()                              # store values of Jk's in (4.3)
```

```
J0[n]<-ssx[n]                                                    #J_n=X_(n)
for(ii in 1:(n-1)) J0[ii]<-ssx[ii]*Sw[ii]^r+sum(LLL[(ii+1):n])
                         # e.g. J_k=X_(k)(S_k)^r+Σ_{i=k+1}^n X_(i){(S_i)^r-(S_{i-1})^r}
M2=M1*(1+r)                                                      # M2=(1+r)β_r
#Get P1 (p_i's ) using el.test() based on Σ_{k=1}^n p_k(J_k-(1+r)β_r)=0
P1<-el.test(J0,mu=M2)$wts/n
#Then use P1 as "P0" to obtain updated P0 using el.test again.
Swn<-array()
Swn[1]<-P1[1]
      for(ii in 2:n) Swn[ii]<-sum(P1[1:ii])
zz<-ssx*(Swn)^r
P2<-el.test(zz,mu=M1)$wts/n
P0<-P2
}
```

Now, we consider that P0 values obtained above are close to theoretical values. The following code computes $X_{(i)}\{(S_i)^{r+1}-(S_{i-1})^{r+1}\}/(r+1)$.

```
Sw<-array()
Sw[1]<-P1[1]                                         # compute Sw[1]=p_1
LLL[1]<-ssx[1]*P1[1]^(r+1)/(r+1)                     # X_(1){(S_1)^(r+1)}/(r+1)
for( ii in 2:n) {
Sw[ii]<-sum(P1[1:ii])                                # compute Sw[ii]=Σ_{j=1}^{ii} p_j
LLL[ii]<-ssx[ii]*(Sw[ii]^(r+1)-Sw[(ii-1)]^(r+1))/(r+1)
}
```

Now, we have an initial value of λ_2 (LambdaI) using the relationship in Equation (4.3).

```
UU<-array()
UU[1]<-0
for(ii in 2:n) UU[ii]<-ssx[ii]*(Sw[ii]^r-Sw[(ii-1)]^r)
LambdaI<-(1/P1[1]-n)/(ssx[1]*P1[1]^r+sum(UU[2:n])-(r+1)*M1)
LambdaI
[1] 6.049043
```

In the following code, we obtain λ_2 in Equation (4.3) using R function "`optimize`". The function "`PP`" has the parameter λ_2 (i.e., u in the function).

```
PP<-function(u){
     p<-array(); S<-array()
     S[n]<-1                                         #S_n=Σ_{j=1}^n p_j=1
     # All pi's can be constructed starting with p_n
     p[n]<-1/(n+u*(xs[n]-M1*(r+1)))                  #calculate p_n
     SS<-0
     for(i in (n-1):1) {
```

```
        S[i]<-S[i+1]-p[i+1]                          # S_i = S_{i+1} - p_{i+1}
        SS<-SS+xs[i+1]*(S[i+1]^r-S[i]^r)
        p[i]<-1/(n+u*(xs[i]*S[i]^r+SS-M1*(r+1)))
    }
    #To obtain Σ_{i=1}^n X_(i){(S_i)^(r+1) - (S_{i-1})^(r+1)}/(r+1)
    ELM<-xs[1]*(S[1]^(r+1))/(r+1)
    for( i in 2:n) {ELM<-ELM+xs[i]*(S[i]^(r+1)-S[i-1]^(r+1))/(r+1)}
    return(ELM)
    }
    PP<-Vectorize(PP)
    PP1<-function(u) (PP(u)-M1)^2 # Σ_{i=1}^n X_(i){(S_i)^(r+1) - (S_{i-1})^(r+1)}/(r+1) = β_r
l0<-optimize(Vectorize(PP1),
     c(LambdaI-2*abs(LambdaI),LambdaI+2*abs(LambdaI)))$minimum
l0
[1] 5.858136
```

We are now ready to obtain the EL likelihood ratio test.

```
  lamb<-l0; p<-array(); S<-array()
  S[n]<-1; p[n]<-1/(n+lamb*(xs[n]-M1*(r+1)))
  SS<-0
  for(i in (n-1):1) {
          S[i]<-S[i+1]-p[i+1]
          SS<-SS+xs[i+1]*(S[i+1]^r-S[i]^r)
          p[i]<-1/(n+lamb*(xs[i]*S[i]^r+SS-M1*(r+1)))
          }
-2*sum(log(p*n))                        #The likelihood ratio test value
[1] 0.1783484
```

R Code to Obtain the Empirical Likelihood Test for Gini Index

1. Code to obtain the true Gini index

```
r<-1; FF<-function(u) u*(pexp(u))^r*dexp(u)
M11<-integrate(Vectorize(FF),-Inf,Inf)[[1]]                    #β_1
FF0<-function(u) u*dexp(u)
M00<-integrate(Vectorize(FF0),-Inf,Inf)[[1]]                   #β_0
Gini<-(2*M11-M00)/M00                           #the true Gini index
Gini
[1] 0.5
```

2. Data generation

```
  set.seed(3)
  n<-50 #sample size
  x<-rexp(n) # generate random sample
```

3. Function to obtain the EL test statistic

   Remark: The program may incorporate a part to make sure p_i values (p) are positive. That part is not provided in the following code:

```
LLRR<-function(M1){
   M0<-2*M1/(1+Gini)
   #PP: Function (below) to calculate $\sum_{i=1}^n X_{(i)}\{(S_i)^2-(S_{i-1})^2\}/2=\beta_1$ in (4.4).
   #u is the vector for $\lambda_1$ and $\lambda_2$.
   PP<-function(u){
    xs<-sort(x)
    p<-array()#p vector of pi's
    S<-array()#S vector of Si's
    S[n]<-1
    p[n]<-1/(n+u[1]*(xs[n]-M1*(r+1))+u[2]*(xs[n]-M0)) #To calculate $p_n$
    SS<-0
    for(i in (n-1):1) {
                    # In this for-loop,$n-1 p_i$'s are sequentially generated.
      S[i]<-S[i+1]-p[i+1]
      SS<-SS+xs[i+1]*(S[i+1]^r-S[i]^r)
      p[i]<-1/(n+u[1]*(xs[i]*S[i]^r+SS-M1*(r+1))+u[2]*(xs[i]-M0))
    }
    ELM<-xs[1]*(S[1]^(r+1))/(r+1)
    for( i in 2:n) {
      ELM<-ELM+xs[i]*(S[i]^(r+1)-S[i-1]^(r+1))/(r+1)
    }
return(ELM)
  }

#PP0: Function (below) to calculate $\sum_{i=1}^n X_{(i)}p_i=\beta_0$ in (4.4)
   PP0<- function(u) {
   p<-array()                                          #p vector of pi's
   S<-array()                                          #S vector of Si's
   S[n]<-1
   p[n]<-1/(n+u[1]*(xs[n]-M1*(r+1))+u[2]*(xs[n]-M0)) #calculate Pn
   SS<-0
   # Following for-loop sequentially generates n-1 Pi's
   for( i in (n-1):1) {
    S[i]<-S[i+1]-p[i+1]
    SS<-SS+xs[i+1]*(S[i+1]^r-S[i]^r)
    p[i]<-1/(n+u[1]*(xs[i]*S[i]^r+SS-M1*(r+1))+u[2]*(xs[i]-M0))
                                         }
   ELM0<- sum(xs*p)
   return(ELM0)
}

# Obtaining $\lambda_1$, $\lambda_2$
   PP1<-function(u) ((PP(u)-M1)^2+(PP0(u)-M0)^2)
   l0<-optim(c(-n,n),PP1)$par
lamb<-l0
```

```
# Obtaining pi's
   p<-array()
   S<-array()
   S[n]<-1
   p[n]<-1/(n+lamb[1]*(xs[n]-M1*(r+1))+lamb[2]*(xs[n]-M0))
   SS<-0
   for(i in (n-1):1) {
    S[i]<-S[i+1]-p[i+1]
    SS<-SS+xs[i+1]*(S[i+1]^r-S[i]^r)
    p[i]<-1/(n+lamb[1]*(xs[i]*S[i]^r+SS-M1*(r+1))+lamb[2]*(xs[i]-M0))
}
L<- -2*sum(log(p*n))
return(L)
}
optimize(LLRR, c(0,M11+0.5))$objective                #EL test statistic
                                             #Inside c() is a range of M1
[1] 0.2928181
```

5

Two-Group Comparison and Combining Likelihoods Based on Incomplete Data

5.1 Introduction

In this chapter, we demonstrate the method for combining likelihood functions in parametric or empirical form in the setting of two-group comparison. Qin (2000) showed an inference on incomplete bivariate data using a method that combines the parametric model and empirical likelihoods (ELs). These types of approaches make it possible to use all information in the form of bivariate data whether completely or incompletely observed. In the context of a group comparison, constraints can be formed based on null and alternative hypotheses and these constraints are incorporated into the EL. Some asymptotic results are presented, which make our technique applicable in inference. In this chapter, we first introduce the combined likelihood for the incomplete and complete data. Then, the likelihood ratio test (LRT) is developed to compare two treatment groups. We will demonstrate that the group comparison based on the EL ratio (ELR) approach is robust to the underlying distribution, and thus a viable alternative for other parametric (e.g., t-test) and nonparametric tests (e.g., Wilcoxon test). In particular, we will show that the ELR test statistic carries out the mean-specific comparisons unlike other available nonparametric tests. In addition, we discuss comparison of multivariate means as a simple extension of univariate two-group comparison, where we discuss the profile analysis. Then, we develop semiparametric and nonparametric approaches to combine the complete and incomplete data, and the asymptotic properties of the likelihood ratio test are examined. We show that the testing power can be augmented by combining relevant information.

5.2 Product of Likelihood Functions Based on the Empirical Likelihood

The definition of the likelihood function allows us to combine different likelihoods. This feature of the likelihood function makes the data analysis flexible and more powerful. In this section, we illustrate the technique for combining likelihood functions. Consider the following motivating example.

Example 5.1: Incomplete Data Issue in Ventilator-Associated Pneumonia Data

Scannapieco et al. (2009) compared two oral treatments (standard of care vs. chlorhexidine [CHX]) for their effects on infection of patients' respiratory system in an intensive care unit (ICU) setting.

Ventilator-associated pneumonia (VAP) is commonly induced by mechanical ventilation and the most common infection in ICUs. It is known that 10%–20% patients receiving mechanical ventilation more than 48 hours develop VAP. VAP can be diagnosed using a composite clinical score, called the clinical pulmonary infection score (CPIS) based on fever, blood leukocyte counts, tracheal secretions, oxygenation index, and chest X-ray. This procedure is reported to have a sensitivity of 72%–77% and a wide range of specificity of 42%–85% for the diagnosis of VAP (Koenig and Truwit, 2006). If CPIS is higher than a threshold value, the diagnosis of VAP is further assured using bronchoalveolar lavage (BAL) fluid culture. BAL is an invasive diagnostic procedure that uses a bronchoscope to collect the specimen directly from lung, thus it cannot be carried out routinely for intubated patients. For each BAL, potential respiratory pathogens greater than 10^4 cfu/mL (colonial forming units per mL) are considered as a likely indicator of infection. BAL is known to have a sensitivity of 73% and a specificity of 82% for the diagnosis of pneumonia in ventilated patients (Dupont et al., 2004). Thus, CPIS and BAL are complementary and both are relevant outcomes to compare the treatment efficacy in VAP studies; however, in a typical clinical setting, BAL data are observed only if CPIS exceeds a threshold. Figure 5.1 describes the relationship between CPIS and BAL. The figure shows a linear relationship between CPIS and BAL.

This example suggests a unique challenge in the data analysis. Both CPIS and BAL contain the relevant information regarding pneumonia diagnosis; incorporating these two variables may increase the power to test the treatment effect. Also, BAL is observed only if CPIS reaches a certain condition, which causes the problem of the limit of detection (LOD). Some relevant discussions regarding the LOD can be found in Vexler et al. (2008a) and (2015).

To explain the approach, let (X, Y) be a bivariate random variable. Suppose that we have independent observations $(X_{11}, Y_{11}),\dots,(X_{1n_1} Y_{1n_1})$ from the control group and $(X_{21}, Y_{21}),\dots,(X_{2n_2}, Y_{2n_2})$ from the intervention group.

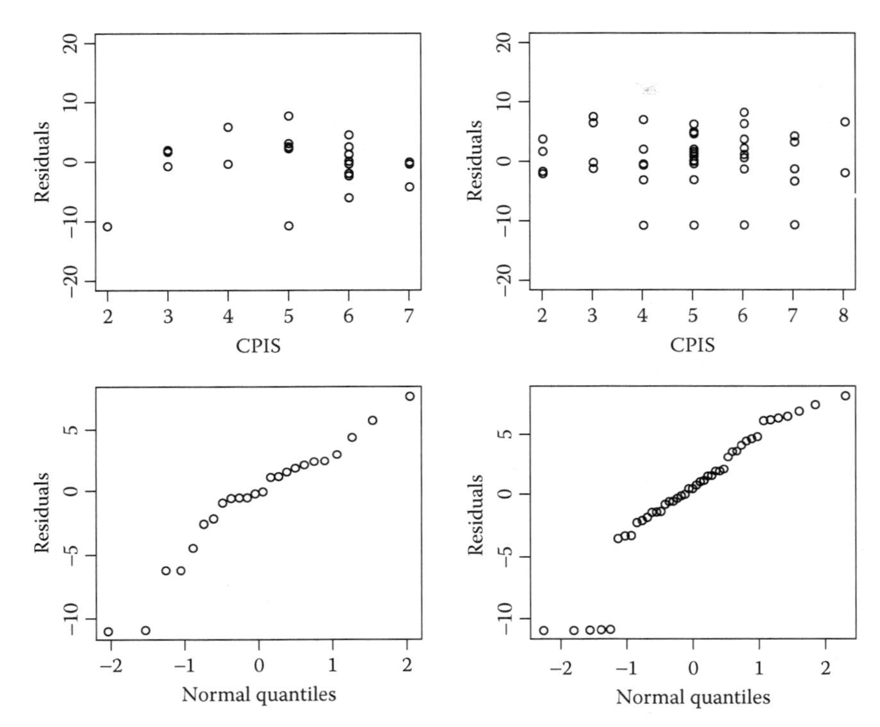

FIGURE 5.1
Residual plots of observed BAL and CPIS based on linear model fitting from R. The figures in the left side are for the control group and those in the right side are for the treatment group.

For both groups, Y (e.g., BAL value) can be observed only if X (e.g., CPIS) exceeds a certain threshold value, c.

A general form of H_0 consists of two parts and can be expressed as

$$H_0 : E[\Upsilon(X_1,\theta)] = E[\Upsilon(X_2,\theta)] \text{ and } E[\Psi(Y_1 \mid X_1,\theta)] = E[\Psi(Y_2 \mid X_2,\theta)], \tag{5.1}$$

where subscripts 1 and 2 indicate group 1 and group 2, θ is a vector of parameters to define the relationship between X and Y, Υ is a function of (X_i,θ) expressing the restriction summarized under H_0 and Ψ is a function of Y_i given (X_i,θ).

Suppose X has the distribution $G(X)$, and Y has the conditional distribution function $F(Y|X,\theta)$. We construct the likelihood, L in the form

$$L = \prod_{i=1}^{2} \prod_{j=1}^{n_i} dG_i(X_{ij}) \prod_{j=1, X_{ij} \geq c}^{n_i} dF_i(Y_{ij}|X_{ij},\theta). \tag{5.2}$$

We will explain two ways to obtain the likelihood function, i.e., semiparametric way and nonparametric way in the later chapter. Since (5.1) consists of two-group mean test statements, we will explain some relevant EL results regarding the mean comparison between two groups in Section 5.3.

5.3 Classical Empirical Likelihood Tests to Compare Means

There have been some discussions of mean comparisons in the EL literature (e.g., Brunner and Munzel, 2000; Jing, 1995; Lin et al. 2008). Consider a comparison of two treatment groups. For each group, $i = 1, 2$, there are n_i experimental units. Let X_{ij} denote the random variable of the j-th unit from group i, satisfying $E|X_{ij}|^3 < \infty$ and has an unknown distribution function, $G(x)$. We construct the likelihood function as

$$L = \prod_{i=1}^{2} \prod_{j=1}^{n_i} dG(x_{ij}) = \prod_{i=1}^{2} \prod_{j=1}^{n_i} p_{ij},$$

where p_{ij} is the probability weight and $\sum_{j=1}^{n_i} p_{ij} = 1$ for $i = 1, 2$. Consider the null hypothesis for two-group comparison,

$$H_0 : E(X_1) = E(X_2).$$

An empirical form of $E(X_i)$ can be expressed as $\sum_{j=1}^{n_i} X_{ij} p_{ij}$. To obtain the maximum of the likelihood function under H_0, $\prod_{i=1}^{2} \prod_{j=1}^{n_i} p_{ij}$ is maximized subject to

$$\sum_{j=1}^{n_1} X_{1j} p_{1j} = \sum_{j=1}^{n_2} X_{2j} p_{2j}, \ \sum_{j=1}^{n_1} p_{1j} = 1, \quad \sum_{j=1}^{n_2} p_{2j} = 1, \quad 0 \le p_{ij} \le 1. \quad (5.3)$$

The corresponding Lagrange function is defined by

$$\begin{aligned} &\sum_{j=1}^{n_1} \log p_{1j} + \sum_{j=1}^{n_2} \log p_{2j} + \lambda_1 \left(1 - \sum_{j=1}^{n_1} p_{1j} \right) \\ &+ \lambda_2 \left(1 - \sum_{j=1}^{n_2} p_{2j} \right) + \lambda_3 \left(\sum_{j=1}^{n_1} X_{1j} p_{1j} - \sum_{j=1}^{n_2} X_{2j} p_{2j} \right), \end{aligned} \quad (5.4)$$

where λ_k, $k = 1, 2, 3$, are Lagrange multipliers. The derivatives of (5.4) with respect to p_{ij} yield equations

$$p_{1j}^{-1} - \lambda_1 + \lambda_3 X_{1j} = 0, \ \text{and} \ p_{2j}^{-1} - \lambda_2 + \lambda_3 X_{2j} = 0. \quad (5.5)$$

Equation (5.5) leads to

$$p_{1j} = (\lambda_1 - \lambda_3 X_{1j})^{-1} \text{ for } j = 1,2,\ldots,n_1, \text{ and } p_{2j} = (\lambda_2 + \lambda_3 X_{2j})^{-1} \text{ for } j = 1,2,\ldots,n_2,$$

where λ_k satisfies the following conditions (C1–C3):

$$\text{C1: } \lambda_1 + \lambda_2 = n_1 + n_2, \text{ C2: } \sum\nolimits_{j=1}^{n_1} (\lambda_1 - 2\lambda_3 X_{1j})^{-1} = 1, \text{ C3: } \sum\nolimits_{j=1}^{n_2} (\lambda_2 + \lambda_3 X_{2j})^{-1} = 1. \quad (5.6)$$

The values of λ_k are found by numerically solving the system of equations (5.6). Under the alternative hypothesis, H_1, maximizing $\prod_{j=1}^{n_i} p_{ij}$ subjected only to $\sum_{j=1}^{n_i} p_{ij} = 1$ yields $\prod_{i=1}^{2} n_i^{-n_i}$. Based on the likelihoods under H_0 and H_1, the Likelihood Ration (LR), say R, is

$$R = \left(\prod\nolimits_{i=1}^{2} n_i^{-n_i} \right)^{-1} \prod\nolimits_{i=1}^{2} \prod\nolimits_{j=1}^{n_i} p_{ij}, \quad (5.7)$$

thus the log-likelihood ratio test statistic is

$$-2\log R = 2\left\{ \log(n_1)^{-n_1} + \log(n_2)^{-n_2} - \sum\nolimits_{j=1}^{n_1} \log p_{1j} - \sum\nolimits_{j=1}^{n_2} \log p_{2j} \right\}. \quad (5.8)$$

We can show the following result.

Proposition 5.1

Under H_0, $-2\log R \to \chi_1^2$ in distribution when both n_1 and n_2 increase.

Proposition 5.1 can be proven by approximating values of λ_3 in the following manner. The equations in (5.5) lead to

$$n_1 - \lambda_1 \sum\nolimits_{j=1}^{n_1} p_{1j} + \lambda_3 \sum\nolimits_{j=1}^{n_1} X_{1j} p_{1j} = 0, \text{ and } n_2 - \lambda_2 \sum\nolimits_{j=1}^{n_2} p_{2j} + \lambda_3 \sum\nolimits_{j=1}^{n_2} X_{2j} p_{2j} = 0,$$

which are equivalent to

$$n_1 - \lambda_1 + \lambda_3 \mu_1 = 0, \text{ and } n_2 - \lambda_2 + \lambda_3 \mu_2 = 0, \quad (5.9)$$

by the related constraints and definitions. By Equation (5.9) and conditions C2 and C3 in (5.6), we obtain $\lambda_1 = n_1 + \lambda_3/\mu_1, \lambda_2 = n_2 + \lambda_3/\mu_2$

$$\sum\nolimits_{j=1}^{n_1} \left(1 - \lambda_3 (X_{1j} - \mu_1)/n_1\right)^{-1} \left(X_{1j} - \mu_1\right) = 0, \text{ and}$$
$$\sum\nolimits_{j=1}^{n_2} \left(1 - \lambda_3 (X_{2j} - \mu_2)/n_2\right)^{-1} \left(X_{2j} - \mu_2\right) = 0. \quad (5.10)$$

Equation in (5.10) can be expanded using the Taylor expansion as

$$n_i^{-1}\sum_{j=1}^{n_i}\left(X_{ij}-\mu_i\right)+(-1)^{i+1}n_i^{-2}\sum_{j=1}^{n_i}\lambda_3\left(X_{ij}-\mu_i\right)^2 + n_i^{-3}\sum_{j=1}^{n_i}\lambda_3^2\left(X_{ij}-\mu_i\right)^3 \cong 0,\ i=1,2. \tag{5.11}$$

In Equation (5.11), we can show $\lambda_3 = O(n^{1/2})$ (Yu et al., 2010), thus the third term is $O(n_1^{-1/2})$ (see Proposition 2.5). By subtracting both sides of the equation for $i=1$ by those for $i=2$ in (5.11) and solving for λ_3, we obtain

$$\lambda_3 \approx \frac{n_2^{-1}\sum_{j=1}^{n_2}X_{2j}-n_1^{-1}\sum_{j=1}^{n_1}X_{1j}}{n_1^{-2}\sum_{j=1}^{n_1}(X_{1j}-\mu_1)^2+n_2^{-2}\sum_{j=1}^{n_2}(X_{2j}-\mu_2)^2}. \tag{5.12}$$

Using (5.9), the log-likelihood ratio test statistic (5.8) can be expressed as

$$2\left[\sum_{j=1}^{n_1}\log\left\{1-n_1^{-1}\lambda_3\left(X_{1j}-\mu_1\right)\right\}+\sum_{j=1}^{n_2}\log\left\{1+n_2^{-1}\lambda_3\left(X_{2j}-\mu_2\right)\right\}\right], \tag{5.13}$$

Now, using the Taylor expansion, the terms inside the bracket of (5.13) become asymptotically to be

$$\sum_{j=1}^{n_1}\left\{-\frac{\lambda_3\left(X_{1j}-\mu_1\right)}{n_1}-\frac{\lambda_3^2\left(X_{1j}-\mu_1\right)^2}{2n_1^2}\right\}+\sum_{j=1}^{n_2}\left\{-\frac{\lambda_3\left(X_{2j}-\mu_2\right)}{n_2}-\frac{\lambda_3^2\left(X_{2j}-\mu_2\right)^2}{2n_2^2}\right\}.$$

The corresponding remaining terms are in an order of $o(1)$ (Yu et al., 2010). By (5.12), we can show that

$$\begin{aligned}
&\sum_{j=1}^{n_1}\lambda_3^2\left(X_{1j}-\mu_1\right)^2\Big/2n_1^2+\sum_{j=1}^{n_2}\lambda_3^2\left(X_{2j}-\mu_2\right)^2\Big/2n_2^2\\
&=\lambda_3^2\left(n_1^{-2}\sum_{j=1}^{n_1}\left(X_{1j}-\mu_1\right)^2+n_2^{-2}\sum_{j=1}^{n_2}\left(X_{2j}-\mu_2\right)^2\right)\Big/2\\
&=\lambda_3\sum_{j=1}^{n_2}X_{2j}\Big/2n_2-\lambda_3\sum_{j=1}^{n_2}X_{1j}/2n_1.
\end{aligned} \tag{5.14}$$

Thus, by Equation (5.14), the log-likelihood ratio test statistic (5.13) under H_0 is approximated by

$$\lambda_3\left(n_2^{-1}\sum_{j=1}^{n_2}X_{2j}-n_1^{-1}\sum_{j=1}^{n_1}X_{1j}\right). \tag{5.15}$$

Now, plugging (5.12) into (5.15), we have

$$\left(\sum_{j=1}^{n_1}(X_{1j}-\mu_1)^2/n_1^2+\sum_{j=1}^{n_2}(X_{2j}-\mu_2)^2/n_2^2\right)^{-1}\left\{\sum_{j=1}^{n_2}X_{2j}/n_2-\sum_{j=1}^{n_1}X_{1j}/n_1\right\}^2, \tag{5.16}$$

which asymptotically has a χ_1^2 distribution. More rigorous proof in the context of the multivariate variables (Proposition 5.2) is provided in the Appendix at the end of this chapter. The formula (5.16) shows that the ELR statistic is equivalent to the two-sample z-test for large samples. For normally distributed data, it has been shown that the Type I error (TIE) rates and power of the ELR test are comparable to those of the two-sample *t*-test (Yu et al., 2010).

5.3.1 Implementation in R

Program packages for Lagrange multiplier method solver are available. Here, we demonstrate how to implement the two-group ELR test. We use an R package called `Rsolnp` (Ye, 1987; Ghalanos and Theussl, 2012). We also explain how to use the R package `emplik2` as well. We note that general optimization function `optim` can be used, in this context too. In programming, the package allows a direct maximization of (5.8) with conditions (5.3). Suppose that we want to compare the following two groups where the sample size for each group is 100:

```
n1<-100; n2<-100;
x1<-rnorm(n1,0,1); x2<-rnorm(n2,0,1.5)
```

The data are generated under the null hypothesis (i.e., equal means). The different standard deviation is used to demonstrate the robustness of the EL method to different distributions.

To accommodate the parse of `Rsolnp` package, we also need a list that combines the two groups' data and probabilities as follows:

```
n<-n1+n2; x1Cx2<-c(x1,x2); p<-array(dim=(n))
```

The following function is the log-likelihood function under H_0, which we need to maximize.

```
fn1=function(p){
sump<-0
for(i in 1:n){
sump<-sump+log(p[i])
}
return(-sump)}
```

In the function `fn1`, returning negative value is necessary for maximization as the package Rsolnp does only minimization. The following functions are to establish conditions (5.3):

```
fn2x1=function(p)
{
sump2<-0
for(i in 1:n1){
sump2<-sump2+p[i]
}
return(sump2)}

fn2x2=function(p)
{
sumq2<-0
for(i in (n1+1):n){
sumq2<-sumq2+p[i]
}
return(sumq2)}

fn3x1=function(p)
{
sump3<-0
for(i in 1:n1){
sump3<-sump3+x1[i]*p[i]
}
return(sump3)}

fn3x2=function(p)
{
sumq3<-0
for(i in (n1+1):n){
sumq3<-sumq3+x1Cx2[i]*p[i]
}
return(sumq3)}
```

Letting the functions `fn2x1` and `fn2x2` be 1 will control the sum of probabilities for each group to be 1. Letting function `eqn1` (below) be 0 will satisfy that the two group means are same (i.e., H_0). The following function corresponds to the collection of those conditions:

```
eqn1=function(p){
z1x1=fn2x1(p)
z1x2=fn2x2(p)
z2=fn3x1(p)-fn3x2(p)
return(c(z1x1,z1x2,z2))
}
```

Now we need to find p such that the returning values of function eqn1 will be (1,1,0).
Initial values for probabilities p are given as

```
p0 <- c(rep((1/n1),n1),rep((1/n2),n2))
```

The maximization of log-likelihood function is carried out using function `solnp`.

```
powell<-solnp(p0, fun = fn1, eqfun = eqn1, eqB = c(1,1,0),
LB = rep(0,n), UB=rep(1,n))
```

Inside the parenthesis of `solnp`, `p0` is the initial values for the probabilities, `fn1` is the function to maximize, `eqn1` and (1,1,0) indicate conditions to be satisfied. The lower bounds for the values in p are given as 0 to make sure positive values. The following code gives the maximized value of `fn1`:

```
lik0<- -(powell$values[length(powell$values)])
```

Then the test statistic (5.8) and the corresponding p-value are obtained as follows:

```
elr<- -2*(lik0+(n1*log(n1)+n2*log(n2)))
elr #The following is an example (e.g.)
[1] 0.1851218
1-pchisq(elr, 1) #e.g.
[1] 0.6670081
```

5.3.2 Implementation Using Available R Packages

The ELR test for two-group comparison can be conveniently obtained using R package `emplik2` (Barton and Zhou, 2012). We note that the package `emplik2` can also handle the censored data. In the package, the statement of H_0 is slightly different from what we have shown in (5.3). Specifically, the empirical form of H_0 is given as

$$\sum_{i=1}^{n_1}\sum_{j=1}^{n_2}\left(X_{1i}-X_{2j}\right)p_{1i}p_{2j}=0.$$

Subsequently, the Lagrange function is defined by

$$\sum_{j=1}^{n_1}\log p_{1j}+\sum_{j=1}^{n_2}\log p_{2j}+\lambda_1\left(1-\sum_{j=1}^{n_1}p_{1j}\right)+\lambda_2\left(1-\sum_{j=1}^{n_2}p_{2j}\right)$$
$$+\lambda_3\sum_{i=1}^{n_1}\sum_{j=1}^{n_2}\left(X_{1i}-X_{2j}\right)p_{1i}p_{2j}. \tag{5.17}$$

The resulting test statistic based on Lagrange function (5.17) has the same χ_1^2 distribution (Barton and Zhou, 2012). The function to carry out the ELR test is as follows:

```
dx1<-rep(1,n1); dx2<-rep(1,n2)
out<-el2.cen.EMs(x1, dx1, x2, dx2, fun=function(x1,x2){x1-x2},
mean=0)
```

The aforementioned variables `dx` and `dy` are indicators for censoring. As we do not assume to have censored data, `dx` and `dy` are simply the list containing 1. For more details, we refer readers to the manual for `emplik2` available in the R website. The p-value is obtained as follows:

```
1-pchisq(out$`-2LLR`,1)
[1] 0.549541
```

Although the settings of hypothesis are different, the test statistics using `solnp` and `el2.cen.Ems` are practically identical.

We also note that R package `EL` features a two-sample EL test as we have seen in Chapter 2.

5.4 Classical Empirical Likelihood Ratio Tests to Compare Multivariate Means

Suppose that we are interested in testing two groups in terms of means of d-variate variables or some combinations of those variables (e.g., Vexler et al., 2006). Let $\mathbf{X}_i = (X_{i1},\dots,X_{id})'$, $i = 1,\dots,n_1$ and $\mathbf{Y}_i = (Y_{i1},\dots,Y_{id})'$, $i = 1,\dots,n_2$ denote $d \times 1$ random vectors from group 1 and group 2, respectively, and the prime indicates the transpose. Consider a contrast matrix $C_{d\times r}$, where each column corresponds to combinations of multivariate vectors to test. For example, if we are interested in the comparison of the first and second elements, then we define

$$C = \begin{pmatrix} 1 & 0 & 0 & \cdots & 0 \\ 0 & 1 & 0 & \cdots & 0 \end{pmatrix}'.$$

In the context of two-group comparison, the null hypothesis to be tested is

$$H_0 : E(C'\mathbf{X}) = E(C'\mathbf{Y}). \tag{5.18}$$

Thus, the relevant constraints are

$$\sum_{j=1}^{n_1} p_{1j}C'\mathbf{x}_j = \sum_{j=1}^{n_2} p_{2j}C'\mathbf{y}_j,\ \sum_{j=1}^{n_1} p_{1j} = 1, \quad \sum_{j=1}^{n_2} p_{2j} = 1, \quad 0 \le p_{ij} \le 1,$$

where $\mathbf{x}_j$ and $\mathbf{y}_j$ and the realizations of $\mathbf{X}_i$ and $\mathbf{Y}_i$.

In a similar manner to (5.4), the Lagrange function is defined by

$$\sum_{j=1}^{n_1} \log p_{1j} + \sum_{j=1}^{n_2} \log p_{2j} + \lambda_1\left(1 - \sum_{j=1}^{n_1} p_{1j}\right)$$
$$+ \lambda_2\left(1 - \sum_{j=1}^{n_2} p_{2j}\right) + \lambda_3'\left(\sum_{j=1}^{n_1} p_{1j} C'\mathbf{X}_j - \sum_{j=1}^{n_2} p_{2j} C'\mathbf{Y}_j\right).$$

Note that λ_3 is $r \times 1$ vector. The Lagrange multipliers can be found numerically similar to the univariate case. Under the alternative hypothesis, H_1, maximizing $\prod_{j=1}^{n_i} p_{ij}$ subjected only to $\sum_{j=1}^{n_i} p_{ij} = 1$ yields $\prod_{i=1}^{2} n_i^{-n_i}$ similarly to the univariate case. Based on the likelihoods under H_0 and H_1, the EL ratio test statistic has the form of (5.7). We can show the following result:

***Proposition* 5.2**

Under H_0 in Equation (5.18), $-2\log R \to \chi_r^2$ in distribution when both n_1 and n_2 increase.

The proof is in the Appendix.

5.4.1 Profile Analysis

We explain how to implement the multivariate test in R in the context of the classical profile analysis. Suppose that there are d different batteries of questions to ask the job satisfaction, and we are ultimately interested in finding out gender difference in terms of the job satisfaction. However, it may be also of interest for a researcher whether these different tests deliver the same conclusions in terms of the gender difference. To answer this question, profile analysis (Johnson and Wichern, 2002) consists of three sequential hypotheses, namely, parallel profile, coincident profile, and level profile. Parallel profile indicates that the differences between groups (e.g., gender) are similar for all variates (e.g., batteries of tests). The corresponding hypothesis to be tested is

$$H_{01}: E(X_i) - E(Y_i) = E(X_j) - E(Y_j), \quad i \neq j,$$

where X_i and Y_i are i-th variates ($i = 1, \ldots, d$) of $\mathbf{X}$ and $\mathbf{Y}$. The next step is to test

$$H_{02}: E(X_i) = E(Y_i), \quad i = 1, \ldots, d,$$

which leads to coincident profile, that is, no group difference for each variate. The next step is to test

$$H_{03}: E(X_i) = E(Y_i) = E(X_j) = E(Y_j), \quad \text{for all } i \neq j,$$

which tells equivalence profile, i.e., there is no difference between groups and no difference between different batteries of tests. These three steps of tests can be carried out sequentially using the contrasts corresponding to each profile tests. For parallel and coincident profiles, we can set the null hypotheses as

$$H_{0i} : E(C_i'\mathbf{X}) = E(C_i'\mathbf{Y}), i = 1,2$$

where C_i's are

$$C_{1_{d\times(d-1)}} = \begin{pmatrix} 1 & -1 & 0 & 0 & \cdots & 0 & 0 \\ 0 & 1 & -1 & 0 & \cdots & 0 & 0 \\ \vdots & \vdots & \vdots & \vdots & \cdots & 0 & 0 \\ 0 & 0 & 0 & 0 & \cdots & 1 & -1 \end{pmatrix}',$$

$$C_{2_{d\times1}} = \begin{pmatrix} 1 & \cdots & 1 \end{pmatrix}'.$$

Keeping both H_{01} and H_{02} means that there is no difference between groups. Thus, the equivalence profile can be tested based on the combined samples, treating the two groups as one group. This leads to one-group test instead of two-group test. Specifically, we test for

$$H_{03} : E(C_3'\mathbf{Z}) = \mathbf{0},$$

where $\mathbf{Z}$ denotes the observations from both groups and $C_3 = C_1$.

The following simulation demonstrates the EL ratio test with the parallel profile test. First, we generate random vectors ($d = 3$) for group 1 and group 2 from the multivariate normal distribution as follows. Note that R library MSBVAR (Brandt, 2012) is used to generate the multivariate random variables.

```
n1<-100; n2<-100; n<-n1+n2 #arbitrary sample sizes for groups 1and2
#Variances of groups 1 and 2
sigma1=matrix(c(1,0.1,0.9,0.1,1.2,1.3,0.9,1.3,0.3),3,3)
sigma2=matrix(c(3,-1.2,2.5,-1.2,9,3.8,2.5,3.8,6),3,3)
x<-rmultnorm(n1, matrix(c(0,0,0),3,1), sigma1)
y<-rmultnorm(n2, matrix(c(0,0,0),3,1), sigma2)
data<-rbind(x,y)
```

In this case, appropriate C_1 is

$$C_{1_{d\times(d-1)}} = \begin{pmatrix} 1 & -1 & 0 \\ 0 & 1 & -1 \end{pmatrix}'.$$

The maximization of the probabilities can be carried out in a similar manner to the univariate two-group comparison. More detailed R code is provided in the Appendix at the end of this chapter. The resulting test statistic has approximately a χ^2 distribution with the degrees of freedom 2.

5.5 Product of Likelihood Functions Based on the Empirical Likelihood

In this section, we discuss the technical details of the combining likelihoods to deal with the information regarding the data structure introduced in the VAP example.

5.5.1 Product of Empirical Likelihood and Parametric Likelihood

Suppose that X has an unknown distribution, $G(x)$, and Y is a parametric function of X, with a conditional density function, $f(y|x,\theta)$, where θ is a vector of parameters. Analogously to (5.2), the likelihood is

$$L_0 = \max_{\theta} \prod_{i=1}^{2} \prod_{j=1}^{n_i} p_{ij} \prod_{i=1, X_{ij} \geq c}^{n_i} f_Y(Y_{ij} \mid X_{ij}, \theta),$$

where p_{ij} is the probability of the EL function. We maximize $\sum_{i=1}^{2} \sum_{j=1}^{n_i} \log p_{ij}$ subjected to the constraints

$$\sum_{j=1}^{n_1} X_{1j} p_{1j} = \sum_{j=1}^{n_2} X_{2j} p_{2j}, \quad \sum_{j=1}^{n_1} p_{1j} = 1, \quad \sum_{j=1}^{n_2} p_{2j} = 1, \quad 0 \leq p_{ij} \leq 1.$$

Suppose

$$Y = \xi(X, \theta) + \varepsilon, \tag{5.19}$$

where ξ is a function defining the relationship between X_i and Y_i, and ε has mean 0 and is independently identically distributed. Typically, ε is assumed to have the normal distribution. Without loss of generality, let us define the linear relationship between X and Y, that is, $E(Y_i) = \alpha + \beta E(X_i)$. Based on the normal residual assumption, the parametric model under H_0 is

$$f_{Y,X}(y \mid x) = (2\pi\sigma^2)^{-1/2} \exp\{-(2\sigma^2)^{-1}(y - \alpha - \beta x)^2\}.$$

Let $\hat{\sigma}_1$ and $\hat{\sigma}_2$ be the maximum likelihood estimators (MLEs) of the standard deviations for each group and $\hat{\sigma}$ be that of the pooled standard deviation.

Incorporating the likelihood ratio for the conditional distribution of Y into the log-likelihood ratio test statistic (5.8), we have the combined likelihood ratio test statistic,

$$(n_1^* + n_2^*)\log\hat{\sigma}^2 - n_1^*\log\hat{\sigma}_1^2 - n_2^*\log\hat{\sigma}_2^2$$
$$+2\left\{\log(n_1)^{-n_1} + \log(n_2)^{-n_2} - \sum_{j=1}^{n_1}\log p_{1j} - \sum_{j=1}^{n_2}\log p_{2j}\right\}, \tag{5.20}$$

where n_1^* and n_2^* are observed numbers of Y for each group. The difference of the parameter dimensions between the null hypothesis and its alternative hypothesis is 3 from the parametric likelihood, since, under H_1, we have the parameters to be estimated, σ^2, α, and β for each group, whereas the same parameters are estimated for the combined sample, that is, the parametric likelihood ratio tests the difference on σ^2, α, and β. Following the Wilks theorem for the likelihood ratio test, when the sample size increases, Statistic (5.20) has χ^2 distribution with the degrees of freedom 4 including 1 degree of freedom from the ELR test. It has been shown that the combined method provides overall very efficient tests (Yu et al., 2010). An example from a simulation is presented in Table 5.1. The first row is the case that the null hypothesis is correct (TIE simulation) and the second row is the case that the null hypothesis is incorrect (Power simulation). The result demonstrates that the combined test of the EL and parametric tests augments the power.

5.5.1.1 Implementation in R

To obtain p_{ij} in (5.20), we refer to Section 5.2. Consider that the following R code is a continuation of the code presented in Section 5.2. Suppose that `ty1` and `tx1` are the observed $Y(> c)$ and corresponding X for group 1, and, `ty2` and `tx2` are those for group 2. In simulation, we obtain those variables as follows. The value of `thres` is 0.

```
tx1<-x1[x1>thres];tx2<-x2[x2>thres]
#thres: threshold value (i.e., c)
ltx1<-length(tx1);ltx2<-length(tx2)
```

TABLE 5.1

The simulations (10,000 simulations) based on $n_1 = n_2 = 100$

$\mu_1,\mu_2,\alpha_1,\alpha_2,\beta_1,\beta_2$	Ave(n_1^*)	Ave(n_2^*)	EL	Parametric	Combined
0,0,2,2,1,1	50	50	0.0495	0.0545	0.0522
0,.2,2,2.2,1,1.2	50	58	0.2851	0.3660	0.4720

Note: Ave(n_1^*) and Ave(n_2^*) are the average numbers of Y observed for groups 1 and 2 ($X_{ij} \sim N(0,1)$, $Y_{ij} = \alpha_i + \beta_i X_{ij} + \varepsilon_{ij}$, $\varepsilon_{ij} \sim N(0,1)$).

In the following code, `c1`, `c2`, `beta1`, `beta2`, `sig1`, and `sig2` are defined as arbitrary numbers for simulation. Under the null hypothesis, we set `c1=c2`, `beta1=beta2`. We use `c1 = 2`, `c2 = 2`, `beta1 = 1`, `beta2 = 1`, `sig1 = 1`, and `sig2 = 1`.

```
ty1<-c1+tx1*beta1+rnorm(ltx1,0,sig1)
ty2<-c2+tx2*beta2+rnorm(ltx2,0,sig2)
```

One can use the following code to obtain `ty1` and `tx1` that we employ.

```
ty1<-ty1[x1>thres]
tx2<-ty2[x2>thres]
```

With the actual dataset related to Example 5.1, the linear relationship seems reasonable as shown in the residual plot (Figure 5.1). Note that the actual dataset is not provided. Using the simulated data, the linear model is fitted for each group as follows:

```
sw1<-lm(ty1~tx1)                                #for group 1
sw2<-lm(ty2~tx2)                                #for group 2
cty<-c(ty1,ty2); ctx<-c(tx1,tx2)
sw<-lm(cty~ctx)                          #for combined sample
```

The necessary maximum likelihood estimators (MLE) of the parameters are obtained as follows:

```
evar1<-sum(sw1$residuals^2)/ltx1                #MLE of σ₁²
evar2<-sum(sw2$residuals^2)/ltx2                #MLE of σ₂²
evar<-sum(sw$residuals^2)/(ltx1+ltx2)           #MLE of σ²
```

The test statistic is obtained as follows:

```
teststat<-elr+((ltx1+ltx2)*log(evar)-ltx1*log(evar1)-ltx2*log(evar2))
teststat
[1] 4.234401
1-pchisq(teststat,4) #p-value
[1] 0.3752116
```

It is notable that the above R code tests not only coefficients but also the difference of the variances on residuals. To some researchers, the difference on the residuals is not of interest as much as the difference on the coefficients of the linear model. In such case, we modify the test as follows. Let us compare the following two models:

$$E(Y_i) = \alpha + \beta E(X_i) \quad vs.$$

$$E(Y_i) = \alpha + \beta E(X_i) + \gamma_1 E(G_i) + \gamma_2 E(X_i G_i), i = 1.2,$$

where G_i is a group variable (0 for group 1 and 1 for group 2). The likelihood ratio can be obtained conveniently as follows. The coefficients γ_1 and γ_2 indicate the changes on the intercept and slope by belonging to a different group.

```
tgrp1<-rep(0,ltx1); tgrp2<-rep(1,ltx2); cgrp<-c(tgrp1,tgrp2)
#group variable
sw1<-lm(cty~ctx)
sw2<-lm(cty~cgrp*ctx)
testlinear<-anova(sw1,sw2,test= "LRT")[[4]][2] #LR test
testlinear
[1] 3.282017
```

The combined test statistic is as follows:

```
teststat<-elr+testlinear
teststat
[1] 3.640161
1-pchisq(teststat,3) #p-value
[1] 0.3752116
```

The above code provides the test that is robust to the difference of the variances in the residuals. As it does not test the difference on σ^2, now the degrees of freedom of the test is 3.

5.5.2 Product of the Empirical Likelihoods

Now, we modify the approach shown in Section 5.4.1 by replacing the parametric likelihood by the EL. This can be meaningful because employing the EL method relaxes the assumption regarding the distribution of data, which gives rise to more flexibility in the practice of the data analysis. Based on the form (5.2), the likelihood function can be written as

$$L = \prod_{i=1}^{2} \prod_{j=1}^{n_i} p_{ij} \prod_{j=1, x_{ij} \geq c}^{n_i} q_{ij}, \tag{5.21}$$

where $dF(x_{ij})$ and $dG(y_{ij} \mid x_{ij})$ are replaced by the empirical probability weights p_{ij} and q_{ij}. The empirical form of the null hypothesis H_0 in (5.1) is expressed as

$$\sum_{j=1}^{n_1} \Upsilon(X_{1j},\theta)p_{1j} = \sum_{j=1}^{n_2} \Upsilon(X_{2j},\theta)p_{2j}, \text{ and}$$
$$\sum_{j=1,X_{1j}\geq c}^{n_1} \Psi(Y_{1j} \mid X_{1j},\theta)q_{1j} = \sum_{j=1,X_{2j}\geq c}^{n_2} \Psi(Y_{2j} \mid X_{2j},\theta)q_{2j}. \tag{5.22}$$

Under H_0, based on relationship (5.19) between X_i and Y_i. Equation (5.22) can be expressed as

$$\sum_{j=1}^{n_1} X_{1j}p_{1j} = \sum_{j=1}^{n_2} X_{2j}p_{2j} \text{ and } \sum_{j=1,X_{1j}\geq c}^{n_1} \varepsilon_{1j}q_{1j} = \sum_{j=1,X_{2j}\geq c}^{n_2} \varepsilon_{2j}q_{2j}, \tag{5.23}$$

where $\varepsilon_{ij} = y_{ij} - \xi(x_{ij},\theta)$. Note that p_{ij} and q_{ij} satisfy restrictions (5.23) under H_0 and $\sum_{j=1}^{n_i} p_{ij} = \sum_{j,x_{ij}\geq c}^{n_i} q_{ij} = 1$. Obtaining p_{ij} and q_{ij} can be accomplished using the Lagrange multipliers. As in Section 5.5.1, assuming the linear relationship between X and Y, the second equation in (5.23) can be expressed as

$$\sum_{j=1,X_{1j}\geq c}^{n_1} \left(Y_{1j} - \alpha - \beta X_{1j}\right)q_{1j} = \sum_{j=1,X_{2j}\geq c}^{n_2} \left(Y_{2j} - \alpha - \beta X_{2j}\right)q_{2j}. \tag{5.24}$$

Since α and β need to be estimated, Equation (5.24) again can be expressed as

$$\sum_{j=1,X_{1j}\geq c}^{n_1} \left(Y_{1j} - \hat{\alpha} - \hat{\beta} X_{1j}\right)q_{1j} = \sum_{j=1,X_{2j}\geq c}^{n_2} \left(Y_{2j} - \hat{\alpha} - \hat{\beta} X_{2j}\right)q_{2j},$$

where the hat indicates the estimates of the parameters based on the pooled sample. The maximum EL estimation can be used for the estimation of α and β. The detailed discussions are found in many EL method-related literature (e.g., Qin and Lawless, 1994). Herein, we apply, for simplicity, the least square estimations of the parameters based on the observed data treating the parameters as nuisance parameters. See Lopez et al. (2009) for more discussion regarding nuisance parameters. Vexler et al. (2010b) showed that such a simple approach gives reasonable performance with the constraints regarding the linear model. The maximization of (5.21) is carried out separately for p_{ij} and q_{ij}. The value of $\prod_{j=1,X_{ij}\geq c}^{n_i^*} q_{ij}$ is maximized subjected to

$$\sum_{j=1,X_{1j}\geq c}^{n_1} (Y_{1j} - \hat{\alpha} - \hat{\beta} X_{1j})q_{1j} = \sum_{j=1,X_{2j}\geq c}^{n_2} (Y_{2j} - \hat{\alpha} - \hat{\beta} X_{2j})q_{2j},$$
$$\sum_{j=1,X_{1j}\geq c}^{n_1} q_{1j} = 1, \sum_{j=1,X_{2j}\geq c}^{n_2} q_{2j} = 1,\ 0 \leq q_{ij} \leq 1.$$

Maximization can be carried out in a similar way to obtaining p_{ij}. Under H_1, $\prod_{j=1,x_{ij}\geq c}^{n_i^*} q_{ij}$ is maximized subjected only to $\sum_{j=1,x_{ij}\geq c}^{n_i^*} q_{ij} = 1$ where $0 \leq q_{ij} \leq 1$. Based on the ELs under H_0 and H_1, the ELR is

$$R = \left(\prod_{i=1}^{2} n_i^{-n_i} n_i^{*-n_i^*} \right)^{-1} \prod_{i=1}^{2} \prod_{j=1}^{n_i} p_{ij} \prod_{j=1}^{n_i^*} q_{ij}.$$

We can directly show that $-2\log R$ has the χ_2^2 distribution as n_1 and $n_2 \to \infty$ for independently distributed x_{ij} and ε_{ij}, with $E(x_{ij}^3) < \infty$, $E(\varepsilon_{ij}^3) < \infty$ under H_0, which basically can be obtained using the similar proof scheme shown in the Appendix for the multivariate cases.

5.5.2.1 Implementation in R (Continued from Section 5.5.1.1)

First, we obtain the residuals as follows:

```
a<-sw$coefficients[[1]]                          #α̂
b<-sw$coefficients[[2]]                          #β̂
r1<-ty1-a-b*tx1                #residuals for group 1
r2<-ty2-a-b*tx2                #residuals for group 2
```

Then, the maximization of $\prod_{j=1,x_{ij}\geq c}^{n_i^*} q_{ij}$ is carried out by:

```
out<-el2.cen.EMs(r1, dx1, r2, dx2, fun=function(x1,x2){x1-x2},
mean=0)
```

The resulting test statistic based on the residuals is

```
teststat2<- out$`-2LLR`
teststat2
[1] 1.239973
```

We note that, although we use the estimates for the coefficients above, the resulting ELR statistic is obtained by maximizing the EL, thus relevant properties of the ELR statistic hold.
The combined test statistic is

```
elr+teststat2
[1] 1.598116
```

Note that `elr` is based on all observations of `x1` and `x2` (Section 5.2). The corresponding p-value is obtained as follows:

```
1-pchisq(elr+teststat2,2)
[1] 0.4497524
```

5.6 Concluding Remarks

The ELR test for two-group comparison is discussed in this chapter. We showed that the relevant null hypothesis for the population means can be built, translated to the empirical form, and tested based on the likelihood ratio test concept. The EL method can also provide straightforward nonparametric extension of other parametric likelihood approach. This convenient feature of the EL method leads to methodological tools handling incomplete data explained in this chapter. Specifically, when two outcomes are relevant surrogate variables to show a treatment effect and closely related while one outcome is substantially missing, the proposed method provides a way to test the difference between two groups utilizing all available observations in the approximate likelihood manner. Handling incomplete data can provide more flexibility in applications to clinical trials that are often carried out in routine care procedures rather than a strictly controlled environment. Finally, we conclude this chapter with an advice when a study has some irregularity issue, that is, the value Y sometimes exists even if corresponding X is not above the threshold. Regardless, the EL is obtained based on the any observations by modifying (5.2) as follows:

$$L = \prod_{i=1}^{2} \prod_{j=1}^{n_i} dG_i(X_{ij}) \prod_{j=1}^{n_i} dF_i(Y_{ij}|X_{ij},\theta)D_{ij},$$

where D_{ij} is 1 if Y_{ij} exists or otherwise 0. The subsequent analysis can be carried out similarly to what is presented in this chapter.

Appendix

Proof of Proposition 5.2

First, let $n = \min(n_1, n_2)$. Also let $p_{1i} = p_i$ and $p_{2i} = q_i$. Empirically, we express $\sum_{i=1}^{n_1} p_i C'\mathbf{x}_i = \mu_\mathbf{x}$ and $\sum_{i=1}^{n_2} q_i C'\mathbf{y}_i = \mu_\mathbf{y}$. Thus, under H_0, we can let $\mu_\mathbf{x} = \mu_\mathbf{y} = \mu$. Under H_0, we maximize the likelihood function $\prod_{i=1}^{n_1} \prod_{j=1}^{n_2} p_i q_j$ by the Lagrange method,

$$H = \sum_{i=1}^{n_1} \log p_i + \sum_{i=1}^{n_2} \log q_i + \lambda_1 \left(1 - \sum_{i=1}^{n_i} p_i \right) + \lambda_2 \left(1 - \sum_{i=1}^{n_2} q_i \right)$$

$$+ \lambda' \left(\sum_{i=1}^{n_1} p_i \, C'\mathbf{x}_i - \sum_{i=1}^{n_2} q_i \, C'\mathbf{y}_i \right),$$

where λ is $d \times 1$ vector, and the prime notation indicates the transpose of a vector or matrix. Thus,

$$\frac{dH}{dp_i} = \frac{1}{p_i} - \lambda_1 + \lambda' C' \mathbf{x}_i \tag{A.5.1}$$

$$\frac{dH}{dq_i} = \frac{1}{q_i} - \lambda_2 - \lambda' C' \mathbf{y}_i \tag{A.5.2}$$

Letting Equations (A.5.1) and (A.5.2) equal to 0, we have

$$p_i = \frac{1}{\lambda_1 - \lambda' C' \mathbf{x}_i} \quad \text{and} \quad q_i = \frac{1}{\lambda_2 + \lambda' C' \mathbf{y}_i}. \tag{A.5.3}$$

Multiplying Equation (A.5.1) by p_i and summing over all p_i $(i = 1, \ldots, n_1)$ gives the λ_1 value, then, p_i in Equation (A.5.3) can be expressed as

$$p_i = \frac{1}{n_1 + \lambda' \Sigma_{\mathbf{x}_i}},$$

where $\Sigma_{\mathbf{x}_i} = C' \mu_{\mathbf{x}} - C' \mathbf{x}_i$. Likewise

$$q_i = \frac{1}{n_2 - \lambda' \Sigma_{\mathbf{y}_i}},$$

where $\Sigma_{\mathbf{y}_i} = C' \mu_{\mathbf{y}} - C' \mathbf{y}_i$. Also, under H_1, $p_i = \dfrac{1}{n_1}, q_i = \dfrac{1}{n_2}$

Thus, the EL ratio test is

$$\begin{aligned} -2\log\text{LR} &= -2\log\left(\frac{\prod_{i=1}^{n_1} p_i \prod_{i=1}^{n_2} q_i}{\left(\frac{1}{n_1}\right)^{n_1} \left(\frac{1}{n_2}\right)^{n_2}} \right) \\ &= 2\left(\underbrace{\sum_{i=1}^{n_1} \left(\log\frac{1}{n_1} - \log p_i \right)}_{A} + \underbrace{\sum_{i=1}^{n_2} \left(\log\frac{1}{n_2} - \log \text{q}_i \right)}_{B} \right) \end{aligned} \tag{A.5.4}$$

For part A in (A.5.4),

$$\sum_{i=1}^{n_1}\left(\log\frac{1}{n_1}-\log p_i\right)=\sum_{i=1}^{n_1}\log\left(1+\frac{\lambda'\Sigma_{\mathbf{x}_i}}{n_1}\right)$$

$$=\sum_{i=1}^{n_1}\left(\frac{\lambda'\Sigma_{\mathbf{x}_i}}{n_1}\right)-\frac{\sum_{i=1}^{n_1}(\lambda'\Sigma_{\mathbf{x}_i})^2}{2n_1^2}+\frac{1}{3}\frac{\sum_{i=1}^{n_1}(\lambda'\Sigma_{\mathbf{x}_i})^3}{n_1^3}+\cdots$$

by the Taylor expansion

$$=\sum_{i=1}^{n_1}\left(\frac{\lambda'\Sigma_{\mathbf{x}_i}}{n_1}\right)-\frac{\sum_{i=1}^{n_1}(\lambda'\Sigma_{\mathbf{x}_i})^2}{2n_1^2}+O(n^{-3/2}).$$

Likewise, for part B in Equation (A.5.4), we have

$$\sum_{i=1}^{n_2}\left(\log\frac{1}{n_2}-\log q_i\right)=-\sum_{i=1}^{n_2}\left(\frac{\lambda'\Sigma_{\mathbf{y}_i}}{n_2}\right)-\frac{\sum_{i=1}^{n_2}(\lambda'\Sigma_{\mathbf{y}_i})^2}{2n_2^2}+O(n^{-3/2}).$$

Thus (A.5.4) is approximated by

$$-2\log LR \simeq 2\left(\sum_{i=1}^{n_1}\left(\frac{\lambda'\Sigma_{\mathbf{x}_i}}{n_1}\right)-\sum_{i=1}^{n_2}\left(\frac{\lambda'\Sigma_{\mathbf{y}_i}}{n_2}\right)-\left(\frac{\sum_{i=1}^{n_1}(\lambda'\Sigma_{\mathbf{x}_i})^2}{2n_1^2}+\frac{\sum_{i=1}^{n_2}(\lambda'\Sigma_{\mathbf{y}_i})^2}{2n_2^2}\right)\right)$$

Also,

$$\sum_{i=1}^{n_i}p_i=1\Leftrightarrow\sum_{i=1}^{n_1}\frac{1}{n_1+\lambda'\Sigma_{x_i}}-\sum_{i=1}^{n_1}\frac{1}{n_1}=0 \tag{A.5.5}$$

$$\Leftrightarrow \sum_{i=1}^{n_1} \left(\frac{\lambda' \Sigma_{x_i}}{n_1 + \lambda' \Sigma_{x_i}} \right) = 0 \Leftrightarrow \sum_{i=1}^{n_1} \frac{\lambda' \Sigma_{x_i}}{n_1} \left(\frac{1}{1 + \frac{\lambda' \Sigma_{x_i}}{n_1}} \right) = 0$$

$$\Leftrightarrow \sum_{i=1}^{n_1} \frac{\lambda' \Sigma_{x_i}}{n_1} \left(1 - \frac{\lambda' \Sigma_{x_i}}{n_1} + \left(\frac{\lambda' \Sigma_{x_i}}{n_1} \right)^2 - \left(\frac{\lambda' \Sigma_{x_i}}{n_1} \right)^3 + \cdots \right) = 0 \text{ by the Taylor expansion}$$

$$\Leftrightarrow \sum_{i=1}^{n_1} \frac{\lambda' \Sigma_{x_i}}{n_1} - \sum_{i=1}^{n_1} \frac{(\lambda' \Sigma_{x_i})(\lambda' \Sigma_{x_i})}{n_1^2} + O(n^{-1}) = 0$$

$$\Leftrightarrow \sum_{i=1}^{n_1} \frac{\lambda' \Sigma_{x_i}}{n_1} = \sum_{i=1}^{n_1} \frac{(\lambda' \Sigma_{x_i})(\lambda' \Sigma_{x_i})}{n_1^2} + O(n^{-1}).$$

Note that double-headed arrow ($\Leftrightarrow$) represents logical equivalence.

Similar to the above we can show

$$\sum_{i=1}^{n_2} \frac{\lambda' \Sigma_{y_i}}{n_2} = \sum_{i=1}^{n_1} \frac{(\lambda' \Sigma_{y_i})(\lambda' \Sigma_{y_i})}{n_2^2} + O(n^{-1}).$$

Thus, we have

$$-2 \log LR \cong \sum_{i=1}^{n_1} \left(\frac{\lambda' \Sigma_{x_i}}{n_1} \right) - \sum_{i=1}^{n_2} \left(\frac{\lambda' \Sigma_{y_i}}{n_2} \right) = \lambda' \left(\frac{\sum_{i=1}^{n_1} \Sigma_{x_i}}{n_1} - \frac{\sum_{i=1}^{n_1} \Sigma_{y_i}}{n_2} \right).$$

Since $\lambda' \neq 0$, (A.5.5), and a similar equation to (A.5.5) for y, the equations

$$\sum_{i=1}^{n_1} \left(\frac{\Sigma_{x_i}}{n_1 + \lambda' \Sigma_{x_i}} \right) = C \text{ and } \sum_{i=1}^{n_2} \left(\frac{\Sigma_{y_i}}{n_2 + \lambda' \Sigma_{y_i}} \right) = 0$$

are obtained. Thus, we have

$$\sum_{i=1}^{n_1} \frac{\Sigma_{\mathbf{x}_i}}{n_1}\left(\frac{1}{1+\dfrac{\lambda'\Sigma_{\mathbf{x}_i}}{n_1}}\right)-\sum_{i=1}^{n_2} \frac{\Sigma_{\mathbf{y}_i}}{n_2}\left(\frac{1}{1+\dfrac{\lambda'\Sigma_{\mathbf{y}_i}}{n_2}}\right)=0$$

$$\Leftrightarrow \sum_{i=1}^{n_1} \frac{\Sigma_{\mathbf{x}_i}}{n_1}\left(1-\frac{\lambda'\Sigma_{\mathbf{x}_i}}{n_1}+\left(\frac{\lambda'\Sigma_{\mathbf{x}_i}}{n_1}\right)^2+\cdots\right)-\sum_{i=1}^{n_2} \frac{\Sigma_{\mathbf{y}_i}}{n_2}\left(1+\frac{\lambda'\Sigma_{\mathbf{y}_i}}{n_2}-\left(\frac{\lambda'\Sigma_{\mathbf{y}_i}}{n_2}\right)^2+\cdots\right)=0$$

$$\Leftrightarrow \sum_{i=1}^{n_1} \frac{\Sigma_{\mathbf{x}_i}}{n_1}-\sum_{i=1}^{n_1} \frac{\Sigma_{\mathbf{x}_i}\Sigma_{\mathbf{x}_i}'}{n_1^2}\lambda+O(n^{-1})-\sum_{i=1}^{n_2} \frac{\Sigma_{\mathbf{y}_i}}{n_2}-\sum_{i=1}^{n_2} \frac{\Sigma_{\mathbf{y}_i}\Sigma_{\mathbf{y}_i}'}{n_2^2}\lambda+O(n^{-1})=0$$

$$\Leftrightarrow -\left(\sum_{i=1}^{n_1} \frac{\Sigma_{\mathbf{x}_i}\Sigma_{\mathbf{x}_i}'}{n_1^2}+\sum_{i=1}^{n_2} \frac{\Sigma_{\mathbf{y}_i}\Sigma_{\mathbf{y}_i}'}{n_2^2}\right)\lambda=-\left(\sum_{i=1}^{n_1} \frac{\Sigma_{\mathbf{x}_i}}{n_1}-\sum_{i=1}^{n_2} \frac{\Sigma_{\mathbf{y}_i}}{n_2}\right)+O(n^{-1})$$

$$\Leftrightarrow \lambda=\left(\sum_{i=1}^{n_1} \frac{\Sigma_{\mathbf{x}_i}\Sigma_{\mathbf{x}_i}'}{n_1^2}+\sum_{i=1}^{n_2} \frac{\Sigma_{\mathbf{y}_i}\Sigma_{\mathbf{y}_i}'}{n_2^2}\right)^{-1}\left(\sum_{i=1}^{n_1} \frac{\Sigma_{\mathbf{x}_i}}{n_1}-\sum_{i=1}^{n_2} \frac{\Sigma_{\mathbf{y}_i}}{n_2}\right)+O(1).$$

Thus,

$$-2\log LR=\left(\sum_{i=1}^{n_1} \frac{\Sigma_{\mathbf{x}_i}}{n_1}-\sum_{i=1}^{n_2} \frac{\Sigma_{\mathbf{y}_i}}{n_2}\right)'\left(\sum_{i=1}^{n_1} \frac{\Sigma_{\mathbf{x}_i}\Sigma_{\mathbf{x}_i}'}{n_1^2}+\sum_{i=1}^{n_2} \frac{\Sigma_{\mathbf{y}_i}\Sigma_{\mathbf{y}_i}'}{n_2^2}\right)^{-1}\left(\sum_{i=1}^{n_1} \frac{\Sigma_{\mathbf{x}_i}}{n_1}-\sum_{i=1}^{n_2} \frac{\Sigma_{\mathbf{y}_i}}{n_2}\right). \tag{A.5.6}$$

Under H_0, the standard multivariate statistics theory (Johnson and Wichern, 2002) leads statistic (A.5.6) to be χ^2 distribution with the degree of freedom r.

The R Code to Carry Out the Empirical Likelihood Profile Analysis

```
c1<-c(1,-1,0); c2<-c(0,1,-1)
p<-array(dim=(n1+n2))         #likelihood to achieve the maximum

fn=function(p){
  sump<-0
  for(i in 1:n){
  sump<-sump+log(p[i])
  }
  return(-sump)
}

fn1x=function(p){
  sump1<-0
  for(i in 1:n1){
```

```
  sump1<-sump1+p[i]
  }
  return(sump1)
}

fn1y=function(p){
  sumq1<-0
  for(i in (n1+1):n){
  sumq1<-sumq1+p[i]
  }
  return(sumq1)
}

fn2x=function(p){
  sump2<-0
  for(i in 1:n1){
  sump2<-sump2+p[i]*sum(c1*data[i,])
  }
  return(sump2)
}

fn2y=function(p){
  sumq2<-0
  for(i in (n1+1):n){
  sumq2<-sumq2+p[i]*sum(c1*data[i,])
  }
  return(sumq2)
}

fn3x=function(p){
  sump3<-0
  for(i in 1:n1){
  sump3<-sump3+p[i]*sum(c2*data[i,])
}
  return(sump3)
}

fn3y=function(p){
  sumq3<-0
  for(i in (n1+1):n){
  sumq3<-sumq3+p[i]*sum(c2*data[i,])
  }
  return(sumq3)
}

#Collection of the constraints
eqn1=function(p){
  z1x=fn1x(p)
  z1y=fn1y(p)
  z2=fn2x(p)-fn2y(p)
```

```
  z3=fn3x(p)-fn3y(p)
  return(c(z1x,z1y,z2,z3))
}

p0 = c(rep((1/n1),n1),rep((1/n2),n2))           #Initial value
lb<-rep(0,n);ub<-rep(1,n)
outcomes<-solnp(p0, fun = fn, eqfun = eqn1, eqB =
c(1,1,0,0),LB=lb)
lik0<--(outcomes$values[length(outcomes$values)])

teststat<- -2*(lik0+(n1*log(n1)+n2*log(n2)))    #test statistic
1-pchisq(teststat,2)                                   #p-value
```

6

Quantile Comparisons

6.1 Introduction

In this chapter we consider comparison of the q-th quantiles between treatment groups. There are many advantages to using quantiles in biomedical research. For example, often, examination of the median is advocated by many elementary textbooks when the distribution of the data is skewed. In fact, many measurements in the biomedical and social science areas have skewed distributions, particularly in cases with low means, large variances, and nonnegative measurements (Limpert et al., 2001). In group comparisons, comparison of medians provides different information than comparing means (Yu et al., 2011). Quantiles, particularly very high ones, provide the relevant information regarding ranges of the outcomes. Investigation into outcome ranges is important in the context of the reference ranges of biomarkers, which provide criteria for classifying the normal and abnormal groups. Also, comparisons of upper quantiles are of great interest in the contexts of receiver operating characteristic curve analyses related to the sensitivity and specificity between different diagnostic tools or biomarkers (e.g., Zhou and Qin, 2005). Comparison of quantiles is often desirable when the population of the case or treatment group differs from that of the control group not only by location but also by the shape of the distribution. Consider the following example.

Example 6.1: Decisions Based on Mean and Median

Information obtained by observing different medians is not same as that obtained by observing different means, as illustrated in Figure 6.1. In each plot, the dashed and solid lines supposedly describe the densities of control and case groups, respectively. Figure 6.1a describes densities with similar medians yet different means and Figure 6.1b describes the opposite scenario. Suppose that someone classifies an individual as a case if the individual has a value (e.g., a biomarker value) beyond the true median of the case group. Based on a preliminary Monte Carlo

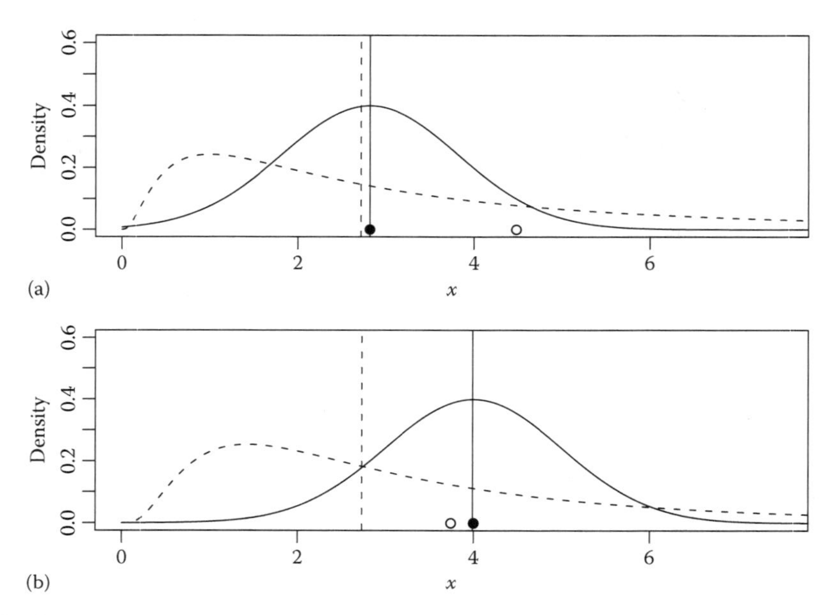

FIGURE 6.1
(a and b) Comparison of two densities. For both figures, the solid vertical line and filled circle are the median and mean of the density of the case group (solid line), and the dashed vertical line and empty circle are those of the control group (dashed line).

power analysis using the two-sample t-test (10,000 data generations), Figures 6.1a and 6.1b show the powers of 0.653 and 0.154, respectively, based on a sample size of 50 per group. Contradicting these powers, in Figure 6.1a, 48.6% of the control group will be incorrectly classified into the case group indicating almost no classification ability, whereas in Figure 6.1b, 31.5% of the control group will be incorrectly classified into the case group indicating some gained classification ability.

Example 6.1 describes cases that the underlying distributions to compare are seemingly different, or put in other terms, violation of the exchangeability assumptions or nonconstant shift (Hutson, 2007; Yu et al., 2011). Although many location-shift tests are available, such tests often do not provide quintile-specific comparisons. Some are testing the distributional difference, wrongfully thinking that they are testing medians (e.g., Wilcoxon rank sum test).

Some research has more keen interest in upper percentiles. See the following examples:

1. Wener et al. (2000) investigated the upper reference limit of serum C-reactive protein (CRP) by different demographic groups. They showed that the sample 95th percentile value of CRP in the overall population was 0.95 mg/dL for males and 1.39 mg/dL for females and varied with age and race as well. They stated that the upper reference limits of CRP should be adjusted by demographic factors.

2. He et al. (2004) investigated the distribution of serum prostate-specific antigen (PSA) in different ethnic groups. The *normal* distribution of serum PSA levels in healthy Chinese men was evaluated. They demonstrated a gradual increase in the sample median and 95th percentiles of serum PSA levels by age.
3. Oremek and Seiffert (1996) showed dramatic changes in PSA levels among men of various ages after 15 minutes of exercise. The investigators presented the sample 95th percentiles of PSA levels before and after exercise for practical usage.
4. Boucai and Surks (2009) showed that reference limits for thyroid-stimulating hormone (TSH) differed between races and with age based on a cross-sectional study of an urban outpatient medical practice. Use of race- and age-specific reference limits was strongly recommended as such practices will decrease misclassification of patients with increased TSH.

Note that, in these examples, investigators' claims were based only on descriptive percentiles without accompanying relevant statistical tests. Now, Figure 6.2 shows some examples that different groups share the same

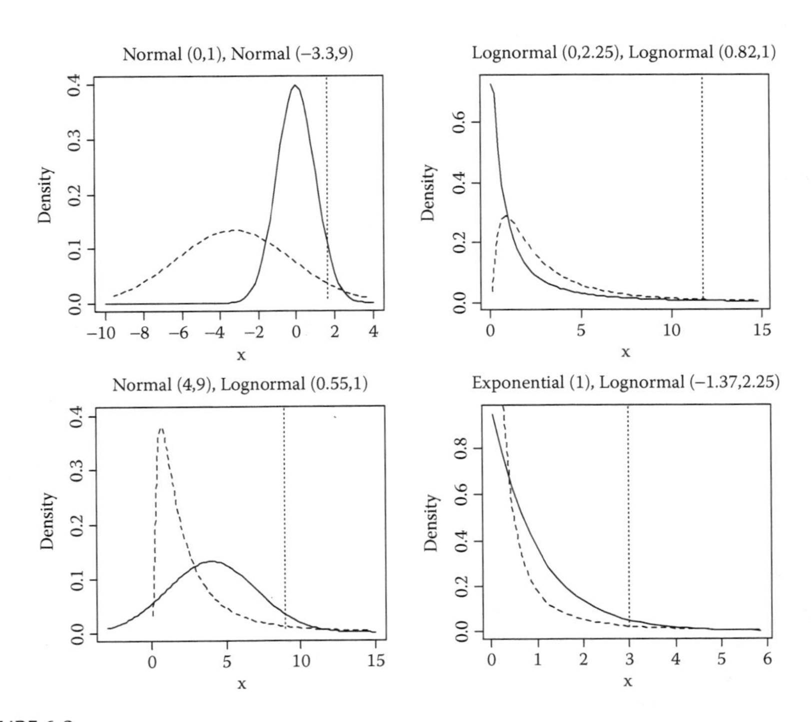

FIGURE 6.2
Descriptions of the same 95th percentiles with different underlying distributions. The vertical dotted lines indicate the 95th percentiles.

quantiles but have vastly different underlying distributions. We need to be careful to check whether a given test can carry out the comparison of a certain quantile regardless of such different distributions with a desirable Type I error (TIE) rate. For example, some are testing the distributional difference, wrongfully thinking that they are testing medians.

In this chapter we show how to construct the tests for percentile-specific group comparisons based on the empirical likelihood (EL) approach. We first illustrate that some existing nonparametric tests for location shift may not be the median-specific test under various underlying distributions. Then, we will construct the test statistics for the two-sample comparisons of the general quantiles.

6.2 Existing Nonparametric Tests to Compare Location Shifts

Several parametric or nonparametric methods are available to test the location shift between two groups. Some tests are based on rank, such as the normal scores test, Wilcoxon rank-sum test, and Cauchy scores test. Tests of distribution homogeneity such as the Kolmogorov–Smirnov (KS) test can also be used to detect location shift (Freidlin and Gastwirth, 2000). With the equal distributions under the null hypothesis, these tests can check the location shift or equivalently the comparison of the medians. However, in general, these tests compare the distributions itself and thus do not provide median-specific comparisons.

To demonstrate that some available tests do not provide median-specific comparisons with different underlying distributions, the Monte Carlo TIE rates of some existing tests such as the KS test, Wilcoxon's test, and Mood's median test (Mood, 1954) are presented in Table 6.1. When the underlying distributions are different despite of equal medians, the KS test is not appropriate for testing location differences as by definition it is constructed to test the homogeneity of distributions. Except for the comparison of lognormal distributions, TIE rates for Wilcoxon's test became uncontrollable with different underlying distributions. This problem does not vanish with a larger sample size (e.g., the TIE rate of Wilcoxon's test is 0.3461 with $n_1 = n_2 = 100$ for comparing $N(1,1)$ and $Lognormal\ (0,1)$). This result confirms that Wilcoxon's test is not suitable in cases with different underlying distributions (Szymczak et al., 2009). Note that Wilcoxon's test (Wilcoxon–Mann–Whitney U-statistic) in fact tests the equal chance that one variable is larger than the other variance (Chapter 7). Unlike the other tests, we observe that the median test shows consistently stable performances regardless of the underlying distributions, thus providing the most reliable test in terms of TIE rate control.

TABLE 6.1

The Monte Carlo Type I error rates of the traditional location shift tests. Entries for each sample size and distribution combination are the results of the Kolmogorov–Smirnov test (KS), Wilcoxon's test (W), and Mood's median test (M), respectively. The significance level is 0.05

		n_1, n_2				
Distributions	**Method**	**15,15**	**15,25**	**50,50**	**100,100**	**100,200**
Normal(0,1) vs.	KS	0.0259	0.0508	0.0386	0.0341	0.0411
Normal(0,1)	W	0.0440	0.0477	0.0518	0.0505	0.0501
	M	0.0231	0.0472	0.0280	0.0355	0.0378
Lognormal(0,1) vs.	KS	0.0314	0.0536	0.0724	0.1189	0.1478
Lognormal(0,1.769)	W	0.0459	0.0470	0.0500	0.0526	0.0399
	M	0.0272	0.0506	0.0274	0.0370	0.0375
Normal(1,1) vs.	KS	0.0378	0.0835	0.1607	0.4995	0.7429
Lognormal(0,1)	W	0.0802	0.1049	0.1970	0.3461	0.4432
	M	0.0293	0.0497	0.0303	0.0384	0.0341
Uniform(0,3) vs.	KS	0.3251	0.5916	0.9970	1.0000	1.0000
Lognormal(0.405,9)	W	0.0770	0.0562	0.1180	0.1663	0.1566
	M	0.0563	0.1047	0.0550	0.0670	0.0816
Exponential(1.5) vs.	KS	0.0288	0.0561	0.0517	0.0738	0.1015
Lognormal(−0.77,1)	W	0.0523	0.0599	0.0672	0.0853	0.0981
	M	0.0256	0.0477	0.0287	0.0365	0.0357

6.3 Empirical Likelihood Tests to Compare Location Shifts

Let us discuss the quantile estimation using the EL in one-group setting first. Let X_i $(i = 1, \ldots, n)$ be univariate random sample of size n from an unknown distribution function F. The q-th quantile is defined as

$$\theta = F^{-1}(q) = \inf\{x : F(x) \geq q\}, \text{ for } 0 < q < 1$$

Suppose that there is a constraint expressed as

$$E(g(X, \eta)) = 0,$$

where the function $g(\cdot)$ is a known scalar or vector function and η is a known parameter. Following the standard technique of the EL, the EL function is expressed as

$$\prod_{i=1}^{n} dF(x_i). \tag{6.1}$$

where we put $p_i = dF(x_i)$ and p_i satisfies

$$\sum_{i=1}^{n} p_i g(X_i, \eta) = 0 \tag{6.2}$$

The likelihood function (6.1) is maximized using the function

$$\sum_{i=1}^{n} \log p_i - \lambda^{*T} \sum_{i=1}^{n} p_i g(X_i, \eta) - \beta\left\{\sum_{i=1}^{n} p_i - 1\right\},$$

where λ^* and β are the Lagrange multipliers. Letting $\lambda^* = n\lambda$, we have

$$p_i = \frac{1}{n[1 + \lambda^T g(X_i, \eta)]}, i = 1, \dots, n,$$

where λ is obtained by solving

$$\sum_{i=1}^{n} \frac{g(X_i, \eta)}{1 + \lambda^T g(X_i, \eta)} = 0.$$

Suppose $\hat{\eta}$ and $\hat{\lambda}$ are the values maximizing the EL (6.1). Subsequently, $p_i = n[1 + \hat{\lambda}^T g(X_i, \hat{\eta})]^{-1}$, and the corresponding empirical distribution function under constraint (6.2) is given as

$$\hat{F}_n(x) = \sum_{i=1}^{n} p_i \, \delta(X_i \le x),$$

where $\delta(\cdot)$ is 1 if the condition inside the parenthesis is satisfied, or otherwise 0. Without the constraint such as (6.2), $\hat{F}_n(x)$ will be the empirical distribution function, that is,

$$\hat{F}(x) = n^{-1} \sum_{i=1}^{n} \delta(X_i \le x).$$

Now, let $\hat{\theta} = \hat{F}_n^{-1}(q)$ be the q-th quantile estimator. With at least twice differentiable $F(x)$, Chen and Chen (2000) showed that $\hat{\theta}$ can be expressed by the Bahadur representation (Bahadur, 1966) as

$$\hat{\theta} = \theta + \frac{q - \hat{F}_n(\theta)}{f(\theta)} + O_p(n^{-3/4}(\log n)^{1/2}), \tag{6.3}$$

where $f(x) = F'(x)$.

Now, we discuss testing for comparison between two groups. Let X_{ij} denote the random variable of the j-th unit from group i ($i = 1, 2$) with the continuous distribution function F_i that is at least two times differentiable in some neighborhood of the q-th quantile. Also, let $f_i(x)$ and $f(x)$ denote the density functions of group i and the pooled data, respectively, and F is the distribution function of the pooled data. We are interested in comparison of the q-th quantile between the two treatment groups, where the q-th quantile of group i is

$$F_i^{-1}(q) = \inf\{x : F_i(x) \geq q\} \text{ for } 0 < q < 1, i = 1,2.$$

Let $F_i^{-1}(q) = \theta_i$. Under H_0, we assume

$$H_0 : \theta_1 = \theta_2. \tag{6.4}$$

The EL ratio (ELR) test is obtained as follows. The relevant likelihood function of X_{ij} is

$$\prod_{i=1}^{2} \prod_{j=1}^{n_i} dF_i(x_{ij}). \tag{6.5}$$

Following the EL concept, (6.5) can be expressed in the nonparametric form

$$\prod_{i=1}^{2} \prod_{j=1}^{n_i} p_{ij}, \tag{6.6}$$

where p_{ij} represents the empirical probabilities replacing $dF_i(x_{ij})$ and satisfies the constraint

$$\sum_{j=1}^{n_1} p_{1j} = \sum_{j=1}^{n_2} p_{2j} = 1, \quad 0 \leq p_{ij} \leq 1. \tag{6.7}$$

In addition to (6.7), under H_0, the probability weights p_{ij} are obtained to maximize the EL function (6.6) subject to relevant constraints with respect to the hypothesis (6.4).

Using the definition of the percentile and the empirical probabilities, for each group i $(i = 1, 2)$, we can establish the empirical equality as $\sum_{j=1}^{n_i} p_{ij}\, \Delta(\theta_i - X_{ij}) = q$ under H_0, where $\Delta(x)$ is an appropriate function for obtaining the empirical distribution. One example of $\Delta(x)$ is an identity function $I(x)$ defined as $I(x) = 0$ if $x < 0$ and $I(x)$ is 1 if $x \geq 0$. Following the conventional EL approach, we have the empirical constraints consistent with (6.4) in a form

$$\sum_{j=1}^{n_1} p_{1j}\left(\Delta(\tilde{\theta} - X_{1j}) - q\right) = 0, \quad \text{and} \quad \sum_{j=1}^{n_2} p_{2j}\left(\Delta(\tilde{\theta} - X_{2j}) - q\right) = 0, \tag{6.8}$$

where $\tilde{\theta}$ is the EL estimator (Chapter 2) of θ that maximizes (6.6). According to constraints (6.7) and (6.8), the log of the likelihood function, $\log \prod_{j=1}^{n_i} p_{ij}$, is maximized subject to

$$\sum_{j=1}^{n_i} p_{ij}\, \Delta(\tilde{\theta} - X_{ij}) = q, \; \sum_{j=1}^{n_i} p_{ij} = 1, 0 \leq p_{ij} \leq 1,$$

for each group $i, i = 1, 2$. Maximization can be achieved based on the Lagrange multiplier method through the function

$$\sum_{j=1}^{n_i} \log p_{ij} + \lambda_{i1}\left(1 - \sum_{j=1}^{n_i} p_{ij}\right) + \lambda_{i2}\left(q - \sum_{j=1}^{n_i} p_{ij}\,\Delta(\tilde{\theta} - X_{ij})\right), \tag{6.9}$$

where λ_{ij} $(i, j = 1, 2)$ are Lagrange multipliers.

Let $\Delta(x) = I(x)$ in (6.9). Following the Lagrange multiplier solutions, we obtain

$$\lambda_{i1} = n_i - \lambda_{i2}\, q, \quad p_{ij} = \left(n_i + \lambda_{i2}\left(I(\tilde{\theta} - X_{ij}) - q\right)\right)^{-1}. \tag{6.10}$$

Using (6.10) and constraint (6.8), we obtain that

$$\lambda_{i2} = (r_i/q - n_i)\,/\,(1 - q),$$

where

$$r_i = n_i \hat{F}_i(\tilde{\theta}) = \sum_{j=1}^{n_i} I(\tilde{\theta} - X_{ij}). \tag{6.11}$$

(See also Section 3.5 in this context.) For the EL function under the alternative hypothesis $H_1 : \theta_1 \neq \theta_2$, we impose the restriction (6.7) only to maximize the EL function, resulting in $L = \prod_{i=1}^{2} \prod_{j=1}^{n_i} 1/n_i = n_1^{-n_1} n_2^{-n_2}$. Consequently, we obtain $-2\log$ of the ELR test,

$$-2\log R = -2\left[\sum_{i=1}^{2} n_i \log n_i - (n_i - r_i)\log\left(n_i - \tfrac{q}{1-q}(r_i/q - n_i)\right) - r_i \log\left(r_i/q\right)\right]. \tag{6.12}$$

Then, we have the following result:

Proposition 6.1

Under H_0 $-2\log R$ in (6.12) *converges in distribution to* χ_1^2 *distribution as* $n_i \to \infty, i = 1, 2$.

Proposition 6.1 can be proven based on the results of Lopez et al. (2009) that address cases with nondifferentiable function $\Delta(\cdot)$. On the other hand, a direct proof of the Proposition 6.1 can be carried out by approximating $-2\log LR$ as

$$-2\log R \simeq (n_1 + n_2)\left(n_1 q(1 - q)\right)^{-1} n_2\left(\hat{F}_2(\tilde{\theta}) - q\right)^2 + o\left(n_*^{-1/2+\alpha}\right), \tag{6.13}$$

for some small α and $n_* = \min(n_1, n_2)$. Also, we can use the expression

$$\hat{F}_2(\tilde{\theta}) - q = \hat{F}_2(\theta) - q + f_2(\theta)(\tilde{\theta} - \theta) + o\left(n_2^{-1/2+\alpha}\right). \tag{6.14}$$

See the proof of Proposition 6.2 for the derivation of (6.13) and (6.14). Based on the arguments shown in Lopez et al. (2009) and Chen and Chen (2000), we can express $\tilde{\theta} - \theta = O_p(n_*^{-1/2})$ and the desired result will be followed when $n_i \to \infty$, $i = 1, 2$.

In actual applications of the test statistic (6.12), the function $I(x)$ can be replaced by a smoothed function using the kernel method (Nadaraya, 1964; Azzalini, 1981) to obtain r_i in (6.11). Specifically, for $\sum_{j=1}^{n_i} I(\tilde{\theta} - X_{ij})$, we can use $\sum_{j=1}^{n_i} K((\tilde{\theta} - X_{ij})/h)$, where $K(u) = \int_{-\infty}^{u} k(u)du$; k is a nonnegative, differentiable function satisfying $\int_{-\infty}^{\infty} k(u)du = 1$, $\int_{-\infty}^{\infty} |u|k(u)du < \infty$, and $\int_{-\infty}^{\infty} |k'(u)|du < \infty$; and h is a bandwidth. It has been shown that the performance of the smoothed version of the ELR test can be improved in terms of the TIE rate and power comparing the ELR test based on the identity function (e.g., Zhou and Jing, 2003b; Yu et al., 2011). For the EL confidence interval, Chen and Hall (1993) showed that the smoothed EL confidence interval for quantiles has faster convergence in terms of the coverage error. The bandwidth h is commonly a function of the sample size and other parameters that are estimated based on the sample (e.g., Altman and Léger, 1995). An extensive Monte-Carlo study demonstrated that the proposed EL ratio tests are robust to the choice of different bandwidths; however, in the context of the approach of Hyndman and Yao (2002), we use a bandwidth of $h = 0.2n_i^{-1/6}$ for group i for actual applications and simulation studies, which showed empirically reasonable performances among many available methodologies. Using the fact that the kernel functions are differentiable, we can show the following:

Proposition 6.2

Let $r_i = n_i\hat{F}_i(\tilde{\theta}) = \sum_{j=1}^{n_i} K((\tilde{\theta} - X_{ij})/h)$. *Under* H_0, $-2\log R$ *in* (6.12) *converges in distribution to a* χ_1^2 *distribution as* $n_i \to \infty, i = 1, 2$.

For a certain kernel function, it can be shown that the smoothed empirical distribution function converges to the distribution function (e.g., Fernholz, 1991). In this case, converges in Proposition 6.2 can be easily proven based on Proposition 6.1. The proof is similar to that of Proposition 6.4.

6.3.1 Plug-in Approach

In application to quantile comparisons, we can replace the EL estimator $\tilde{\theta}$ by the sample $100q$-th percentile estimator $\hat{\theta}$ based on the pooled sample, and subsequently we define

$$r_i = n_i\hat{F}_i(\hat{\theta}) = \sum_{j=1}^{n_i} I(\hat{\theta} - X_{ij}). \tag{6.15}$$

This replacement gives rise to a change in the asymptotic distribution of the test statistic given in (6.12).

Proposition 6.3

When $n_i \to \infty$, $i=1,2$ *and* $n_1/(n_1+n_2) \to \eta$, *under* H_0 *the statistic* $-2\log R/v$ *based on* (6.12) *with* r_i *in* (6.15) *converges in distribution to a* χ_1^2 *distribution, where* $v = \eta \frac{1}{f(\theta)}(f_1(\theta)^2 + f_2(\theta)^2(\frac{1}{\eta}-1))$.

The proof is in the Appendix

In the application of Proposition 6.3, the density functions need to be estimated using the kernel density estimation (Sheather and Jones, 1991). For the plug-in approach, we can replace the indicator function by the smoothed function similar to the test statistic for Proposition 6.2. Although the plug-in method is developed by the framework of the EL, the test statistic is not based on the maximization of the EL, and is simplified by using the indicator function in the development of (6.12), making it a unique test to investigate. We can show the following result.

Proposition 6.4

Define $r_i = n_i\hat{F}_i(\hat{\theta}) = \sum_{j=1}^{n_i} K((\hat{\theta}-X_{ij})/h)$. *When* $n_i \to \infty$, $i=1,2$ *and* $n_1/(n_1+n_2) \to \eta$, *under* H_0 *the statistic* $-2\log R/v$ *based on* (6.12) *with* r_i *converges in distribution to a* χ_1^2 *distribution, where* $v = \eta \frac{1}{f(\theta)}(f_1(\theta)^2 + f_2(\theta)^2(\frac{1}{\eta}-1))$.

The proof is in the Appendix

Overall, the EL methods show viable accuracies in terms of TIE rate control, and their powers respond well with the various alternative hypotheses presented even for small sample sizes. Tables 6.2 and 6.3 show the simulated TIE rates and powers of the proposed ELR test statistics for median comparisons, respectively, through a Monte Carlo study with various underlying distributions for groups with vastly different distributions. The TIE rates of the statistics with the indicator function and kernel function behave similarly. With the small sample size, the kernel function improves the power of the proposed tests across the board. Note that these ELR test statistics with the kernel or indicator function generally outperform Mood's median test (Yu et al., 2011). The plug-in test statistic with the kernel function is the most powerful test in a majority of cases including cases with the small sample sizes.

The performance of the ELR test statistics with the kernel function to compare upper quantiles such as the 95th percentile is presented in Table 6.4 (TIE rates) and Table 6.5 (Power). Since there are no well-established general test statistics for quintile-specific comparisons, in the simulations, the EL methods are compared to the test statistic using the sample percentile constructed in the following way (say, sample percentile test). Let $\hat{\theta}_i$ and $\hat{\theta}$ define q-th sample percentiles for the group i and the pooled sample,

TABLE 6.2

The Monte Carlo Type I error rates in median comparisons. Entries for each sample size and distribution combination are the results of the classic approach (classic), the classic approach with the kernel function (classic, K), the plug-in approach (plug-in), the plug-in approach with the kernel function (plug-in, K). The significance level is 0.05

		n_1, n_2				
Distributions	**Method**	**15,15**	**15,25**	**50,50**	**100,100**	**100,200**
Uniform(0,3) vs. Lognormal(0.405,9)	Classic	0.0402	0.0424	0.0508	0.0478	0.0493
	Classic, K	0.0342	0.0347	0.0482	0.0485	0.0492
	Plug-in	0.0491	0.0543	0.0443	0.0498	0.0478
	Plug-in, K	0.0504	0.0533	0.0466	0.0473	0.0465
Exponential(1.5) vs. Lognormal(−0.77,1)	Classic	0.0271	0.0249	0.0318	0.0393	0.0378
	Classic, K	0.0206	0.0285	0.0254	0.0306	0.0312
	Plug-in	0.0264	0.0518	0.0691	0.0593	0.0485
	Plug-in, K	0.0233	0.0233	0.0325	0.0343	0.038

TABLE 6.3

The Monte Carlo powers in median comparisons. The significance level is 0.05

		n_1, n_2				
Distributions	**Method**	**15,15**	**15,25**	**50,50**	**100,100**	**100,200**
Uniform(0,6) vs. Lognormal(0.405,9)	Classic	0.0826	0.1095	0.2363	0.4041	0.6626
	Classic, K	0.0662	0.1024	0.2296	0.4041	0.6498
	Plug-in	0.0959	0.1755	0.2614	0.4511	0.7179
	Plug-in, K	0.1018	0.1673	0.2726	0.4626	0.7266
Exponential(1.5) vs. Lognormal(−0.4,1)	Classic	0.0765	0.0823	0.2426	0.4663	0.5860
	Classic, K	0.0819	0.1003	0.2571	0.507	0.6169
	Plug-in	0.0784	0.131	0.3342	0.5515	0.6328
	Plug-in, K	0.0839	0.109	0.2786	0.5197	0.6289

$\hat{f}(x)$ define the estimated density at x with the pooled sample. Based on the asymptotic distribution of $\hat{\theta}_i$ (Serfling, 1980), we have that

$$\frac{(\hat{\theta}_1 - \hat{\theta}_2)}{\sqrt{q(1-q)}\sqrt{\left(n_1(\hat{f}(\hat{\theta}))^2\right)^{-1} + \left(n_2(\hat{f}(\hat{\theta}))^2\right)^{-1}}} \tag{6.16}$$

has asymptotically the standard normal distribution, under $H_0 : \theta_1 = \theta_2$. With the relatively small sample sizes (i.e., $n_1 = n_2 = 15$ or 30), the sample percentile test was not reliable as many simulated TIE rates are much

TABLE 6.4

The Monte Carlo Type I error rates to compare *95th Percentiles*. For the method column, sample, classic, and plug-in indicate the sample percentile test, classical ELR test using kernel function and the plug-in ELR test using kernel function. The significance level is 0.05

		n_1, n_2			
Distributions	**Method**	**15,15**	**30,30**	**50,100**	**200,200**
Normal(4,9) vs. Lognormal(0.5451,1)	Sample	0.1004	0.0494	0.0476	0.0430
	Classic	0.0000	0.0666	0.0478	0.0458
	Plug-in	0.0132	0.0544	0.0560	0.0468
Exponential(1) vs. Lognormal(−1.3701,2.25)	Sample	0.1760	0.0914	0.0792	0.0582
	Classic	0.0000	0.0222	0.0370	0.0366
	Plug-in	0.0386	0.0504	0.0458	0.0480

TABLE 6.5

The Monte Carlo powers to compare *95th Percentiles*. The significance level is 0.05

		n_1, n_2			
Distributions	**Method**	**15,15**	**30,30**	**50,100**	**200,200**
Normal(4,9) vs. Lognormal(0.7451,1)	Sample	0.1412	0.0800	0.0934	0.3136
	Classic	0.0000	0.1066	0.1502	0.2446
	Plug-in	0.0178	0.0746	0.1834	0.2838
Exponential(1) vs. Lognormal(−1.0701,2.25)	Sample	0.1958	0.1168	0.1068	0.2538
	Classic	0.0000	0.0472	0.1008	0.1986
	Plug-in	0.0448	0.0666	0.1410	0.2356

higher than 0.05 (Table 6.4). On the contrary, although it is not consistent, the classical EL has overall much lower simulated TIE rates as too few were rejected in some scenarios. On the other hand, the plug-in ELR test shows viable TIE control even with the small sample sizes. The plug-in ELR test shows the better simulated power than classical EL test with relatively small sample sizes (Table 6.5). The differences in the power between the two ELR methods decrease when the sample sizes increase, showing that, with a large sample size, the two methods are comparable.

Overall, when comparing upper percentiles, the simulation results show that the plug-in ELR performs very well with various underlying distributions and sample sizes.

Since the plug-in approach allows us to use the sample statistics for nuisance parameters, we can use other types of constraints corresponding to H_0 than Equation (6.8). For example, Yu et al. (2011) considered the following two equivalent constraints to test two groups' medians:

$$\sum_{j=1}^{n_1} p_{1j}\Delta\{X_{1j}-\widehat{\theta}\}=\sum_{j=1}^{n_2} p_{2j}\Delta\{X_{2j}-\widehat{\theta}\}, \tag{6.17}$$

or

$$\sum_{j=1}^{n_1} p_{1j}\Delta\{X_{1j} - \hat{\theta}_2\} = \sum_{j=1}^{n_2} p_{2j}\Delta\{X_{2j} - \hat{\theta}_1\}, \tag{6.18}$$

where $\hat{\theta}_i$ is the sample quantile of group i and Δ can be either the indicator function or smoothed function.

Yu et al. (2011) showed the limiting distributions of the ELR test based on the constraints (6.17) and (6.18), respectively, which have quite complex forms. Yu et al. (2011) demonstrated that the ELR test statistics based on the constraints (6.8) outperform those based on (6.17) and (6.18). We note that, when the data distribution is skewed to right, the proposed ELR tests may not work well to compare the lower quartiles such as fifth quantile. When lower quantiles are compared with right-skewed underlying distributions, data points are densely accumulated around the lower quantiles causing the poorer performance of the proposed ELR tests than that with upper quantiles.

6.4 Computation in R

Suppose that x and y are the lists of the data, which contain the observations from groups 1 and 2, respectively. The sample sizes are n1 and n2 for groups 1 and 2, respectively.

```
alpha<-0.5           #For testing median, alpha is set as 0.5
n1<-50;n2<-50
y<-rlnorm(n2,0,1);x<-rnorm(n2,exp(0),1)
                                        #equal median under the null
rm(list=".Random.seed", envir=globalenv());
sx<-sort(x); sy<-sort(y)
```

In the following function ELR, q is the quantile estimate that minimizes the ELR statistic. Corresponding to (6.12), the EL ratio test can be constructed as a function:

```
ELR<-function(q){
  F1<-length(sx[sx<q])/n1 +0.00000001 #0.00000001 is to prevent 0.
  F2<-length(sy[sy<q])/n2 +0.00000001
  w<- -2*(n1*((1-F1)*log(1-alpha)+F1*log(alpha)-
        F1*log(F1)-(1-F1)*log(1-F1))+n2*((1-F2)*log(1-alpha)+
            F2*log(alpha)-F2*log(F2)-(1-F2)*log(1-F2)))
return(w)}
```

The minimization of the ELR function can be carried out by running the optimize function in R:

For one-dimensional optimization, we define interval that contains the list of boundaries of q to find the maximum of the ELR function. The boundaries can be given as the neighborhood of the sample quantile such as

```
interval<-c(0,(quantile(c(x, y),alpha)+2*sd(c(x, y))))
```

For the lower bound of interval, we use 0 because it is reasonably expected that the median cannot be less than 0. A careful boundary definition is needed not to produce NaN for the object of the optimization. Boundary needs to be within the convex hull of the data. The optimization is carried out as follows. The outcome will provide the quantile estimation and the corresponding likelihood ratio value that follows a χ_1^2 distribution under H_0.

```
out<-optimize(ELR, interval, maximum=FALSE)
```

The ELR statistics and p-value are as follows:

```
teststat<-out$objective
teststat #e.g.
[1] 0.08002143
1-pchisq(teststat,1) #e.g.                              #p-value
[1] 0.7772684
```

The estimated quantile by EL is as follows:

```
out$minimum #e.g.
[1] 1.218902
```

We note that the sample median of the data from the two groups is 1.204. The estimated quantile using the EL is commonly close to a reasonable estimate such as the sample quantile. If the estimate is substantially different, it may be an indication that the optimization may not reach a convergence.

When the kernel function is used in the function ELR (Proposition 6.2), the estimation of the distribution function will be simply replaced by:

```
h1<-n1^(-1/6)*0.2; h2<-n2^(-1/6)*0.2
F1<-sum(pnorm((q-x)/h1,0,1))/n1; F2<-sum(pnorm((q-y)/h2,0,1))/n2
```

The values h1 and h2 are the bandwidths as noted earlier.

For the plug-in approach, the optimization step is not necessary. Instead, we obtain the sample alpha-th quantile, then F1, F2, and the EL ratio statistic are obtained as follows:

```
q<-quantile(c(x,y), alpha)                          #sample quantile
F1<-length(sx[sx<q])/n1
F2<-length(sy[sy<q])/n2
w<--2*(n1*((1-F1)*log(1-alpha)+F1*log(alpha)-
       F1*log(F1)-(1-F1)*log(1-F1))+n2*((1-F2)*log(1-alpha)+
       F2*log(alpha)-F2*log(F2)-(1-F2)*log(1-F2)))
```

The densities used in Propositions 6.3 and 6.4 are estimated using the `density` function in R:

```
z<-c(x,y); sz<-sort(z)
f1<-density(x, from=sz[(n1+n2)*alpha],
to=sz[(n1+n2)*alpha])[[2]][[1]]
f2<-density(y, from=sz[(n1+n2)*alpha],
to=sz[(n1+n2)*alpha])[[2]][[1]]
f<-density(z, from=sz[(n1+n2)*alpha],
to=sz[(n1+n2)*alpha])[[2]][[1]]
```

The test statistic is obtained by

```
eta<-n1/(n1+n2)
teststat<-w/(eta*(f1^2+f2^2*(1/eta-1))/f^2)
[1] 0.164569
1-pchisq(teststat,1)                                       #p-value
[1] 0.6849843
```

The kernel function can be used in a similar way to that of the classical approach.

Example 6.2: Application to Cytokine Treatments for Analysis of Signaling

Cells are constantly exposed to irritants and pathogens that may cause inflammation of the cells and such damage may propel tumor growth. It is hypothesized that constant damages to the cells alter cell proliferation and growth cessation processes and eventually lead to cell abnormalities. To test this hypothesis, normal and abnormal (metaplastic or dysplastic) lung cell cultures were treated by various signaling molecules (i.e., cytokines), and phosphorylation of biomarkers was measured using Western blot analysis. Quantified responses of a biomarker called ERK after cytokine treatments are shown in Figure 6.3. The cytokines shown in Figure 6.3 include leukemia inhibitory factor (LIF), oncostatin M (OSM), IL-6, and no treatment (control). We look for an increased sensitivity of such stimulants (cytokines), which will demonstrate the growth-stimulatory activity giving rise to tumor progression. For more technical details of these treatments, we refer to Loewen et al. (2005).

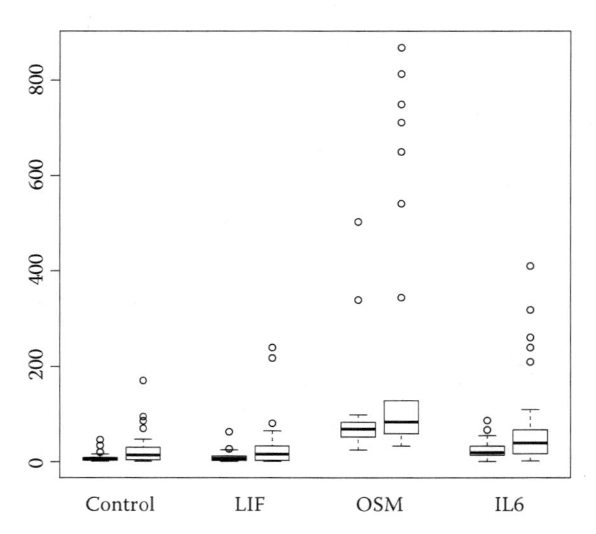

FIGURE 6.3
Boxplots to show the relative standings of the quantified level (arbitrary units) of ERK activations. For each cytokine treatment, the plot on the left is for normal cells and the plot on the right is for abnormal cells.

A total of 48 subjects are available (18 normal, 30 abnormal). At first glance, some elevations of the expressions after cytokine treatments are observed for both the normal and tumor cells, although tumor cells seem to react more. Distributions of all the biomarkers are right skewed and possibly nonconstant shifts are observed. The ratios of medians for tumor versus normal cells are 3.8, 3.9, 1.7, and 4.7 for control, LIF, OSM, and IL-6, respectively, suggesting that IL-6 treatment causes the greatest alterations in biomarkers.

The data analysis results are presented in Table 6.6. Overall, test results based on the indicator and the kernel functions are similar. Somewhat distinctive differences between Wilcoxon's test and the ELR methods are observed in OSM, possibly the result of nonconstant shift. If nonconstant shift, Wilcoxon's test may not test the median difference. At the level of 0.05, all presented tests show a significant difference in IL-6, whereas the ELR tests show lower p-values. For testing LIF, the ELR tests consistently lower p-values compared to Wilcoxon or Mood's median tests.

TABLE 6.6

P-values of Wilcoxon's Test, Mood's median test, and the ELR methods based on the biomarker data

Treatment	Wilcoxon	Mood	Classic	Classic, K	Plug-in	Plug-in, K
Control	0.0589	0.1351	0.0716	0.0829	0.0922	0.0922
LIF	0.1381	0.0729	0.0382	0.0653	0.0513	0.0449
OSM	0.0863	0.3715	0.1533	0.3102	0.2562	0.2562
IL-6	0.0487	0.0355	0.027	0.027	0.0175	0.0175

For interested readers, we provide the generated dataset for the control treatment. The data were generated to have similar features to the original data. To start, use the following code:

```
disease
<-c(0,0,0,0,0,0,0,0,0,0,0,0,0,0,0,0,0,0,1,1,1,1,1,1,1,1,1,1,1,
1,1,1,1,1,1,1,1,1,1,1,1,1,1,1,1,1,1,1)
control<-c(4.9,5.8,1.6,5.7,2.4,8.6,5.0,17.8,46.9,5.3,17.3,
5.8,4.5,5.4,2.4,5.7,9.8,9.4,41.0,5.3,12.5,7.9,19.1,13.1,23.4,
8.1,4.5,2.7,22.5,12.8,40.2,2.3,23.9,3.3,3.1,10.6,22.8,19.4,
8.8,2.0,87.4,3.2,2.2,1.7,0.6,21.6,3.4,17.2)
x<-control[disease==0];n1<-length(x)
y<-control[disease==1];n2<-length(y)
```

You can use the R codes explained already to carry out the EL tests. The p-values with the data are 0.0716, 0.1386, 0.0942, and 0.0942 for classic, classic with kernel, plug-in, and plug-in with kernel methods, respectively.

Example 6.3: Oral Health Data

The data are obtained from oral health and ventilator-associated pneumonia study (OHP study) at University at Buffalo, State University of New York (Scannapieco et al., 2009). The primary objective of the OHP study was to determine the effects of oral decontamination with chlorhexidine (CHX) on reducing the colonization of potential respiratory pathogens in the oral cavity. The target group for this study is patients admitted to an intensive care unit (ICU) who were mechanically ventilated. A total of 175 patients met the eligibility requirements and consented to participate in the study. These 175 patients were randomized into three treatment groups (control: 59, CHX once: 58, CHX twice: 58). We investigate the early colonization (at day 6) of potential respiratory pathogens among the ICU patients. The aggregated and log-transformed values of the potential pathogens (*S. aureus, P. aeruginosa, Acinetobacter sps.*, and enteric organisms) are obtained according to the study protocol. We carry out the 90th percentile comparisons between the control group and CHX-treated group. The comparison of the upper percentile is meaningful as a highly concentrated colonization of specific pathogens is evidence of lung infection, which may not be properly tested based on the center of the distributions such as the mean or median. The final sample includes 23 controls and 51 CHX-treated patients. Visual inspection of the histogram and box plots for the two groups shows that the distributions between the two groups are different (Figure 6.4). Also note that the standard deviations for the control and CHX groups are 4.92 and 5.67, respectively, and the interquartile ranges for the control and CHX groups are 6.28 and 12.22, respectively, indicating the differences in the distributions. The sample 90th percentiles for control and CHX groups are 14.24 and 13.74, suggesting not much difference in the percentiles. The p-values with the data are 0.2909, 0.6545, 0.4572, and 0.4763 for classic, classic with kernel, plug-in, and plug-in with kernel methods, respectively. Both the test results indicate that there is not enough evidence of different 90th percentiles between the two treatment groups. The data are not provided for readers to check. The data analysis technique is same as what we previously described. For 90th percentile, the readers make sure to use `alpha=0.9` in the R code.

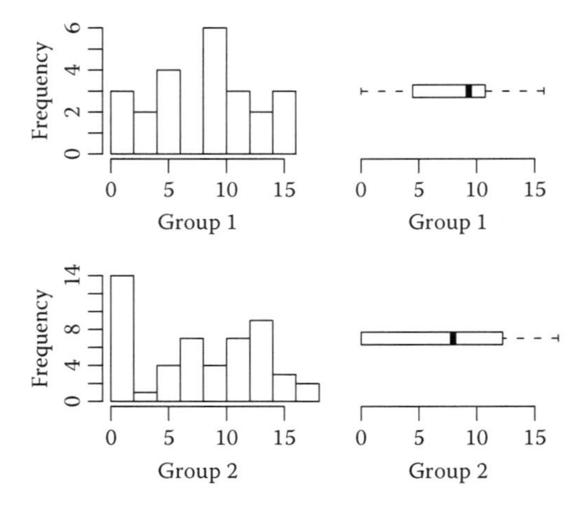

FIGURE 6.4
The histograms and boxplots for the distributions of pathogens of control (group 1, top) and CHX-treated groups (group 2, bottom) in the OHP study.

6.5 Constructing Confidence Intervals on Quantile Differences

The confidence interval estimations based on an application of the EL approach has demonstrated robust performances on various underlying distributions (e.g., Owen, 1990; Qin and Wong, 1996; Peng and Qi, 2006). To construct EL confidence regions, the construction of a pivotal quantity is not necessary and the EL preserves the range of the parameter space (Hall and La Scala, 1990).

We are interested in the difference of q-th quantiles between two groups,

$$\delta = F_2^{-1}(q) - F_1^{-1}(q),$$

Let $F_1^{-1}(q) = \theta$, then the q-th quantile of group 2 is $\theta + \delta$. Letting $L(\delta)$ present the likelihood function based on the observations from the two groups, we can construct the likelihood ratio test as

$$R(\delta_0) = \max_{\delta=\delta_0} L(\delta) / \max_{\delta \neq \delta_0} L(\delta),$$

where δ_0 is the value of δ under the null hypothesis, H_0. The $100(1-\alpha)\%$ confidence interval is the collection of δ_0 that satisfies

$$\{\delta_0 : R(\delta_0) \notin c_\alpha\},$$

where c_α is the rejection region for the size α test corresponds to the relevant asymptotic distribution of $R(\delta_0)$. The ELR test statistic (6.12) is used for $R(\delta_0)$. The restriction $\delta = \delta_0$ is equivalent to

$$\delta = F_2^{-1}(q,\delta_0) - F_1^{-1}(q) = 0,$$

where $F^{-1}(q,\delta_0) = \inf\{x : F(x-\delta_0) > q\}$. Thus, $R(\delta_0)$ is obtained based on X_{1j} and $X_{2j} - \delta_0$, and whether $R(\delta_0)$ is in c_α will be determined. For the confidence interval construction, using the indicator function to obtain r_i in (6.11) may not be recommended as a resulting interval is oftentimes not a single interval due to the discreteness of the indicator function. An example of the changes of $R(\delta_0)$ by different δ_0 values is described in Figure 6.5. The lower and upper bounds are obtained at the points where the 0.95th quantile of the χ_1^2 distribution crosses $R(\delta_0)$. Note that $R(\delta_0)$ is obtained using the classical EL with the kernel function. The data used for Figure 6.5 are generated from two different lognormal distributions using the following code:

```
mu1<-0.8; sd1<-0.8; mu2<-0.5; sd2<-0.5
alpha<-0.9 #quantile probability

n1<-200;n2<-200
x<-rlnorm(n1,mu1,sd1); y<-rlnorm(n2,mu2,sd2)
```

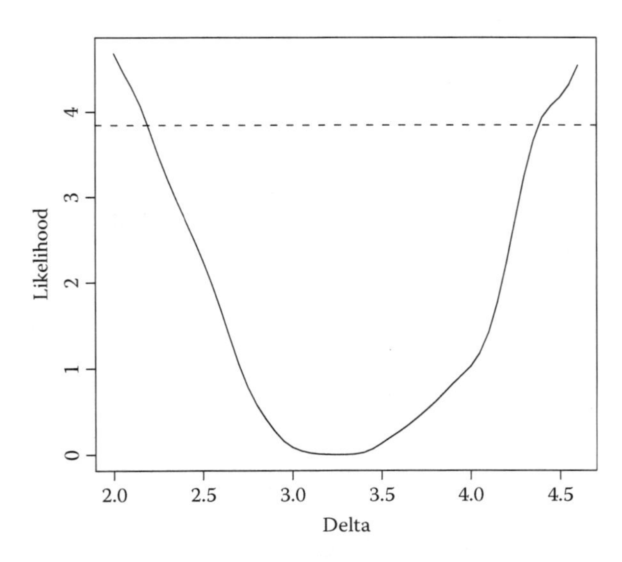

FIGURE 6.5
An example of δ_0 versus $R(\delta_0)$ (solid line). The dashed line indicates the 0.95-th quantile of the χ_1^2 distribution.

In this setting, the true difference of 0.9th quantile is 3.075.

```
qlnorm(alpha,mu1,sd1) - qlnorm(alpha,mu2,sd2) #e.g.
[1] 3.075097
```

In Figure 6.5, we use the following function to produce the likelihood ratio of the EL quantile estimate (q) where the data are adjusted by "candidate" difference (`diffest`) between two groups (i.e., `x-diffest` and y). "Candidate" difference indicates δ value that could be included in the confidence interval.

```
Likelihood<-function(q){
    h1<-n1^(-1/6)*0.2
    h2<-n2^(-1/6)*0.2
    F1<-sum( pnorm((q-(x-diffest))/h1,0,1))/n1-0.00000001
    F2<-sum( pnorm((q-y)/h2,0,1))/n2-0.00000001
    w<--2*(n1*((1-F1)*log(1-alpha)+F1*log(alpha)-
       F1*log(F1)-(1-F1)*log(1-F1))+n2*((1-F2)*log(1-alpha)+
       F2*log(alpha)-F2*log(F2)-(1-F2)*log(1-F2)))
return(w)}
```

For the x-axis of Figure 6.5, we use

```
diffests<-seq(2.0, 4.6, 0.05)     #differences (δ) for the x-axis
```

The following code gives the ELR values corresponding to `diffests`:

```
liks<-array()          #variable to contain the likelihood value
for(i in 1:length(diffests)){
   diffest<-diffests[i]
   lik<-optimize(Likelihood,interval=c(quantile(c((x-
        diffest),y),alpha)-sd2,quantile(c((x-
        diffest),y),alpha)+sd2),maximum=FALSE)$objective
   if(is.na(lik))break;
liks[i]<-lik}
plot(diffests,liks, type='l', xlab='delta', ylab='likelihood')
abline(qchisq(0.95,1),0,lty=2)
```

The lower and upper bounds are the x values where the likelihood ratio curve and the horizontal line of the 95th quantile of χ_1^2 distribution meet. The exact point is obtained by giving a narrower interval to search for the value (δ) that minimizes the square distance between the 95th quantile of the χ_1^2 distribution and $R(\delta)$. The following code carries out that task:

```
detailCIs<-function(diffest){
     Likelihood<-function(q){
         h1<-n1^(-1/6)*0.2
         h2<-n2^(-1/6)*0.2
```

```
        F1<-sum( pnorm((q-(x-diffest))/h1,0,1))/n1-0.00000001
        F2<-sum( pnorm((q-y)/h2,0,1))/n2-0.00000001
        w<--2*(n1*((1-F1)*log(1-alpha)+F1*log(alpha)-
           F1*log(F1)-(1-F1)*log(1-F1))+n2*((1-F2)*log(1-alpha)+
           F2*log(alpha)-F2*log(F2)-(1-F2)*log(1-F2)))
     return(w)}
   lik<-optimize(Likelihood,interval=c(quantile(c((x-
        diffest),y),alpha)-(sd2),quantile(c((x-
        diffest),y),alpha)+(sd2)),maximum=FALSE)$objective
return((lik-qchisq(0.95,1))^2)}
lb<-optimize(detailCIs,interval=c(2,2.5),maximum=FALSE)$minimum
ub<-optimize(detailCIs,interval=c(4,4.5),maximum=FALSE)$minimum
c(lb,ub)
[1] 2.189313 4.380300      #lower and upper bound of 95% conf.
interval
```

We note that when the sample size is small or we search for the confidence interval of extreme quantiles (e.g., 95th quantile), the likelihood ratio may not be monotone increasing or decreasing. In general, the strategy explained earlier finds upper and lower bounds of the confidence interval that provides reasonable coverage rates as shown in Table 6.7. The confidence interval using the normal approximation in Table 6.7 is constructed based on (6.16). The results show that the quantile confidence interval based on the normal approximation may perform poorly even with fairly large sample sizes. With unbalanced sample sizes, it becomes more erratic. On the other hand, EL methods provide better coverage rates, especially EL with the plug-in method.

TABLE 6.7

The simulated coverage rates of the 95% confidence intervals using the normal approximation (normal), classical EL method with the kernel function (classic, K) and EL method with the plug-in and kernel function (plug-in, K). Inside the parenthesis is the average lengths of intervals

		n_1, n_2		
Distribution	**Method**	**30,30**	**50,100**	**200,200**
Normal(−2.06,9) vs. Normal(0,1)	Normal	0.775 (2.529)	0.679 (1.464)	0.824 (1.021)
	Classic, K	0.97 (4.464)	0.957 (3.152)	0.964 (1.534)
	Plug-in, K	0.95 (9.080)	0.946 (3.407)	0.955 (1.533)
Lognormal(0.5,0.5^2) vs. Lognormal(0.8,0.8^2)	Normal	0.831 (5.196)	0.679 (1.464)	0.915 (2.416)
	Classic, K	0.895 (8.512)	0.951 (4.431)	0.945 (2.651)
	Plug-in, K	0.961 (9.638)	0.957 (4.477)	0.963 (2.633)

6.6 Concluding Remarks

In this chapter, we illustrate that EL tests have good power characteristics while at the same time maintaining the appropriate TIE rate control. In general, the EL approach outperforms traditional nonparametric location shift tests for cases that violate the exchangeability assumption. Although the plug-in approach uses the same EL principle as the classical ELR test to maximize the nonparametric likelihood function, the resulting distribution of the plug-in approach was different from that of the classical ELR test. Also, the plug-in ELR test shows well-controlled TIE rates and better (or comparable) powers even based on relatively small sample sizes, where the other tests were unstable.

Some investigations regarding inference for percentiles based on the EL approach are found in the literature. Chen and Hall (1993) showed that smoothed EL confidence intervals show an excellent coverage rate. Chen and Chen (2000) investigated the properties of EL quantile estimation in large samples, Zhou and Jing (2003a) proposed an alternative smoothed EL approach in which the EL ratio has an explicit form based on the concept of M-estimators. Lopez et al. (2009) investigated testing general parameters that are determined by the expectation of nonsmooth functions. Chen and Lazar (2010) investigated the quantile estimation for discrete distributions. Zhou and Jing (2003b) investigated the confidence interval estimation of the quantile difference within one group, for example, interquantile range.

Several articles discussing plug-in approaches in the construction of EL are available in the literature (e.g., Qin and Jing, 2001; Wang and Jing, 2001; Li and Wang, 2003). In the context of one sample problem, Hjort et al. (2009) showed that the limit distribution of −2 log of the ELR test is a sum of weighted χ^2 distributions, where the weights are often intractable because of the complexity of the asymptotics. Recently, for median comparisons between two groups, Yu et al. (2011) obtained the analytic form of the asymptotic distribution of −2 log of the ELR test based on the plug-in EL approach, which has a weighted χ^2 distribution. Yu et al. (2014b) investigated the properties of the EL approach on the upper quantiles showing the viability of the approach.

Appendix

Proof of Proposition 6.3

By the definition in (6.15), we can show that

$$\hat{F}_1(\hat{\theta}) = \left((n_1 + n_2)q - n_2\hat{F}_2(\hat{\theta})\right)\Big/ n_1. \tag{A.6.1}$$

The plug-in ELR statistic can be obtained in a similar manner to (6.12) and has the form of

$$-2\log R = -2\left[\sum_{i=1}^{2} n_i \left\{ \begin{matrix} \left(1-\hat{F}_i(\hat{\theta})\right)\log(1-q)+\hat{F}_i(\hat{\theta})\log(q)- \\ \hat{F}_i(\hat{\theta})\log(\hat{F}_i(\hat{\theta}))-(1-\hat{F}_i(\hat{\theta}))\log(1-\hat{F}_i(\hat{\theta})) \end{matrix} \right\}\right]. \quad \text{(A.6.2)}$$

Incorporating (A.6.1) into (A.6.2), and using Taylor's expansion about $\hat{F}_i(\hat{\theta}) = q$ up to the order of $(\hat{F}_i(\hat{\theta})-q)^2$, we have

$$-2\log R = (n_1+n_2)\left(n_1 q(1-q)\right)^{-1} n_2\left(\hat{F}_2(\hat{\theta})-q\right)^2 + O_p\left(n_*^{-1/2}\right)$$

We can express $\hat{F}_2(\hat{\theta})-q = \{\hat{F}_2(\hat{\theta})-\hat{F}_2(\theta)-(F_2(\hat{\theta})-q)\}-2q+\hat{F}_2(\theta)+F_2(\hat{\theta})$ where the first curly bracket has the order of $O_p(n_2^{-3/4}(\log n_2)^{1/2})$ by virtue of $\hat{\theta}-\theta = O_p((n_1+n_2)^{-1/2})$ and the well-known fact,

$$\sup_{|s-\theta|<c\sqrt{n}} \left|\left(\hat{F}(s)-\hat{F}(\theta)\right)-\left(F(s)-F(\theta)\right)\right| = O_p(n^{-3/4}(\log n)^{1/2})$$

(Chen and Chen, 2000), for a sample size n. Approximating $F_2(\hat{\theta})-q$ by $(\hat{\theta}-\theta)f_2(\theta)+O_p((n_1+n_2)^{-1})$, we have

$$\hat{F}_2(\hat{\theta})-q = n_2^{-1}\sum_{j=1}^{n_2}\left(I(x_{2i}<\theta)-q\right)+f_2(\theta)(\hat{\theta}-\theta)+O_p\left(n_2^{-3/4}(\log n_2)^{1/2}\right). \quad \text{(A.6.3)}$$

Since

$$\hat{\theta}-\theta = \left(q(n_1+n_2)-n_1\hat{F}_1(\theta)-n_2\hat{F}_2(\theta)\right)/\left((n_1+n_2)f(\theta)\right)+O_p\left(n_2^{-3/4}\log n_2\right) \quad \text{(A.6.4)}$$

by the Bahadur representation of the sample quantiles (Bahadur, 1966; Chen and Chen, 2000), (A.6.3) can be expressed as

$$\begin{aligned}\hat{F}_2(\hat{\theta})-q = n_2^{-1/2}&\left[\left(1-(1-\eta)\tfrac{f_2(\theta)}{f(\theta)}\right)\left(\hat{F}_2(\theta)-q\right)-\left(\tfrac{f_2(\theta)}{f(\theta)}\eta\left(\hat{F}_1(\theta)-q\right)\right)\right] \\ &+O_p\left(n_2^{-3/4}\log n_2\right).\end{aligned} \quad \text{(A.6.5)}$$

Based on (A.6.5) and applying the central limit theorem, the result of Proposition 6.3 follows.

Proof of Proposition 6.4

The proof is similar to that of Proposition 6.3 except establishment of the relationships (A.6.1) and (A.6.4). Consider

$$\hat{F}_i(\hat{\theta}) - q = \left\{\hat{F}_i(\hat{\theta}) - \hat{F}_i(\theta) - (F_i(\hat{\theta}) - q)\right\} - 2q + \hat{F}_i(\theta) + F_i(\hat{\theta}), i = 1,2,$$

where the first curly bracket has the order of $o(n_2^{-1/2+\alpha})$ for some $\alpha > 0$, and $\hat{F}_i(\theta) = F(\theta) + o(n_i^{-1/2+\alpha})$ (Winter, 1979) and $F_i(\hat{\theta}) = F(\theta) + o(n_i^{-1/2+\alpha})$ (Serfling, 1980) under H_0. Thus we obtain the relationship (A.6.1) asymptotically. Also, by Azzalini (1981), we have

$$E\left((n_1 + n_2)(\hat{F}(\theta) - q)\right)^2 \sim (n_1 + n_2)q(1-q),$$

where $\hat{F}(\theta) \simeq \hat{F}_1(\theta)\frac{n_1}{n_1+n_2} + \hat{F}_2(\theta)\frac{n_2}{n_1+n_2}$. The variance of the q-th sample quantile is approximately $(n_1 + n_2)q(1-q)\frac{1}{(n_1+n_2)^2 f(\theta)^2}$, thus, the variance of $\hat{\theta}$ can be substituted by $(q(n_1 + n_2) - n_1\hat{F}_1(\theta) - n_2\hat{F}_2(\theta)) / ((n_1 + n_2)f(\theta))$. By substituting $\hat{\theta} - \theta$ with $(q(n_1 + n_2) - n_1\hat{F}_1(\theta) - n_2\hat{F}_2(\theta))/((n_1 + n_2)f(\theta))$, we obtain the relationship (A.6.5).

7

Empirical Likelihood for a U-Statistic Constraint

7.1 Introduction

In this chapter, we discuss the empirical likelihood ratio (ELR) test with the constraints in the form of U-statistics. U-statistics belong to a general class of statistics including the sample mean and the popular Wilcoxon rank sum test statistic. A U-statistic is known to be a uniformly minimum variance-unbiased estimator under the assumption that the vector of order statistics is sufficient and complete (Fraser, 1954; Serfling, 1980).

Consider a parameter in a form of the expectation

$$\theta = E(h(X_1, \ldots, X_m)), \tag{7.1}$$

where $h(X_1, \ldots, X_m)$ is a symmetric function, i.e., the different permutation of $X_1, \ldots, X_m$ does not change the value of $h(X_1, \ldots, X_m)$. The function h is called a *kernel* of order m. The corresponding U-statistic based on n independent and identically distributed observations $(X_1, \ldots, X_n)$ is

$$\mathrm{U}_n = \binom{n}{m}^{-1} \sum\nolimits_C h(X_{i_1}, \ldots, X_{i_m}), \tag{7.2}$$

where C indicates all possible combinations of m distinct elements of the data points from n observations. The U-statistic (7.2) is known to be an unbiased estimator of θ (Serfling, 1980). By definition (7.2), the sample mean is a U-statistic with $h(X_{i_1}, \ldots, X_{i_m}) = X_i$ and $m = 1$. The sample variance is a U-statistic with $h(X_{i_1}, \ldots, X_{i_m}) = (X_{i_1} - X_{i_2})^2/2$ and $m = 2$. Assuming that θ in (7.1) exists, the U-statistic (7.2) corresponding to $\theta\,(<\infty)$ is an unbiased estimator.

Let us define

$$h_c(X_1, \ldots, X_c) = E(h(X_1, \ldots, X_m) \mid X_1 = x_1, \ldots, X_c = x_c) \text{ for } c \le m.$$

Also, let

$$\tilde{h} = h(X_1,\ldots,X_m) - \theta, \quad \tilde{h}_c = h_c(X_1,\ldots,X_c) - \theta.$$

The variance of U_n is given as

$$Var(U_n) = \binom{n}{m}^{-1} \sum_{c=1}^{m} \binom{m}{c}\binom{n-m}{m-c} \eta_c^2, \tag{7.3}$$

where $\eta_c^2 = E(\tilde{h}_c^2)$.

Example 7.1

Let μ_c^i define the i-th central moment. Consider the variance $\mu_c^2 = \int (x-\mu)^2 dF(x)$ where μ is the mean. The corresponding U-statistic is

$$\binom{n}{2}^{-1} \sum_{1 \le i_1 < i_2 \le n} (X_{i_1} - X_{i_2})^2/2.$$

with the kernel $h(x_1,x_2) = (x_1 - x_2)^2/2$. Thus, $E(h(X_1,X_2)|X_1 = x_1) = (x_1-\mu)^2/2 + \mu_c^2/2$ and $\tilde{h}_1(x_1) = \{(x_1-\mu)^2 - \mu_c^2\}/2$. Since $E(X_1 - X_2)^4 = E((X_1-\mu)-(X_2-\mu))^4 = 2\mu_c^4 + 6\{\mu_c^2\}^2$,

$$\eta_2^2 = E(h^2) - \{\mu_c^2\}^2 = [\mu_c^4 + \{\mu_c^2\}^2]/2, \tag{7.4}$$

and

$$\eta_1^2 = E(\tilde{h}_1^2) = [\mu_c^4 - \{\mu_c^2\}^2]/4. \tag{7.5}$$

Applying (7.3), the results (7.4) and (7.5) lead to

$$\mathrm{Var}(U_n) = \frac{2}{n(n-1)}\{2(n-2)\eta_1^2 + \eta_2^2\} = \frac{\mu_c^4 - \{\mu_c^2\}^2}{n}.$$

7.2 Empirical Likelihood Statistic for a U-Statistics Constraint

Some recent investigations dealing with the empirical likelihood (EL) statistics for U-statistics are found in the literature. Wood et al. (1996) considered the EL approach to U-statistics via a bootstrap calibration. A comprehensive investigation of the EL method involving U-statistics in a one-sample setting was carried out by Yuan et al. (2012). Main discussions of relevant EL statistics in two-sample setting are often found in the analysis of the receiver operating characteristic (ROC) curves (Claeskens et al., 2003; Qin and Zhou, 2006; Zou et al., 2011); however, the proposed methods may not provide an EL approach for general U-statistics. For example, Qin and Zhou (2006), in their investigation of the test of the area under an ROC curve, constructed a constraint for one group so that the test could be performed in a similar manner to the one-sample EL method via sample estimates of specificity and the *plug-in* method (e.g., Hjort et al., 2009). For an application to more general U-statistics, Jing et al. (2009) obtained an EL based on jackknife pseudovalues that were conjectured to be independent.

In this chapter, we first discuss the EL test statistic with general U-statistics (Yu et al., 2016). Obtaining the EL statistics follows the common approach that we explained in the previous chapters (e.g., Chapter 5). However, constraints in U-statistics are not a summation of independent observations, thus the resulting EL statistic does not follow a χ^2 distribution.

The framework of obtaining the EL statistic in one sample setting is as follows. Let $X_1,\ldots,X_n$ be n independent observations with unknown identical distribution function $F(x)=P_r(X_i<x)$. Suppose a constraint under H_0,

$$E(h(X_1,\ldots,X_m)\,|\,\theta_0)=0, \tag{7.6}$$

where θ_0 is a fixed value under H_0 and $m\le n$. We will also express the expectation in (7.6) as $E(h(X_1,\ldots,X_m,\theta_0)$. Using Definition (7.2), the corresponding empirical constraint to (7.6) is

$$\sum\nolimits_{\mathbf{i}\in C} w_{\mathbf{i}}\, h(\mathbf{X}_{\mathbf{i}},\theta_0)=0,$$

where $\mathbf{i}=(i_1,\ldots,i_m)$ indicates a set of combination in C, $\mathbf{X}_{\mathbf{i}}=(X_{i_1},\ldots,X_{i_m})$, and $w_{\mathbf{i}}$ is a nonnegative weight satisfying.

$$\max\left\{\prod\nolimits_{\mathbf{i}\in C} w_{\mathbf{i}} : \sum\nolimits_{\mathbf{i}\in C} w_{\mathbf{i}}=1,\ \sum\nolimits_{\mathbf{i}\in C} w_{\mathbf{i}}\, h(\mathbf{X}_{\mathbf{i}},\theta_0)=0\right\}. \tag{7.7}$$

Under H_0, the EL function is $\prod_{\mathbf{i}\in C} w_{\mathbf{i}}$. The weight $w_{\mathbf{i}}$ may not be directly interpreted as a probability point mass if $m\ge 2$. For example, if $m=2$,

$$\sum\nolimits_{\mathbf{i}\in C} w_{\mathbf{i}}=1 \Leftrightarrow \sum\nolimits_{i_1=1}^{n}\sum\nolimits_{i_2>i_1}^{n} w_{\mathbf{i}}=1. \tag{7.8}$$

However, a bivariate probability mass satisfies

$$\sum\nolimits_{i_1=1}^{n}\sum\nolimits_{i_2=1}^{n} P_r(X_{i_1},X_{i_2})=1. \tag{7.9}$$

Equations (7.8) and (7.9) indicate $w_i \neq P_r(X_{i_1}, X_{i_2})$. Maximization in (7.7) can be carried out using the Lagrange method, which leads to give the weight as

$$w_i = \left\{ \binom{n}{m} (1 + \lambda h(\mathbf{X}_i, \theta_0)) \right\}^{-1},$$

where λ satisfies

$$\sum_{i \in C} \frac{h(\mathbf{X}_i, \theta_0)}{1 + \lambda h(\mathbf{X}_i, \theta_0)} = 0. \tag{7.10}$$

Under H_1, the EL function is $\binom{n}{m}^{-\binom{n}{m}}$. Thus, $-2 \log \text{ELR}$ has the form

$$-2 \log LR = -2 \sum_{i \in C} \log \left\{ w_i \binom{n}{m} \right\}.$$

The step to find the asymptotic distribution of the ELR statistic starts with approximating λ using the Taylor expansion of the denominator of (7.10), which gives

$$\lambda \simeq \frac{\sum_{i \in C} h(\mathbf{X}_i, \theta_0)}{\sum_{i \in C} h(\mathbf{X}_i, \theta_0)^2}. \tag{7.11}$$

With the approximated λ in (7.11), the log-EL ratio test statistic is

$$l(\theta_0) = -2 \log LR \simeq \frac{\left\{ \sum_{i \in C} h(\mathbf{X}_i, \theta_0) \right\}^2}{\sum_{i \in C} h(\mathbf{X}_i, \theta_0)^2}. \tag{7.12}$$

Since $E(h(\mathbf{X}_i, \theta_0)) = 0$, if the denominator in (7.12) is the variance estimator of $\sum_{i \in C} h(\mathbf{X}_i, \theta_0)$, that may lead to a χ_1^2 distribution; however, the variance of $\sum_{i \in C} h(\mathbf{X}_i, \theta_0)$ has the form $\sum_{c=1}^{m} \binom{m}{c} \binom{n-m}{m-c} \eta_c^2$ based on (7.3). This leads to the following result:

Assume that $E|h(\mathbf{X}), \theta_0|^{\alpha}$ exists up to some positive α, and θ_0 is inside the convex hull of points given by the set of points $h(\mathbf{X}_i, \mathbf{Y}_j)$, $i, j \in S$.

Proposition 7.1

Under H_0, $\gamma(\theta_0)l(\theta_0)$ converges in distribution to a χ_1^2 distribution, where

$$\gamma(\theta_0) = \frac{\sum_{\mathbf{i}\in C} h(\mathbf{X}_\mathbf{i}, \theta_0)^2}{\binom{n}{m}\sum_{c=1}^{m}\binom{m}{c}\binom{n-m}{m-c}\eta_c^2}.$$

Example 7.2

Consider the U-statistic with $m = 1$ (e.g., the sample mean). Then, under H_0

$$\sum_{c=1}^{m}\binom{m}{c}\binom{n-m}{m-c}\eta_c^2 = \eta_1^2 = E\{(h(X)-\theta_0)^2\}$$

Also,

$$\binom{n}{m}^{-1}\sum_{\mathbf{i}\in C} h(X_i, \theta_0)^2 = n^{-1}\sum_{i=1}^{n}(h(X)-\theta_0)^2$$

is an unbiased estimator of $E\{(h(X)-\theta_0)^2\}$. Thus, $\gamma(\theta_0)$ is asymptotically 1.

Example 7.3: Variance Confidence Interval

The EL statistic based on the U-statistic to estimate the variance may provide the confidence interval estimate for the variance. By Proposition 7.1, the EL statistic is $\gamma(\theta)l(\theta)$ where

$$\gamma(\theta) = \frac{\sum_{1\le i_1<i_2\le n}\{(X_{i_1}-X_{i_2})^2/2-\theta\}^2}{\binom{n}{2}^2 \frac{\hat{\mu}_c^4 - \{\hat{\mu}_c^2\}^2}{n}}. \tag{7.13}$$

In (7.13), the estimates of the central moments are obtained by

$$\hat{\mu}_c^k = \frac{\sum_{i=1}^{n}(X_i-\bar{X})^k}{n}.$$

The statistic $\gamma(\theta)l(\theta)$ has a χ_1^2 distribution with the correct specification of θ. The confidence interval of the variance is

$$\{\theta : \gamma(\theta)l(\theta) \le \chi_{1,\alpha}^2\}, \tag{7.14}$$

where $\chi^2_{1,\alpha}$ is the quantile of the χ^2_1 distribution corresponding to the probability $1-\alpha$. R code can be created using the functions in the R package, `emplik` as follows.

```
n<-100;
x<-rnorm(n); #data are generated from the standard normal distribution.
varx<-var(x)
varx #e.g.                                              #Sample variance
[1] 1.062097
```

The following code produces the values of $\sum_{1\le i_1<i_2\le n}\{(X_{i_1}-X_{i_2})^2-\hat{\mu}_c^2\}$ (`sumval`) and $\sum_{1\le i_1<i_2\le n}\{(X_{i_1}-X_{i_2})^2-\hat{\mu}_c^2\}^2$ (`sumval2`):

```
Sumval<-matrix(NA, nrow=n, ncol=n)
Sumval2<-matrix(NA, nrow=n, ncol=n)
Mval<-matrix(NA, nrow=n, ncol=n)
Mcenterval<-matrix(NA, nrow=n, ncol=n)
for(ii in 1:n){ for(jj in ii:n){
                    #ii=jj cases are not counted by the kernel
  Sumval[ii,jj]<-(x[ii]-x[jj])^2/2-varx
  Mcenterval[ii,jj]<-Sumval2[ii,jj]<-((x[ii]-x[jj])^2/2-varx)^2
  Mval[ii,jj]<-(x[ii]-x[jj])^2/2 }}
sumval<-sum(Sumval[upper.tri(Sumval,diag=FALSE)])
sumval2<-sum(Sumval2[upper.tri(Sumval2,diag=FALSE)])
```

The following code used the initial value:

$$\frac{\sum_{1\le i_1<i_2\le n}\{(X_{i_1}-X_{i_2})^2-\hat{\mu}_c^2\}}{\sum_{1\le i_1<i_2\le n}\{(X_{i_1}-X_{i_2})^2-\hat{\mu}_c^2\}^2}.$$

```
inilamval<-sumval/sumval2                               #Initial value
```

In the following, `notcenterval` is the collection of kernels of the U-statistic.

```
notcenterval<-Mval[upper.tri(Mval, diag = FALSE)]    #(X_i1 - X_i2)^2/2
rvalnume<- sumval2
m4<-sum((x-mean(x))^4)/n
m2<-sum((x-mean(x))^2)/n
v<-(m4-m2^2)/n
rvaldenom<-(n*(n-1)/2)^2*v
rval<- rvalnume/rvaldenom                                        #γ(θ)
```

We use the function `findUL` from `emplik` package to obtain the EL confidence interval. The function `varfun` produces a list where the first element produces the EL test statistic depending on θ. The `varx` is used as a center value for the confidence interval.

TABLE 7.1

Comparison of the variance confidence intervals

Method	$n = 100$	$n = 400$	$n = 500$
Normal based (1) in (7.15)	80.2%	77.2%	79.1%
Normal based (2) in (7.15)	87.4%	92.5%	93.1%
Bootstrap (percentile)	87.4%	92.4%	93.2%
EL method for U-statistics	92.5%	92.8%	94.6%

```
varfun <- function(theta, x) {
outval<-el.test(x, mu=theta, inilamval)
outval[[1]]<-outval$`-2LLR`* rval
return(outval)}
out<-findUL(step=0.1, fun=varfun, MLE=varx, x=notcenterval)
c(out$Low, out$Up) #lower and upper bounds of the confidence interval, e.g.,
[1] 0.7750364 1.5957376
```

In Table 7.1, the performance of the confidence interval (7.14) is compared to the confidence interval based on the normal approximation assumptions,

$$\text{(1)} \quad \left(\frac{(n-1)\hat{\theta}}{\chi^2_{1-\alpha/2,n-1}}, \; \frac{(n-1)\hat{\theta}}{\chi^2_{\alpha/2,n-1}} \right),$$

$$\text{(2)} \quad \left(\hat{\theta} - z_\alpha \sqrt{\frac{\hat{\mu}_c^4 - \{\mu_c^2\}^2}{n}}, \; \hat{\theta} + z_\alpha \sqrt{\frac{\hat{\mu}_c^4 - \{\mu_c^2\}^2}{n}} \right), \tag{7.15}$$

where $\chi^2_{p,n-1}$ and z_p are quantiles corresponding to the probability $1-p$ for the χ^2_{n-1} distribution and standard normal distribution, respectively. Table 7.1 includes the bootstrap percentile confidence interval (e.g., Vexler and Hutson, 2018). The underlying distribution for the simulation is $Gamma(2, 0.8)$. The result clearly shows that the EL method demonstrates an excellent performance. It is notable that the normal distribution-based interval (1) in (7.15) shows a poor performance that is not improved with increasing sample sizes n.

7.3 Two-Sample Setting

Let $X_1, \ldots, X_{n_1}$ be n_1 independent observations from group 1 with unknown distribution function $F(x) = P_r(X_i < x)$, and let $Y_1, \ldots, Y_{n_2}$ be n_2 independent observations from group 2 with unknown distribution function $G(y) = P_r(Y_j < y)$. Let $m_1 \le n_1, m_2 \le n_2$, and $h(X_1, \ldots, X_{m_1}, Y_1, \ldots, Y_{m_2}) = h(\mathbf{X}, \mathbf{Y})$ be a symmetric kernel of a U-statistic for the two groups. Also, let $E_{F,G}(h(\mathbf{X}, \mathbf{Y})) = \theta$ and $E_{F,G}(h(\mathbf{X}, \mathbf{Y}) - \theta)^2 = \eta^2$, where $E_{F,G}$ denotes the expectation with respect to the true underlying distributions F and G. The corresponding U-statistic estimator of θ is given as

$$\hat{\theta} = \frac{1}{\binom{n_1}{m_1}\binom{n_2}{m_2}} \sum_{i,j \in S} h(\mathbf{X}_i, \mathbf{Y}_j), \tag{7.16}$$

where $i = (i_1, \ldots, i_{m_1})$, $j = (j_1, \ldots, j_{m_2})$, and $S = \{i, j\colon 1 \le i_1 < \ldots < i_{m_1} \le n_1,\ 1 \le j_1 < \ldots < j_{m_2} \le n_2\}$ denote all permutations of the m_k indices for group k $(k = 1, 2)$. Note that, given all $h(\mathbf{X}_i, \mathbf{Y}_j) = 1$, we have

$$\left[\binom{n_1}{m_1}\binom{n_2}{m_2}\right]^{-1} \sum_{i,j \in S} 1 = 1.$$

Following a conventional notation (Lee, 1990), let us define

$$\begin{aligned} h_{c_1,c_2}(X_1, \ldots, X_{c_1}, Y_1, \ldots, Y_{c_2}) &= \int \ldots \int h(u_1, \ldots, u_{m_1}, v_1, \ldots, v_{m_2}) \prod_{i=1}^{c_1} (d\delta_{x_i}(u_i) \\ &\quad - dF(u_i)) \prod_{i=c_1+1}^{m_1} dF(u_i) \prod_{j=1}^{c_2} (d\delta_{y_j}(v_j) \\ &\quad - dG(v_j)) \prod_{j=c_2+1}^{m_2} dG(v_j) \\ &= E[h(\mathbf{X}, \mathbf{Y}) \mid X_1, \ldots, X_{c_1}, Y_1, \ldots, Y_{c_2}] - E[h(\mathbf{X}, \mathbf{Y})], \end{aligned} \tag{7.17}$$

for some integers $c_1 (\le m_1)$ and $c_2 (\le m_2)$, where δ_x takes value 1 at $u_i = x_i$ and 0 otherwise. In (7.17), if $c_i = 0$, the product involving δ_x is omitted. The asymptotic variance of $(n_1 + n_2)^{1/2} \hat{\theta}$ (Lee, 1990) has the form

$$\frac{m_1^2 (n_1 + n_2)}{n_1} \sigma_{1,0}^2 + \frac{m_2^2 (n_1 + n_2)}{n_2} \sigma_{0,1}^2, \tag{7.18}$$

where

$$\begin{aligned} \sigma_{c_1,c_2}^2 = Cov\{ & h(X_1, \ldots, X_{c_1}, X_{c_1+1}, \ldots, X_{n_1}, Y_1, \ldots, Y_{c_2}, Y_{c_2+1}, \ldots, Y_{n_2}), \\ & h(X_1, \ldots, X_{c_1}, X'_{c_1+1}, \ldots, X'_{n_1}, Y_1, \ldots, Y_{c_2}, Y'_{c_2+1}, \ldots, Y'_{n_2})\}. \end{aligned} \tag{7.19}$$

Example 7.4

Consider the Wilcoxon rank sum statistic, where $h(X, Y) = I(X > Y)$ where I is an indicator function. Then, by (7.19),

$$\begin{aligned} \sigma_{1,0}^2 &= Cov(I(X > Y), I(X > Y')) \\ &= E(I(X > Y), I(X > Y')) - E(I(X > Y))E(I(X > Y')) \\ &= P_r(X > Y, X > Y') - \{P_r(X > Y)\}^2. \end{aligned} \tag{7.20}$$

Under the assumption of an equal distribution of X and Y, $P_r\{X > Y, X > Y'\} = 1/3$ and $P_r\{X > Y\} = 1/2$, giving $\sigma_{1,0}^2 = 1/12$ by (7.20). Likewise, $\sigma_{0,1}^2 = 1/12$. Thus, the variance in (7.18) is $(n_1 + n_2)^2/(12\, n_1 n_2)$. The Wilcoxon rank sum test statistic is equivalent to the area under the ROC curve that will be discussed in a later example, where a more general form of the variance estimator will be used.

Consider the null hypothesis of interest:

$$H_0 : \ \mathrm{E}_{F,G}(h(\mathbf{X}, \mathbf{Y})) = \theta_0. \tag{7.21}$$

For the empirical constraint corresponding to (7.21), we use a weight w_{ij} instead of $\left[\binom{n_1}{m_1}\binom{n_2}{m_2}\right]^{-1}$ in (7.16) as

$$\sum_{i,j \in S} w_{ij} h(\mathbf{X}_i, \mathbf{Y}_j) = \theta_0, \tag{7.22}$$

where $\sum_{i,j \in S} w_{ij} = 1$, and $w_{ij} \geq 0$. If $m_1 = m_2 = 1$, w_{ij} has a direct interpretation as a probability point mass for (x_i, y_j), that is, w_{ij} is the estimated probability mass $\hat{P}_r(X = x_i, Y = y_j)$. For the other values of m_1 and m_2, the correspondence of w_{ij} to a probability point mass is generally not true. The EL function under H_0 is defined as

$$L_{\theta_0} = \max_{w_{ij}} \prod_{i,j \in S} w_{ij}, \tag{7.23}$$

which is subjected to $\sum_{i,j \in S} w_{ij} = 1$, $0 \leq w_{ij} \leq 1$, and Constraint (7.22). The EL function under the alternative hypothesis H_1 (i.e., not H_0) is

$$L_{\theta_1} = \left[\binom{n_1}{m_1}\binom{n_2}{m_2}\right]^{-\binom{n_1}{m_1}\binom{n_2}{m_2}}. \tag{7.24}$$

Obtaining (7.23) is carried out by maximizing $\sum_{i,j \in S} \log w_{ij}$ using the method of Lagrange multipliers with conditions $\sum_{i,j \in S} w_{ij} = 1$ and (7.22). This step gives us

$$w_{ij} = \left\{\binom{n_1}{m_1}\binom{n_2}{m_2}(1 + \lambda(h(\mathbf{X}_i, \mathbf{Y}_j) - \theta_0))\right\}^{-1}, i, j \in S, \tag{7.25}$$

where λ satisfies

$$\sum_{i,j \in S} \frac{h(\mathbf{X}_i, \mathbf{Y}_j) - \theta_0}{1 + \lambda(h(\mathbf{X}_i, \mathbf{Y}_j) - \theta_0)} = 0. \tag{7.26}$$

By Equations (7.23) through (7.25), we obtain the ELR-type statistic as

$$R(\theta_0) = \prod_{i,j \in S} \{1 + \lambda (h(\mathbf{X}_i, \mathbf{Y}_j) - \theta_0)\}^{-1},$$

and then the corresponding EL log-likelihood ratio statistic is

$$l(\theta_0) = -2 \log R(\theta_0) = 2 \sum_{i,j \in S} \log(1 + \lambda (h(\mathbf{X}_i, \mathbf{Y}_j) - \theta_0)). \tag{7.27}$$

Assume that $E_{F,G} |h(\mathbf{X}, \mathbf{Y})|^{\alpha}$ exists up to some positive α, and θ_0 is inside the convex hull of points given by the set of points $h(\mathbf{X}_i, \mathbf{Y}_j)$, $i, j \in S$. Also, assume that $n = (n_1 + n_2) \to \infty$ and $\frac{n_1}{n_1 + n_2} \to r$ for asymptotic results. Let $V(\hat{\theta}) = \sigma^2 = \frac{m_1^2}{r} \sigma_{1,0}^2 + \frac{m_2^2}{1-r} \sigma_{0,1}^2$. Then, we have the following result:

Proposition 7.2

Under H_0, $\gamma(\theta_0) l(\theta_0)$ converges in distribution to a χ_1^2 distribution, where $\gamma(\theta_0) = \eta^2 / \left[\binom{n_1}{m_1}\binom{n_2}{m_2}\sigma^2\right]$.

The proof of Proposition 7.2 is shown in the Appendix of this chapter.

To compute w_{ij} at (7.25), we need to solve the nonlinear equation given in (7.26), which can be carried out using commonly available optimization packages (Section 7.4).

The extension of the ELR test to multivariate random variables follows the univariate development outlined above. Now, consider $X_1, \ldots, X_{n_1}$ and $Y_1, \ldots, Y_{n_2}$ as the p-variate random vectors. We have that $E_{F,G}((h(\mathbf{X}, \mathbf{Y}) - \theta)(h(\mathbf{X}, \mathbf{Y}) - \theta)^T) = \mathrm{H}$ and Σ is the covariance matrix of $\hat{\theta}$. Note that the null hypothesis is given as $H_0: \mathrm{E}_{F,G}(h(\mathbf{X}, \mathbf{Y})) = \theta_0$, where θ_0 is a $q \times 1$ vector ($q \le p$). The corresponding log-likelihood ratio test has the form of

$$l(\theta_0) = 2 \sum_{i,j \in S} \log(1 + \lambda^T (h(\mathbf{X}_i, \mathbf{Y}_j) - \theta_0)), \tag{7.28}$$

where $q \times 1$ vector λ satisfies

$$\sum_{i,j \in S} \frac{h(\mathbf{X}_i, \mathbf{Y}_j) - \theta_0}{1 + \lambda^T (h(\mathbf{X}_i, \mathbf{Y}_j) - \theta_0)} = 0, \tag{7.29}$$

where 0 is the $q \times 1$ zero vector. As in the univariate setting, assume that $E_{F,G} \|h(\mathbf{X}, \mathbf{Y})\|^{\alpha}$ exists, and θ_0 is inside the convex hull given by the set of points $h(\mathbf{X}_i, \mathbf{Y}_j)$, $i, j \in S$. Then, we have the following result:

Proposition 7.3

Under H_0, $l(\theta_0)\left[\binom{n_1}{m_1}\binom{n_2}{m_2}\right]^{-1}$ *in (7.28) converges in distribution to* $\sum_{k=1}^{q} c_k \chi_{1k}^2$ *where* c_k*'s are the eigenvalues of* $H^{-1}\Sigma$ *and* χ_{1k}^2*'s are independent* χ_1^2 *distributed random variables.*

A brief sketch of the proof is given in this chapter's Appendix.

7.4 Various Applications

The following examples demonstrate that, if the analytical form of the variance estimate can be obtained, a straightforward application of the proposed method is possible.

7.4.1 Receiver Operating Characteristic Curve Analysis

The ROC curve has been used as an important tool to examine the discriminant ability of a biomarker for separating individuals with a certain disease from those without the disease. The ROC curve analysis looks at the probability $P_r(Y > X)$, where X and Y are random variables representing two different populations. More details regarding the ROC curve analysis will be provided in Chapter 8. Suppose $X_1,\ldots,X_{n_1}$ are n_1 independent observations from population 1 and $Y_1,\ldots,Y_{n_2}$ are n_2 independent observations from population 2. Also, let $X_i \sim X$ and $Y_i \sim Y$ where $\sim$ indicates the same distribution. The corresponding U-statistic for estimating the probability $\varsigma = P_r(Y > X)$ is given by

$$\hat{\varsigma}_{X,Y} = \frac{1}{n_1 n_2}\sum_{i=1}^{n_1}\sum_{j=1}^{n_2}\phi(X_i, Y_j), \tag{7.30}$$

where $\phi(X_i, Y_j) = I(X_i < Y_j)$ and I denotes the indicator function. The statistic $\hat{\varsigma}_{X,Y}$ is essentially the Wilcoxon–Mann–Whitney U-statistic, which estimates the area under the estimated ROC curve (referred to as AUC). Let ς_0 denote the AUC under H_0. We construct the ELR statistic as

$$R(\varsigma_0) = \frac{\prod_{i=1}^{n_1}\prod_{j=1}^{n_2} w_{ij}}{(n_1 n_2)^{-n_1 n_2}}, \tag{7.31}$$

where w_{ij}'s satisfy

$$\sup\left\{\prod_{i=1}^{n_1}\prod_{j=1}^{n_2} w_{ij} : \sum_{i=1}^{n_1}\sum_{j=1}^{n_2} w_{ij}=1,\ \sum_{i=1}^{n_1}\sum_{j=1}^{n_2} w_{ij}(\phi_{ij}-\varsigma_0)=0\right\},$$

and $\phi_{ij}=\phi(X_i,Y_j)$. Sen (1967) provided a consistent estimate of the variance for the U-statistic $\hat{\varsigma}$, which we can incorporate in our development. Let

$$S_{10}^2=\frac{1}{n_1-1}\sum_{i=1}^{n_1}\left(V_{10}(X_i)-\hat{\varsigma}_{X,Y}\right)^2,\text{ and } S_{01}^2=\frac{1}{n_2-1}\sum_{j=1}^{n_2}\left(V_{01}(Y_j)-\hat{\varsigma}_{X,Y}\right)^2, \quad (7.32)$$

where $V_{10}(X_i)=1/n_2\sum_{j=1}^{n_2}\phi(X_i,Y_j)$ for $i=1,\cdots,n_1$ and $V_{01}(Y_j)=1/n_1\sum_{i=1}^{n_1}\phi(X_i,Y_j)$ for $j=1,\cdots,n_2$. Then, the variance estimate of $\hat{\varsigma}_{X,Y}$ (Sen, 1967) is given as

$$\hat{V}(\hat{\varsigma}_{X,Y})=\frac{n_1+n_2}{n_1n_2}\left(\frac{n_2S_{10}^2+n_1S_{01}^2}{n_1+n_2}\right). \quad (7.33)$$

Based on Proposition 7.2 and Equation (7.33), we have the following result:

Corollary 7.1

Under $H_0:\varsigma=\varsigma_0$, $-2\log R(\varsigma_0)\sum_{i=1}^{n_1}\sum_{j=1}^{n_2}(\phi_{ij}-\varsigma_0)^2/(n_1n_2)^2\hat{V}(\hat{\varsigma}_{X,Y})$ converges in distribution to a χ_1^2 distribution.

The value $\hat{\varsigma}_{X,Y}$ in (7.32) can be replaced by ς_0 under H_0.

7.4.1.1 R Code

We use the data generated from Group 1: $X\sim$ *lognormal*(0,0.25) and Group 2: $Y\sim$ *lognormal* (0.4705, 0.5), which give the true $\varsigma=0.8$ (d0).

```
d0<-0.8
x_ln_mu=0                                    #location parameter of X
x_ln_sd=0.25                                    #scale parameter of X
y_ln_mu=sqrt(0.25^2+0.5^2)*qnorm(0.8)  #location parameter of Y
y_ln_sd=0.5                                     #scale parameter of Y
n1<-100; n2<-100     #sample sizes. n1 and n2 can be different.
n<-n1+n2;m<-n1*n2
x<-rlnorm(n1, x_ln_mu,x_ln_sd)
```

```
y<-rlnorm(n2, y_ln_mu,y_ln_sd)
```

The variable `indicators_v` contains the values ϕ_{ij}.

```
indicators<-matrix(data=NA, n1, n2)
for ( u in 1:n1) {for ( z in 1:n2) {
  indicators[u,z]<-as.numeric(x[u]<y[z])}}
indicators_v<-c(indicators)
```

The estAUC contains $\hat{\varsigma}_{X,Y}$.

```
estAUC<-mean(indicators_v)
```

An initial value of λ can be given by equating the first-order expansion of the left-sided equation of (7.26) to 0 (see (A.7.6) in the Appendix for details). The appropriate solution may be given within some neighborhood of the initial value.

```
inilamval<-sum(centerval)*m/sum(centerval^2)
```

Obtaining the value minimizing `fn.Lamda` in the following will produce the desirable Lagrange multiplier:

```
centerval<-indicators_v-d0
fn.Lamda<-function(lamval){
  returnval<-(sum(centerval/(m+lamval*centerval)))^2
return(returnval)}
```

Optimization to obtain λ can be done as follows:

```
lamval<-optimize(fn.Lamda,interval=c((inilamval-1*abs(inilamval)),
(inilamval+1*abs(inilamval))),maximum=FALSE)$minimum
```

The weights w_{ij} are obtained as follows:

```
wijs<-1/(m+lamval*centerval)
```

In some rare cases, w_{ij} values obtained are not positive. Then, we consider that λ is not appropriate and look for a new λ. More intricate R code needs to be used. We present the code in the Appendix that tries to find λ with a different initial value. The function `fn1.2` returns the sum of log of w_{ij}.

```
fn1.2<-function(p){sump<-0;for(j in 1:m)
{sump<-sump+log(p[j])};return(-sump)}
```

$R(\varsigma_0)$ is obtained as follows:

```
lr<--2*(m*log(n1)+m*log(n2)-fn1.2(wijs))
lr #e.g.
[1] 4.351325
```

The following code is to compute $\hat{V}(\hat{\varsigma}_{X,Y})$:

```
v10<-apply(indicators,1,mean)
s10<-sum((v10-d0)^2)/(n1-1)
v01<-apply(indicators,2,mean)
s01<-sum((v01-d0)^2)/(n2-1)
v<-((n2*s10+n1*s01)/(n1+n2))/(n1*n2/(n1+n2))          #V̂(ς̂X,Y)
v #e.g.
[1] 0.001019111
```

The following code gives $\sum_{i=1}^{n_1}\sum_{j=1}^{n_2}(\phi_{ij}-\varsigma_0)^2/\{(n_1n_2)^2\hat{V}(\hat{\varsigma}_{X,Y})\}$ (`factor1`)

```
sum_phi<-sum((indicators_v-d0)^2)
factor1<-(v*m^2)/sum_phi
```

The test statistic and p-value are as follows:

```
teststat<-lr/factor1
teststat #e.g.
[1] 0.06618929
1-pchisq(teststat,1) #e.g.
[1] 0.7969682
```

We note that the optimization to obtain $R(\varsigma_0)$ can be carried out using `el.test` in `emplik` package. Note that emplik works for one-group setting; however, obtaining w_{ij} in the EL for U-statistics is much like obtaining the probability masses of the data points in the EL for the one group. The centered kernel values (i.e., $\phi_{ij}-\varsigma_0$) can be treated as the data points for the one-group EL. The resulting *probability mass* is not a probability in this case.

```
out<-el.test(centerval,0, inilamval)
lr<-out$`-2LLR` #e.g.
lr
[1] 4.351325
```

7.4.2 Generalization for Comparing Two Correlated AUC Statistics

Suppose that individuals from population 1 provide independent observations $X_i = (X_{1i},\ldots,X_{pi})^T$, $i = 1,\ldots,n_1$ and individuals from population 2 provide independent observations $Y_j = (Y_{1j},\ldots,Y_{pj})^T$, $j = 1,\ldots,n_2$. Then we may be interested in testing generalized differences in AUCs given by the hypothesis,

$$H_0 : P_r(\ell_1^T X < \ell_2^T Y) - P_r(\ell_3^T X < \ell_4^T Y) = \delta_0, \tag{7.34}$$

where $X \sim X_i$ and $Y \sim Y_i$, and ℓ_i's are some known contrast vectors. The corresponding U-statistic $\hat{\delta}$ is

$$\hat{\delta} = \frac{1}{n_1 n_2} \sum_{i=1}^{n_1} \sum_{j=1}^{n_2} \{\phi(l_1^T X_i, l_2^T Y_j) - \phi(l_3^T X_i, l_4^T Y_j)\},$$

under the notation used in Section 7.4.1. We construct the ELR test statistics as

$$R(\delta_0) = \frac{\prod_{i=1}^{n_1} \prod_{j=1}^{n_2} w_{ij}}{(n_1 n_2)^{-n_1 n_2}}, \tag{7.35}$$

where w_{ij}'s satisfy

$$\sup\left\{ \prod_{i=1}^{n_1} \prod_{j=1}^{n_2} w_{ij} : \sum_{i=1}^{n_1} \sum_{j=1}^{n_2} w_{ij} = 1, \ \sum_{i=1}^{n_1} \sum_{j=1}^{n_2} w_{ij} (\phi_{12_{ij}} - \phi_{34_{ij}} - \delta_0) = 0 \right\},$$

and $\phi_{kk'_{ij}} = I({\ell_k}^T X_i < {\ell_{k'}}^T Y_j)$. Since ${\ell_i}^T X$ and ${\ell_j}^T Y$ result in new variables given as linear combinations of X's and Y's, without loss of generality, let us consider bivariate outcomes $X_i = (X_{1i}, X_{2i})^T$ and $Y_j = (Y_{1j}, Y_{2j})^T$, and set $l_1 = l_2 = (1,0)^T$ and $l_3 = l_4 = (0,1)^T$ in (7.34). DeLong et al. (1988) extended Sen's variance estimate (7.33) to covariance estimates for correlated variables. Specifically, following Delong's approach, Equations in (7.32) can be redefined as

$$\begin{aligned} S_{10}^{kl} &= \frac{1}{n_1 - 1} \sum_{i=1}^{n_1} \left(V_{10}(X_{ki}) - \hat{\varsigma}_{X_k,Y_k}\right)\left(V_{10}(X_{li}) - \hat{\varsigma}_{X_l,Y_l}\right), \\ \text{and } S_{01}^{kl} &= \frac{1}{n_2 - 1} \sum_{j=1}^{n_2} \left(V_{01}(Y_{kj}) - \hat{\varsigma}_{X_k,Y_k}\right)\left(V_{01}(Y_{lj}) - \hat{\varsigma}_{X_l,Y_l}\right) \text{ for } k,l = 1,2, \end{aligned} \tag{7.36}$$

where $V_{10}(X_{ki})=1/n_2\sum_{j=1}^{n_2}\phi(X_{ki},Y_{kj})$ for $i=1,\ldots,n_1$, $V_{01}(Y_{kj})=1/n_1\sum_{i=1}^{n_1}\phi(X_{ki},Y_{kj})$ for $j=1,\ldots,n_2$, and $\hat{\varsigma}_{X_k,Y_k}$ as in (7.30). Then the variance estimate of $\hat{\delta}$ can be given as

$$\hat{V}(\hat{\delta})=(S_{10}^{11}-2S_{10}^{12}+S_{10}^{22})/n_1+(S_{01}^{11}-2S_{01}^{12}+S_{01}^{22})/n_2. \qquad (7.37)$$

Based on Proposition 7.2 and Equation (7.37), we have the following result:

Corollary 7.2

Under $H_0:\delta=\delta_0$, $-2\log R(\delta_0)\left(\sum_{i=1}^{n_1}\sum_{j=1}^{n_2}(\phi_{12_{ij}}-\phi_{34_{ij}}-\delta_0)^2/(n_1n_2)^2\hat{V}(\hat{\delta})\right)$ converges in distribution to the χ_1^2 distribution.

7.4.2.1 Implementation in R

In the following code and results, we use data with a setting as

$$\begin{pmatrix}\log X\\ \log W\end{pmatrix}\sim N_2\left(\begin{pmatrix}0\\0\end{pmatrix},\begin{pmatrix}1&1\\1&4\end{pmatrix}\right),\ \begin{pmatrix}\log Y\\ \log Z\end{pmatrix}\sim N_2\left(\begin{pmatrix}1.882\\3.764\end{pmatrix},\begin{pmatrix}4&4\\4&16\end{pmatrix}\right).$$

where Np indicates p-variate multinormal distribution. This statement provide $P_r(Y>X)=P_r(Z>W)=0.8$, whereas X and W are correlated, Y and Z are correlated, and (X,W) and (Y,Z) are independent and have the multivariate lognormal distribution. Thus, the null value $\delta_0=0$. We provide a code based on a generated data set as follows.

```
require("mvtnorm")

#Parameter setting
normmean_xw=c(0,0)
ncov_xw=matrix(c(1,1,1,4),byrow=T,nrow=2)
normmean_yz=c(1.882,3.764)
ncov_yz=matrix(c(4,4,4,16),byrow=T,nrow=2)

#Sample sizes
n1<-n2<-100
n<-n1+n2;m<-n1*n2

#Data generation
xw=exp(rmvnorm(n=n1, mean=normmean_xw, sigma=ncov_xw))
yz=exp(rmvnorm(n=n2, mean=normmean_yz, sigma=ncov_yz))
x=xw[,1];w=xw[,2];y=yz[,1];z=yz[,2]
```

`indicator_vxy` and `indicator_vwz` contain the kernels of the AUC U-statistics for (X, W) and (Y, Z), respectively.

```
indicator_xy<-matrix(data=NA, n1, n2)
for(a in 1:n1){for(b in 1:n2){
indicator_xy[a,b]=as.numeric(x[a]<y[b])}}
indicator_wz<-matrix(data=NA, n1, n2)
for(p in 1:n1){for(q in1:n2){
indicator_wz[p,q]=as.numeric(w[p]<z[q])}}
indicator_vxy=c(indicator_xy);indicator_vwz=c(indicator_wz)
```

The values in `centerval` correspond to the kernels of $\hat{\delta}$.

```
centerval<-indicator_vxy-indicator_vwz
```

In rare cases, it is possible that all centerval values are 0. It can be considered to be a strong evidence in favor of the null hypothesis, thus we give the test statistic = 0. Otherwise, we obtain the Lagrange multiplier (lamval) by optimization.

```
lamval_0<-optimize(fn.Lamda,
interval=c((inilamval-1*abs(inilamval)),
(inilamval+1*abs(inilamval))),maximum=FALSE)$minimum
```

The function `fn.Lamda` is same as that of the one mentioned in Section 7.4.1. The function `el.test` can also be used for this optimization as mentioned in the previous section (Section 7.4.1). Now, the weights and the initial ELR are as given in the following:

```
wijs<-1/(m+lamval_0*centerval)
lr<- -2*(m*log(n1)+m*log(n2)-fn1.2(wijs))
lr #e.g.
[1] 35.32965
```

In the case that some `wijs` elements are negative, re-optimization can be carried out in a similar manner to that used in Section 7.4.1. The next step is to obtain $\hat{V}(\hat{\delta})$ and $\sum_{i=1}^{n_1}\sum_{j=1}^{n_2}(\phi_{12_{ij}} - \phi_{34_{ij}} - \delta_0)^2/\{(n_1 n_2)^2 V(\delta)\}$ (`factor1`). The relevant code is provided in the Appendix. The test statistic and p-value are given as follows:

```
Teststat<-lr/factor1
teststat #e.g.
[1,] 0.5815071
1-pchisq(teststat,1) #e.g.
[1,] 0.4457222
```

7.4.3 Comparison of Two Survival Curves

A few generalizations of the two-sample Wilcoxon rank sum test statistic given censored data are available (Letón and Zuluaga, 2005). The most commonly used generalization is Gehan's test (Gehan, 1965), which is known to have a higher power than the log rank test when the proportional hazards' assumption is violated (Lee et al., 1975). Suppose that we observe $(X_1,C_1),\cdots,(X_{n_1},C_{n_1})$ that are n_1 independent observations from population 1 and $(X_{n_1+1},C_{n_1+1}),\cdots,(X_{n_1+n_2},C_{n_1+n_2})$ that are n_2 independent observations from population 2, where C_i is 1 if the observation is censored, 0 if the observation is uncensored. We assume noninformative censoring. Gehan's test statistic estimates the difference between the two distributions (say τ), which can be expressed in the form of $\hat{\tau}=\sum_{i=1}^{n_1}U_i$ where $U_i=\sum_{j=1}^{n_1+n_2}\phi_{ij}$,

$$\phi_{ij}=I\{(X_i,0)>(X_j,0) \text{ or } (X_i,1)\geq(X_j,0)\}-I\{(X_i,0)<(X_j,0) \text{ or } (X_i,1)\leq(X_j,0)\},$$

and the inequality is applied only to the first element. Gehan's test statistic can be expressed as

$$\hat{\tau}=\sum_{i=1}^{n_1}\sum_{j=n_1+1}^{n_1+n_2}\phi_{ij}. \tag{7.38}$$

Under $H_0:\tau=\tau_0=0$, the variance of $\hat{\tau}$ is estimated by

$$\hat{V}(\hat{\tau})=\frac{n_1n_2}{(n_1+n_2)(n_1+n_2-1)}\sum_{i=1}^{n_1+n_2}U_i^2.$$

It can be shown that $\sum_{i=1}^{n_1}\sum_{j=1}^{n_1}\phi_{ij}=0$, since, e.g., if $\phi_{ij}=I((X_i,C_i)>(X_j,C_j))=1$, then $\phi_{ji}=-1$. Thus, we express $\tau=\sum_{i=1}^{n_1}\sum_{j=1}^{n_2}\phi_{ij}$. Considering that $I\{(X_i,0)>(X_j,0) \text{ or } (X_i,1)\geq(X_j,0)\}$ and $I\{(X_i,0)<(X_j,0) \text{ or } (X_i,1)\leq(X_j,0)\}$ in ϕ_{ij} are correlated, we can obtain $\hat{V}(\hat{\tau})$ the same way as Section 7.4.2. We can construct the ELR test statistic $R(\tau_0)$, similar to (7.31) and (7.35), where now w_{ij}'s satisfy

$$\sup\left\{\prod_{i=1}^{n_1}\prod_{j=1}^{n_2}w_{ij}:\sum_{i=1}^{n_1}\sum_{j=n_1+1}^{n_2}w_{ij}=1,\sum_{i=1}^{n_1}\sum_{j=n_1+1}^{n_2}w_{ij}\phi_{ij}=0\right\}.$$

We have the following result:

Corollary 7.3

Under $H_0:\tau=0$, $-2\log R(\tau_0)\sum_{i=1}^{n_1}\sum_{j=n_1+1}^{n_2}\phi_{ij}{}^2/\hat{V}(\hat{\tau})$ converges in distribution to a χ_1^2 distribution.

7.4.3.1 R Code

In the following R code, we use a simulated dataset considering cases with nonconstant hazard functions using *Weibull*(0.5,1) versus *Weibull*(0.5,1) for respective groups. Each individual is assumed to enter the study based on the standard exponential distribution (rate parameter = 50), and overall censoring rate set at 20%. Censoring occurs with 20% chance.

```
n1<-100;n2<-100;n<-n1+n2;m<-n1*n2

#Each individual's survival time
x<-rweibull(n1, shape=0.5, scale = 1)
y<-rweibull(n2, shape=0.5, scale = 1)

#Time to enter a study
dx<-rexp(n1,rate =50);dy<-rexp(n2,rate =50)

#Time to terminate from the study if not censored
tx<-array();ty<-array()
for (m1 in 1:n1) {tx[m1]=sum(dx[1:m1])+x[m1]}
for (m2 in 1:n2) {ty[m2]=sum(dy[1:m2])+y[m2]}

#Cutoff time that the study will end at
cutoffx=min(sum(dx)+0.000001,quantile(tx,0.8))
cutoffy=min(sum(dy)+0.000001,quantile(ty,0.8))

#Observed values
cx<-array();cy<-array()
for (m1 in 1:n1) {if (tx[m1]<=cutoffx) {
cx[m1]=x[m1]} else if (tx[m1]>cutoffx)
{cx[m1]=x[m1]-(tx[m1]-cutoffx)}}
for (m2 in 1:n2) {if (ty[m2]<=cutoffy) {
cy[m2]=y[m2]} else if (ty[m2]>cutoffy)
{cy[m2]=y[m2]-(ty[m2]-cutoffy)}}

#Censoring indication
censorx =as.numeric(tx>cutoffx)
censory =as.numeric(ty>cutoffy)
```

By executing the following code, `centerval` contains ϕ_{ij}.

```
indicator1_xy=matrix(data=0, n1, n2)
indicator2_xy=matrix(data=0, n1, n2)
for(a in 1:n1){for(b in 1:n2){
  if((cx[a]>cy[b] & censorx[a]==0 & censory[b]==0)|
  (cx[a]>=cy[b] & censorx[a]==1 & censory[b]==0))
{indicator1_xy[a,b]=1
  }else if ((cx[a]<cy[b] & censorx[a]==0 & censory[b]==0)|
```

```
  (cx[a]<=cy[b] & censorx[a]==0 & censory[b]==1))
indicator2_xy[a,b]=1
}}
indicator1_vxy=c(indicator1_xy)
indicator2_vxy=c(indicator2_xy)
centerval<-indicator1_vxy-indicator2_vxy
```

The data analysis after obtaining centerval can be carried out in the same way as Section 7.4.2. We leave the rest of the data analysis to readers. The resulting test statistic is 0.0721 and p-value is 0.7882.

7.4.4 Multivariate Rank-Based Tests

An extension of the univariate rank procedures to multivariate problems can be carried out in a straightforward manner using Proposition 7.3. Particular definitions of the kernel function $h(\mathbf{X},\mathbf{Y})$ can give rise to various U-statistic-based multivariate tests (e.g., Choi and Marden, 1997). In this subsection, we illustrate an application of the proposed method based on multivariate variables via a simple extension of the univariate Wilcoxon–Mann–Whitney statistic to that for multivariate variables. Consider independent continuous random vectors $X_i=(X_{1i},\ldots,X_{pi})^T$, $i=1,\ldots,n_1$ from population 1 and $Y_j=(Y_{1j},\ldots,Y_{pj})^T$, $j=1,\ldots,n_2$ from population 2. A null hypothesis in consideration is

$$H_0:(P_r(X_1<Y_1),\ldots,P_r(X_p<Y_p))^T=(0.5,\ldots,0.5)^T. \tag{7.39}$$

The probabilities in the left-hand side of (7.39) are estimated by $\hat{\varsigma}=(\hat{\varsigma}_{X_1,Y_1},\ldots,\hat{\varsigma}_{X_p,Y_p})$ using the Definition (7.30). By (7.36), let

$$\frac{1}{n_1}\begin{pmatrix} S_{10}^{kk} & S_{10}^{kl} \\ S_{10}^{lk} & S_{10}^{ll} \end{pmatrix}+\frac{1}{n_2}\begin{pmatrix} S_{01}^{kk} & S_{01}^{kl} \\ S_{01}^{lk} & S_{01}^{ll} \end{pmatrix}=\begin{pmatrix} C_{kk} & C_{kl} \\ C_{lk} & C_{ll} \end{pmatrix}. \tag{7.40}$$

The covariance matrix of $\hat{\varsigma}$ is estimated by

$$\hat{V}(\hat{\varsigma})=(C_{ij}),\, i,j=1,\ldots,p,$$

where (C_{ij}) is a matrix with C_{ij} in (7.40) for its (i,j)-th element. Let $\varsigma_0=(0.5,\ldots,0.5)^T$. Under H_0 in (7.39), we can construct the ELR test statistic $R(\varsigma_0)$ similar to (7.31). Specifically, w_{ij}'s satisfy

$$\sup\left\{\prod_{i=1}^{n_1}\prod_{j=1}^{n_2} w_{ij}:\sum_{i=1}^{n_1}\sum_{j=n_1+1}^{n_2} w_{ij}=1,\ \sum_{i=1}^{n_1}\sum_{j=n_1+1}^{n_2} w_{ij}(\phi_{ij}-\varsigma_0)=0\right\},$$

where $\phi_{ij} = (\phi(X_{i1}, Y_{j1}), \ldots, \phi(X_{ip}, Y_{jp}))^T$ by the definition used in (7.30), and 0 is the $p \times 1$ zero vector. Let

$$\hat{H} = \frac{1}{n_1 n_2} \sum_{i=1}^{n_1} \sum_{j=1}^{n_2} (\phi_{ij} - \varsigma_0)(\phi_{ij} - \varsigma_0)^T,$$

which is a nonsingular matrix. Let us define $\lim_{n\to\infty, n_1/n\to r} \hat{H}^{-1}\hat{V}(\hat{\varsigma}) = K$. Then, by Proposition 7.3, we have the following result:

Corollary 7.4

Under H_0 defined in (7.39), $-2\log R(\hat{\varsigma}_0)/(n_1 n_2)$ converges in distribution to $\sum_{k=1}^{p} c_k \chi_{1k}^2$ where c_k's are the eigenvalues of K.

7.4.4.1 Implementation in R

We illustrate the method to carry out a multivariate test on $P_r(X < Y)$ and $P_r(W < Z)$ simultaneously in the following code. Under the null hypothesis, $\hat{\varsigma}_0 = (0.5, 0.5)^T$. The data are provided in ch7-multivariate.csv, where the data are based on distributions

$$\begin{pmatrix} \log X \\ \log W \end{pmatrix} \sim N_2\left(\begin{pmatrix} 0 \\ 0 \end{pmatrix}, \begin{pmatrix} 4 & 1.5 \\ 1.5 & 2.25 \end{pmatrix} \right), \begin{pmatrix} \log Y \\ \log Z \end{pmatrix} \sim N_2\left(\begin{pmatrix} 0 \\ 0 \end{pmatrix}, \begin{pmatrix} 1 & 0.25 \\ 0.25 & 0.25 \end{pmatrix} \right).$$

Use the following code.

```
require("mvtnorm")
#Parameter setting
normmean _ xw=c(0,0)
ncov _ xw=matrix(c(4,1.5,1.5,2.25),byrow=T,nrow=2)
normmean _ yz=c(0,0)
ncov _ yz=matrix(c(1,0.25,0.25,0.25),byrow=T,nrow=2)
#Sample sizes
n1<-n2<-100
n<-n1+n2;m<-n1*n2
#Data generation
xw=exp(rmvnorm(n=n1, mean=normmean _ xw, sigma=ncov _ xw))
yz=exp(rmvnorm(n=n2, mean=normmean _ yz, sigma=ncov _ yz))
x=xw[,1];w=xw[,2];y=yz[,1];z=yz[,2]
diffmu _ xy<-0.5  #overall mean value under H0: E(y)-E(x)
diffmu_wz<-0.5  #overall mean value under H0: E(z)-E(w)
```

Now, we obtain U-statistic kernels of $P_r(X < Y)$ (indicator_v1) and $P_r(W < Z)$ (indicator_v2) and centralized kernels by respective parameters of ς_0 (centerval1, centerval2).

```
indicator_xy=matrix(data=NA, n1, n2)
for(a in 1:n1){for(b in 1:n2){
indicator_xy[a,b]=as.numeric(x[a]<y[b])}}
indicator_wz=matrix(data=NA, n1, n2)
for(p in 1:n1){for(q in 1:n2){indicator_wz[p,q]=
as.numeric(w[p]<z[q])}}
indicator_vxy<-c(indicator_xy); indicator_vwz<-c(indicator_wz)
centerval1<-indicator_vxy-diffmu_xy;
centerval2<-indicator_vwz-diffmu_wz
```

To obtain the vector of the Lagrange multipliers, we need to optimize the function

```
fn.Lamda<-function(lamvals)
{lamval1<-lamvals[1];lamval2<-lamvals[2];
  returnval1<-(sum(centerval1/(m+lamval1*centerval1+
lamval2*centerval2)))^2
  returnval2<-(sum(centerval2/(m+lamval1*centerval1+
lamval2*centerval2)))^2
return(returnval1+returnval2)}
```

Now, we obtain $\hat{H}$.

```
Hval<-cov(cbind(centerval1,centerval2))*(m-1)/m #Ĥ
```

An initial value vector for the Lagrange multiplier is given as:

```
inilamval<-c(solve(Hval*m)%*%matrix(c(sum(centerval1),
sum(centerval2)),2)*m)
```

We use optim function that carries out the multivariate optimization.

```
awH0<-optim(inilamval,fn.Lamda)
lam1<-awH0$par[1];lam2<-awH0$par[2] #The Lagrange multiplers
```

The weights are given as:

```
wijs<-1/(m+lam1*centerval1+lam2*centerval2)
```

The ELR is as follows:

```
lr=-2*(m*log(n1)+m*log(n2)-fn1.2(wijs))
lr #e.g.
[1] 183.1258
```

To estimate Σ in Proposition 7.3, use the R code and obtain s in the Appendix. Now, we proceed

```
Sigmaval<-s
Sigma #e.g.
[,1]    [,2]
[1,] 0.0018410164 0.0007616806
[2,] 0.0007616806 0.0018919457
prefactor<-solve(Hval)%*%Sigmaval*m                              #H^-1Σ
cofs<-eigen(prefactor)$values
cofs #e.g.
[1] 81.37236 64.51757
cof1<-cofs[1]; cof2<-cofs[2]                   #eigenvalues of H^-1Σ
```

Now, the p-value is calculated based on simulation.

```
psim<-cof1*rchisq(50000,1)+cof2*rchisq(50000,1)
mean((psim>lr)*1) #approximated p-value #e.g.
[1] 0.28242
```

Since the p-value is based on simulation, p-value will be slightly different for each simulation; however, readers should obtain the very close value to 0.28.

7.4.4.2 Comments on the Performance of the Empirical Likelihood Ratio Statistics

Yu et al. (2016) compared the ELR test statistics with other methods through an extensive Monte Carlo study. The EL test for the AUC under the ROC curve in Corollary 7.1 was compared to the method by Qin and Zhou (2006), jackknife EL method (2009), and the normal approximation based on Sen's variance estimator (1967). The EL test for the AUC was consistently more robust toward maintaining the specified Type I error (TIE) rates in decision making under various circumstances, whereas other compared methods have inflated TIE rates. The TIE rate control is particularly important in the nonparametric setting where various underlying distributions are possible and generally unknown in real data analysis. The EL test to compare two correlated ROC curves in Corollary 7.2 was compared to the normal approximation approach by DeLong et al. (1988). Overall, both the normal approximation and the EL test show reasonable TIE rate control in many of the considered cases; however, the EL test maintains the nominal TIEs across different values of AUC better than the other approach. The power of the proposed method responds well when sample sizes are increased and is comparable to the normal approximation method. The robust characteristic of the EL test in terms of TIE rates control is shown with the two-group survival analysis test in Corollary 7.3 as well. Overall, the performance of the proposed method is similar to that of Gehan's test, that is, both Gehan's test and the proposed method show comparable TIE rate control and comparable values for power. The multivariate extension of the Wilcoxon–Mann–Whitney test in Corollary 7.4 also showed the robustness in the TIE rate control even with relatively small sample sizes (e.g., $n_1 = 20$, $n_2 = 20$), when it was compared to a test statistic based on the normal theory, that is, $(\hat{\varsigma} - \varsigma_0)^T \hat{V}(\hat{\varsigma})^{-1}(\hat{\varsigma} - \varsigma_0) \sim \chi_2^2$.

7.5 An Application to Crossover Designs

In this section, we demonstrate the diverse applicability of the proposed methods by applying the proposed approach to data analyses in the context of crossover designs. Crossover designs are commonly used in areas with outcomes that evaluate responses with relatively short-term effects and chronic conditions. To name a few, we observe that crossover designs are used to study pharmacokinetic parameters (e.g., Milán-Segovia et al., 2014), performance of cognitive tasks (e.g., finger tapping in Wylie et al., 2013), and air quality improvement (Rosbach et al., 2013). We note that the crossover designs may have a methodological limitation in handling the long-term carryover effect. More detailed discussions are found in Fleiss (1989) and Senn (2006).

Although crossover designs are commonly used in bioequivalence studies based on pharmacokinetic parameters, the results derived under normality assumptions can be affected by some outlying observations, which in turn may lead to incorrect decisions regarding the bioequivalence of two or more agents (Huang and Ke, 2013). Herein, we apply the methods previously explained to the 2×2 crossover design and the 2×2 crossover design with baseline and washout period data. The washout period is defined to be the time between treatment periods to remove the carryover effects from the previous treatment (Jung and Koch, 1999).

We use the peak heart rate data analyzed by Jung and Koch (1999). The peak heart rate data are based on a study comparing a novel treatment (say B) and an active control (say A) for patients with ventricular arrhythmia and organic heart disease. In the study, a total of 20 patients were randomly assigned to the two sequence groups (9 in the A:B group and 11 in the B:A group). The response variable in the dataset was the peak heart rate during the bicycle exercise test in four different periods (baseline, first treatment, washout, and second treatment). We note that the sample size may not be sufficiently large; however, we use this dataset for the purpose of demonstrating that the proposed methods can be easily adapted for diverse sets of hypothesis tests. The data found in Jung and Koch (1999) are recorded in ch7-crossover.txt for readers. Simply copy and execute on R's console.

The 2×2 crossover design (Grizzle, 1965) compares two treatments in the form of two different sequences (A:B and B:A) during two periods. Let Y_{ijk} be the outcome variable where subscript i is 1 for the sequence A:B and 2 for the sequence B:A, subscript j is for the period (1 or 2), and subscript k indicates independent subjects. Using the similar notations of Kenward and Jones (1987), the response in the 2×2 crossover design is expressed as:

$$\begin{aligned} Y_{11k} &= \mu - \gamma + \pi_1 - \tau + \varepsilon_{11k}, Y_{21k} = \mu + \gamma + \pi_1 + \tau + \varepsilon_{21k}, \\ Y_{12k} &= \mu - \gamma + \pi_2 + \tau - \theta + \varepsilon_{12k}, Y_{22k} = \mu + \gamma + \pi_2 - \tau + \theta + \varepsilon_{22k}, \end{aligned} \tag{7.41}$$

where μ, γ, π_j, τ, and θ are the overall mean, the sequence effect, the j-th period effect (where $\pi_1 + \pi_2 = 0$), the treatment effect, and the carryover effect, respectively, and ε_{ijk} is an independent random effect with a mean of 0 and the same distribution within the sequence i and period j. For notational ease, let $Y_{ijk} \sim Y_{ij}$. In case of an equal carryover effect (including a case of no carryover effect) between the two sequences, θ is 0 as π_2 can replace the carryover effect in such cases. The standard procedure of hypothesis testing consists of two steps:

Step 1: Test the carryover effect.

Step 2: If the carryover effect is significant at the first step, the treatment effect is tested based only on the outcomes of the first period. Otherwise, the treatment effect is tested based on the outcomes of all periods.

The *relative effect* between two groups can be defined by a probability $P_r(Z_i > Z_j)$, where Z_i indicates the outcome variable from Group i (Schacht et al., 2008). No difference between the two treatment groups is expressed by $P_r(Z_i > Z_j) = 0.5$, which is the null hypothesis of the Wilcoxon–Mann–Whitney test (Wilcoxon, 1945; Mann and Whitney, 1947). In the crossover design, the treatment effects are tested based on contrasts of Y_{ij}'s (e.g., Jung and Koch, 1999).

For the first step, the carryover effect is commonly tested based on the null hypothesis $H_0 : E(Y_{11} + Y_{12}) = E(Y_{21} + Y_{22})$ or $H_0 : E(Y_{11} - Y_{21}) = E(Y_{22} - Y_{12})$, which can be interpreted that the relative effect between Y_{11} and Y_{21} is same as that between Y_{22} and Y_{12}. In this spirit, a null hypothesis can be rewritten as

$$H_0 : P_r(Y_{11} > Y_{21}) = P_r(Y_{22} > Y_{12}), \tag{7.42}$$

based on the definition of the relative effect. The hypothesis in (7.42) can be tested by the direct application of Corollary 7.2, which tests two correlated cases. We note that, as there are many tied values to calculate $I(Y_{ijk} > Y_{i'j'k'})$ in the peak heart rate dataset, the value of 0.5 is assigned in cases of tied values, and the variances are estimated accordingly. See the Appendix for the tied value treatment.

For the second step, on the decision of no carryover effect, we look into the treatment effect in both periods. The null hypothesis to indicate no relative treatment effect in either of the two periods is

$$H_0 : P_r(Y_{11} > Y_{21}) = 0.5 \text{ and } P_r(Y_{12} > Y_{22}) = 0.5. \quad (7.43)$$

On the other hand, upon deciding the existence of the carryover effect, the treatment effect is tested based only on the first period as

$$H_0 : P_r(Y_{11} > Y_{21}) = 0.5. \quad (7.44)$$

Both the hypotheses (7.43) and (7.44) are tested by the direct application of Corollary 7.4.

Based on the peak heart rate dataset from the first and second treatment periods, the estimated values of $P_r(Y_{11} > Y_{21})$ and $P_r(Y_{22} > Y_{12})$ are 0.732 and 0.899, respectively. The test statistic to test the carryover effect has the value of 1.0889 (p-value = 0.297 based on the χ_1^2 distribution), indicating no strong evidence of the carryover effect. Thus, we test the treatment effect based on the hypothesis (7.43) as the next step. The estimated values of $P_r(Y_{11} > Y_{21})$ and $P_r(Y_{12} > Y_{22})$ are 0.727 and 0.101, respectively, showing sizable deviations from the probability 0.5 in the both periods. The log-likelihood ratio statistic $-2\log R(\varsigma_0)$ in Corollary 7.4 is 929.538, and the corresponding Monte Carlo p-value based on the estimated variances (i.e., $\hat{H}$ and $\hat{V}(\hat{\varsigma})$) is smaller than 0.0001, strongly indicating a treatment difference. We note for readers that there are some discussions related to keeping the size of the overall test under the nominal value (Freeman, 1989; Senn, 2006) for this multiple testing scheme in the crossover designs, although it may not be a specific interest of this chapter as our analysis example is more toward illustrating the testing methodology.

Now let us consider the 2 × 2 crossover design with baseline and washout periods. Herein, we follow the analytical scheme of Kenward and Jones (1987) to illustrate how hypothesis tests can be carried out using the proposed methods. We note that some discussions indicate that the usage of differences between baseline and treatment outcomes may decrease the study power in some cases (Senn, 2006). Nevertheless, it is also common that the change from the baseline is of specific interest in many studies (e.g., Guzman et al., 2014). In such cases, it may be more desirable to use the differences themselves as outcome variables. Due to the baseline and washout periods, besides the responses in (7.41), we have additional observations as

$$X_{11k} = \mu - \gamma + \pi_b + \varepsilon_{1bk}, \; X_{21k} = \mu + \gamma + \pi_b + \varepsilon_{2bk},$$

$$X_{12k} = \mu - \gamma + \pi_w - \lambda + \varepsilon_{1wk}, \; X_{22k} = \mu + \gamma + \pi_w + \lambda + \varepsilon_{2wk},$$

where the subscripts b and w indicate the effects in baseline and washout periods, λ indicates the first-order carryover effect, and $\sum_{i\in\{1,2,b,w\}}\pi_i = 0$. Note that Jung and Koch (1999) considered $\gamma = 0$ in their analysis. The value θ in the responses (7.41) now indicates the second-order carryover effect. Three steps of tests are now the part of our testing procedure: (1) the first-order carryover effect, (2) the second-order carryover effect, and (3) the treatment effect. The ordinary least squares estimator of the first-order carryover effect has the structure of the contrast of the observations, $\{X_{11} - X_{21} - (X_{12} - X_{22})\}/2$, which allows us to test the null hypothesis $H_0 : \lambda = 0$ (Kenward and Jones, 1987). This contrast can be interpreted as comparing the relative effect between X_{11} and X_{21} and that between X_{12} and X_{22}. Thus, the null hypothesis can be rewritten as

$$H_0 : P_r(X_{11} > X_{21}) = P_r(X_{12} > X_{22}), \tag{7.45}$$

which can be tested by the direct application of Corollary 7.2. When we fail to reject the hypothesis (7.45), the second-order carry-over effect is tested as the next step. Let us define $Z_{ij} = Y_{ij} - X_{ij}$, the difference between the treatment and baseline (or washout) for the respective sequence group i and period j. The second-order carryover effect is tested based on the contrast of the observations, $\{Z_{11} - Z_{21} - (Z_{22} - Z_{12})\}/2$, which is indeed the estimator of the treatment-by-period interaction (Kenward and Jones, 1987). The corresponding null hypothesis can be rewritten as

$$H_0 : P_r(Z_{11} > Z_{21}) = P_r(Z_{22} > Z_{12}), \tag{7.46}$$

which is equivalent to $H_0 : \theta = 0$ (θ indicates the second carryover effect), and can be tested by an application of Corollary 7.2. Upon deciding that there is no carryover effect, the treatment effect is suggested to be tested based on the hypothesis (7.43). If either (7.45) or (7.46) is rejected, the test is based on the first period only as

$$H_0 : P_r(Z_{11} > Z_{21}) = 0.5.$$

For the heart peak dataset, the estimated values of $P_r(X_{11} > X_{21})$ and $P_r(X_{12} > X_{22})$ are exactly the same as 0.293, indicating no first-order carryover effect. The corresponding test statistic is 0 as the maximum of the EL function under H_0 is same as that under H_1. For the second-order carryover effect, the estimated values of $P_r(Z_{11} > Z_{21})$ and $P_r(Z_{22} > Z_{12})$ are 0.919 and 0.778, respectively. The test statistic is 1.196 (p-value = 0.274) indicating no strong evidence of the second-order carryover effect. Upon deciding no first or second-order carryover effect, the treatment effect is tested based on the hypothesis (7.43), which we already presented earlier.

7.6 Concluding Remarks

It was shown that U-statistics can be used as constraints in the framework of the EL approach. The limiting distributions of the considered EL likelihood ratio test statistics are weighted χ^2 distributions or combinations of weighted χ^2 distributions. It was demonstrated that the application of the proposed approach to any U-statistic type of tests can be carried out in a straightforward manner. The proposed approaches are generally more robust in TIE control than the other test statistics based on U-statistics for various situations, including a violation of exchangeability under the null hypotheses.

One reason for such robustness is that the proposed approaches are in essence based on the principle of the ratio of the EL functions, which accommodate different shapes of underlying distributions better than the normal approximation-based U-statistics that rely on symmetry of their limiting distributions. In a typical one-sample EL problem or two-sample EL problem, the Lagrange multiplier convergence rate is the inverse of the square root of the overall sample size or the sample size of one group (e.g., Qin and Zhou, 2006; Jing et al., 2009); however, in our approach for two groups, the convergence rate is based on the product of two-group sample sizes giving rise to a fast convergence (for more details, see the Appendix). Overall, the results presented in this chapter demonstrate that the EL approaches based on U-statistic constraints have workable properties and may improve the performance of traditional U-statistics approximation as shown in the examples.

Appendix

We need the following lemma for the proof of Proposition 7.2.

Lemma 7.1 (Arvesen, 1969; Lee, 1990)

1. Assume that $E|h(\mathbf{X},\mathbf{Y})|<\infty$. Then $\hat{\theta}\xrightarrow{a.s.}\theta$ as $n\to\infty$.
2. Assume that $Eh^2(\mathbf{X},\mathbf{Y})<\infty$. Suppose $\frac{n_1}{n_1+n_2}\to r$ as $n\to\infty$, where $n=n_1+n_2$, then we have $\sqrt{n}(\hat{\theta}-\theta)\xrightarrow{d}N(0,v^2)$, where $v^2=\frac{m_1^2}{r}\sigma_{1,0}^2+\frac{m_2^2}{1-r}\sigma_{0,1}^2$ as in (7.18).

Proof of Proposition 7.2

As $\min_{i,j\in S} h(\mathbf{X}_i,\mathbf{Y}_j)<\theta<\max_{i,j\in S} h(\mathbf{X}_i,\mathbf{Y}_j)$, there is a solution of λ^* that satisfies

$$\frac{1}{N}\sum_{i,j\in S}\frac{h(\mathbf{X}_i,\mathbf{Y}_j)-\theta}{1+\lambda^*(h(\mathbf{X}_i,\mathbf{Y}_j)-\theta)}=0, \quad \text{(A.7.1)}$$

where $N=\binom{n_1}{m_1}\binom{n_2}{m_2}$. Let $\psi_{ij}^c=h(\mathbf{X}_i,\mathbf{Y}_j)-\theta$. From (A.7.1), we have

$$\begin{aligned}0&=\frac{1}{N}\left|\sum_{i,j\in S}\psi_{ij}^c-\lambda^*\sum_{i,j\in S}\frac{(\psi_{ij}^c)^2}{1+\lambda^*\psi_{ij}^c}\right|\geq\frac{|\lambda^*|}{N}\sum_{i,j\in S}\frac{(\psi_{ij}^c)^2}{1+\lambda^*\psi_{ij}^c}-\left|\sum_{i,j\in S}\frac{\psi_{ij}^c}{N}\right|\\&\geq\frac{|\lambda^*|}{1+|\lambda^*|K}\left[\sum_{i,j\in S}\frac{(\psi_{ij}^c)^2}{N}\right]-\left|\sum_{i,j\in S}\frac{\psi_{ij}^c}{N}\right|,\end{aligned} \quad \text{(A.7.2)}$$

where $K=\max_{i,j}\left\{|\psi_{ij}^c|:\ i,\ j\in S\right\}$. It can be shown that $K=o(N^{1/\alpha})$ as $E(h(\mathbf{X}_i,\mathbf{Y}_j))^\alpha<\infty$ for some integer α (≥ 2) (Owen, 1991; Yuan et al., 2012).

By Lemma 7.1, the second term of the right side of Inequality (A.7.2) is $O_p(n_1^{-1/2})$, and the value inside the bracket in the first term is $O(1)$, that is, it has the upper bound less than ∞ as it is a U-statistic and $E(h(\mathbf{X}_i,\mathbf{Y}_j)-\theta)^2<\infty$. Thus, $|\lambda^*|/(1+|\lambda^*|K)=O_p(n_1^{-1/2})$, and it follows that

$$|\lambda^*|=O_p(N^{-1/2}). \quad \text{(A.7.3)}$$

Expanding (A.7.1), we have

$$0=\frac{1}{N}\sum_{i,j\in S}\psi_{ij}^c-\frac{\lambda^*}{N}\sum_{i,j\in S}(\psi_{ij}^c)^2+\frac{(\lambda^*)^2}{N}\sum_{i,j\in S}\frac{(\psi_{ij}^c)^3}{1+\lambda^*\psi_{ij}^c} \quad \text{(A.7.4)}$$

Note $\max_{i,j}\left\{\lambda^*|\psi_{ij}^c|\right\}=O_p(N^{-1/2})o(N^{1/\alpha})=o_p(1)$ for $\alpha\geq 2$. And,

$$\sum_{i,j\in S}\frac{(\psi_{ij}^c)^3}{N}\leq K\sum_{i,j\in S}\frac{(\psi_{ij}^c)^2}{N}=o(N^{1/\alpha})O(1)=o(N^{1/\alpha}). \quad \text{(A.7.5)}$$

Thus, the last term of (A.7.4) has an order of $O_p(N^{-1})o(N^{1/\alpha})o_p(1)=o_p(N^{-1/2})$ for $\alpha\geq 2$. This leads to

$$\lambda^*=\sum_{i,j\in S}\psi_{ij}^c\Big/\sum_{i,j\in S}(\psi_{ij}^c)^2+o_p(N^{-1/2}). \quad \text{(A.7.6)}$$

Now,

$$l(\theta_0) = -2\log R(\theta_0) = -2\left[\sum_{i,j\in S}(\log w_{ij} + \log N)\right] = 2\left[\sum_{i,j\in S}\log\left\{1+\lambda^*\psi_{ij}^c\right\}\right]$$
$$= 2\left[\sum_{i,j\in S}\lambda^*\psi_{ij}^c - \frac{1}{2}\sum_{i,j\in S}\lambda^{*2}(\psi_{ij}^c)^2 + \frac{1}{3}\sum_{i,j\in S}\left|\lambda^*\right|^3\xi(\psi_{ij}^c)^3\right], \tag{A.7.7}$$

for some $\xi < \infty$, thus the last term of the bracket is $O_p(N^{-3/2})o(N^{1+1/\alpha}) = o_p(1)$ by letting $\alpha = 2$ and using (A.7.3) and (A.7.5). By (A.7.6) and (A.7.7), we have

$$-2\log R(\theta_0) = 2\cdot\frac{\left[\sum_{i,j\in S}\psi_{ij}^c\right]^2}{\sum_{i,j\in S}(\psi_{ij}^c)^2} - \frac{\left[\sum_{i,j\in S}\psi_{ij}^c\right]^2}{\sum_{i,j\in S}(\psi_{ij}^c)^2} + o_p(1) = \frac{(\hat{\theta}-\theta)^2\cdot N^2}{\sum_{i,j\in S}(\psi_{ij}^c)^2} + o_p(1).$$

Since $\sum_{i,j\in S}(\psi_{ij}^c)^2/N$ is a consistent estimator of η^2, by Lemma 7.1 and Slutsky's theorem, we have

$$-2\log R(\theta_0)\frac{\eta^2}{N\sigma^2}\xrightarrow{d}\chi_1^2,$$

where $\sigma^2 = \frac{m_1^2}{r}\sigma_{1,0}^2 + \frac{m_2^2}{1-r}\sigma_{0,1}^2$. We remark that the first term of the right-hand side of (A.7.6) multiplied by $\binom{n_1}{m_1}\binom{n_2}{m_2}$ is used for the initial value to obtain the solution of (7.26).

Proof of Proposition 7.3

The proof of Proposition 7.3 is similar to that of Proposition 7.2, thus we only give an outline in the following scheme. Let $K = \max_{i,j}\{|d^T\psi_{ij}^c| : i, j\in S\}$ for a fixed vector d. As $E|d^Th(\mathbf{X},\mathbf{Y})|^\alpha < \infty$, $K = o(N^{1/\alpha})$ for some integer $\alpha(\geq 2)$ (Owen, 1991; Yuan et al., 2012). Similarlly to (A.7.2), we expand $1/N|\sum_{i,j\in S}d^T\psi_{ij}^c/1+\lambda^*\psi_{ij}^c|$, which leads to $\|\lambda^*\| = O_p(N^{-1/2})$. Also, expanding the left-hand side of (7.29) similarly to (A.7.4) and solving for λ^*, we have $\lambda^* = \left(\sum_{i,j\in S}\psi_{ij}^c\psi_{ij}^{c\,T}\right)^{-1}\sum_{i,j\in S}\psi_{ij}^c + o_p(N^{-1/2})$. Expanding $l(\theta_0)$ in (7.28) similarly to (A.7.7), plugging λ^*, and using $\|\lambda^*\| = O_p(N^{-1/2})$, we have that $l(\theta_0)$ asymptotically has the form

$$N\left(\sum_{i,j\in S}\psi_{ij}^c/N\right)^T\Sigma^{-1/2}\Sigma^{1/2}\left(\sum_{i,j\in S}\psi_{ij}^c\psi_{ij}^{c\,T}/N\right)^{-1}\Sigma^{1/2}\Sigma^{-1/2}\left(\sum_{i,j\in S}\psi_{ij}^c/N\right),$$

where $\sum_{i,j\in S}\psi_{ij}^{c}\psi_{ij}^{c\,T}/N$ is the unbiased U-statistic of H and $\sum^{-1/2}\left(\sum_{i,j\in S}\psi_{ij}^{c}/N\right)$ has q-variate multinormal distribution $N_q(0,I)$. Thus, the desired result follows.

R Code When w_{ij} Is Not Positive in Section 7.4.1

The following is the optimization to obtain λ:

```
lamval<-optimize(fn.Lamda,interval=c((inilamval-1*abs(inilamval)),
(inilamval+1*abs(inilamval))),maximum=FALSE)$minimum
wijs<-1/(m+lamval*centerval)
```

In the following, the code is written to look for a new λ.

```
if(length(wijs[wijs<=0])>0){
  xxxx<-matrix(seq((lamval-1*abs(lamval)),
  (lamval+1*abs(lamval)),0.1),1)
  yyyy<-apply(xxxx,2,fn.Lamda)
  posit<-match(min(yyyy),yyyy)
  inilamval2<-xxxx[posit]
  lamval<-optimize(fn.Lamda,interval=c((inilamval2-0.2),
(inilamval2+0.2)),maximum=FALSE)$minimum
  wijs<-1/(m+lamval*centerval)
     if(length(wijs[wijs<=0])>0){
    xxxx<-matrix(seq((inilamval-1*abs(inilamval)),(inilamval),
0.01),1)
    yyyy<-apply(xxxx,2,fn.Lamda)
    posit<-match(min(yyyy),yyyy)
    inilamval2<-xxxx[posit]
    lamval<-optimize(fn.Lamda,interval=c((inilamval2-0.02),
(inilamval2+0.02)),maximum=FALSE)$minimum
    wijs<-1/(m+lamval*centerval)}}
```

R Code to Obtain $\hat{V}(\hat{\delta})$ and $\sum_{i=1}^{n_1}\sum_{j=1}^{n_2}(\phi_{12_{ij}}-\phi_{34_{ij}}-\delta_0)^2/\{(n_1n_2)^2\hat{V}(\hat{\delta})\}$ in Section 7.4.2.

You can use this code to estimate Σ (s) in Section 7.4.4, as well

```
auc_xy<-mean(indicator_vxy); auc_wz<-mean(indicator_vwz)
v10_x=apply(indicator_xy,1,mean)
v01_y=apply(indicator_xy,2,mean)
v10_w=apply(indicator_wz,1,mean)
v01_z=apply(indicator_wz,2,mean)
s10_12=sum((v10_x-auc_xy)*(v10_w-auc_wz))/(n1-1)
s10_11=sum((v10_x-auc_xy)^2)/(n1-1)
s10_22=sum((v10_w-auc_wz)^2)/(n1-1)
s01_12=sum((v01_y-auc_xy)*(v01_z-auc_wz))/(n2-1)
```

```
s01_11=sum((v01_y-auc_xy)^2)/(n2-1)
s01_22=sum((v01_z-auc_wz)^2)/(n2-1)
s<-matrix(c(s10_11,s10_12,s10_12,s10_22),nrow=2,ncol=2,
byrow=T)/n1+matrix(c(s01_11,s01_12,s01_12,s01_22),nrow=2,
ncol=2,byrow=T)/n2
v=matrix(c(1,-1),nrow=1)%*%s%*%t(matrix(c(1,-1),nrow=1))  #V̂(δ̂)
sum_phi=sum((centerval)^2)
factor1=(v*m^2)/sum_phi                  #∑_{i=1}^{n1} ∑_{j=1}^{n2}(φ_{12ij} − φ_{34ij} − δ_0)^2/{(n1n2)^2 V̂_k(δ̂)}
```

Tied Values Treatment to Estimate *P*(*Y*>*X*)

```
indicators<-matrix(data=NA, n1, n2)
for(u in 1:n1){for(z in 1:n2){
 indicators[u,z]<-as.numeric(x[u]<y[z])
 if(x[u]==y[z])indicators[u,z]<-0.5 }}
```

8

Empirical Likelihood Application to Receiver Operating Characteristic Curve Analysis

8.1 Introduction

In this chapter, we introduce the empirical likelihood (EL) application to receiver operating characteristic (ROC) curve analysis. Based on the fact that the nonparametric estimator of the area under the ROC curve (AUC) has a form of the U-statistic, the material introduced in Chapter 7 will be applied for constructing the corresponding EL statistics. As discussed previously, the main task of constructing the EL statistic is to incorporate the correct variance estimate to the EL statistic. In this context, we further discuss estimation of the variance of the U-statistic type estimator of the partial area under the ROC curve (pAUC) to construct the corresponding EL statistic, where a typical variance formula for U-statistics (e.g., Sen, 1967) is inaccurate to estimate the variability of the pAUC estimator up to the point that the inference based on the estimate is impractical.

ROC curve analysis is a popular tool for visualizing, organizing, and selecting classifiers based on their classification accuracy. The methodology has been extensively adapted to medical areas that are heavily dependent on screening and diagnostic tests (Lloyd, 1998; Pepe and Thompson, 2000; Zhou, Mcclish and Obuchowski, 2009; Pepe, 2003; Ma and Huang, 2005; Ma and Huang, 2007; Pepe et al., 2006). The area under the ROC curve for a biomarker has an interpretation as the sensitivities corresponding to the respective specificities allowing treating false positives and false negatives in an efficient and relatively simple manner. A large area under the ROC curve is a result of generally high sensitivity over the range of the specificity value, indicating a good classification ability of the biomarker. ROC-based methods are handedly used to evaluate the various diagnostic tools. For example, based on the retrospective study, the carotid artery stenting scoring system called Buffalo Risk Assessment Scale (BRASS) was devised to predict complications risk in symptomatic patients undergoing the stenting, where the best scoring system among many combinations of score items was selected comparing the area under ROC curves (Fanous et al., 2015).

In health-related studies, the ROC curve methodology is commonly related to case-control studies. As a type of observational study, case-control studies differentiate and compare two existing groups differing in outcome on the basis of some causal attributes. For example, based on factors that may contribute to a medical condition, subjects can be grouped as cases (subjects with a condition/disease) and controls (subjects without the condition/disease), e.g., cases could be subjects with breast cancer and controls may be health subjects. For independent populations, various parametric and nonparametric approaches have been proposed to evaluate the performance of biomarkers (Bamber, 1975; Wieand et al., 1989; Hsieh and Turnbull, 1996; Pepe, 1997; Metz et al., 1998; Pepe and Thompson, 2000; McIntosh and Pepe, 2002).

8.2 Receiver Operating Characteristic Curve

Assume that $X_1,\ldots,X_{n_1}$ and $Y_1,\ldots,Y_{n_2}$ are independent identically distributed (i.i.d.) observations from nondiseased and diseased populations, respectively, and let F and G denote the corresponding cumulative distribution functions of X and Y. The ROC curve $R(t)$ is defined as $R(t)=1-G(F^{-1}(1-t))$, where $t\in[0,1]$ (Pepe, 1997). The ROC curve is a plot of sensitivity (true positive rate, $1-G(t)$) against 1 minus specificity (true negative rate, $1-F(t)$) for various values of the threshold t. Note that the ROC curve is a special case of a probability–probability plot (P–P plot). As an example, we consider three biomarkers with their corresponding ROC curves presented in Figure 8.1, whose underlying distributions are $F_1\sim N(0,1)$, $G_1\sim N(0,1)$ for biomarker A (the diagonal line); $F_2\sim N(0,1)$, $G_2\sim N(1,1)$ for biomarker B (in a dashed line); and $F_3\sim N(0,1)$, $G_3\sim N(10,1)$ for biomarker C (in a dotted line), respectively.

It can be seen that farther apart the two distributions F and G are in terms of location, the more the ROC curve shifts to the top-left corner. A near perfect biomarker would have an ROC curve coming close to the top-left corner, and a biomarker without any discriminability would result in a ROC curve that is a diagonal line from the points (0,0) to (1,1).

There exists extensive research on estimating ROC curves from the parametric and nonparametric perspectives (Wieand et al., 1989; Hsieh and Turnbull, 1996; Pepe, 1997). Assuming both the nondiseased and diseased populations are normally distributed, that is, $F\sim N(\mu_1,\sigma_1^2)$ and $G\sim N(\mu_2,\sigma_2^2)$, the corresponding ROC curve can be expressed as

$$R(t)=\Phi(a+b\Phi^{-1}(t)),$$

where $a=(\mu_2-\mu_1)/\sigma_2$, $b=\sigma_1/\sigma_2$, and Φ is the standard normal cumulative distribution function. This is oftentimes referred to as the binormal

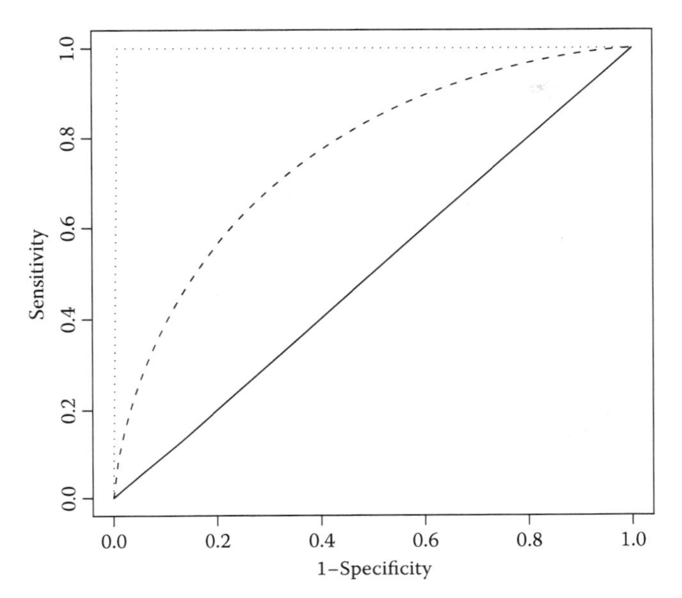

FIGURE 8.1
The ROC curves related to the biomarkers. The solid diagonal line corresponds to the ROC curve of biomarker A, where $F_1 \sim N(0,1)$ and $G_1 \sim N(0,1)$. The dashed line displays the ROC curve of biomarker B, where $F_2 \sim N(0,1)$ and $G_2 \sim N(1,1)$. The dotted line close to the upper left corner plots the ROC curve for biomarker C, where $F_3 \sim N(0,1)$ and $G_3 \sim N(10,1)$.

ROC curve. The estimated ROC curve can be obtained by substituting the maximum likelihood estimators (MLE) of the normal parameters μ_1, μ_2, σ_1, and σ_2 into the formula above. The nonparametric estimation of the ROC curve incorporates empirical distribution functions (Wieand et al., 1989; Hsieh and Turnbull, 1996) in place of their parametric counterparts. Toward this end, define the empirical distribution function of F as

$$\hat{F}_{n_1}(t) = \frac{1}{n_1}\sum_{i=1}^{n_1} I\{X_i \le t\},$$

where $I\{\cdot\}$ denotes the indicator function. The empirical distribution function $\hat{G}_{n_2}$ of G can be defined similarly. Estimating F and G by their corresponding empirical estimates $\hat{F}_{n_1}$ and $\hat{G}_{n_2}$, respectively, gives the empirical estimator of the ROC curve as

$$\hat{R}(t) = 1 - \hat{G}_{n2}(\hat{F}_{n1}^{-1}(1-t)),$$

which can be shown theoretically to converge to $R(t)$ for large sample sizes (Hsieh and Turnbull, 1996).

8.3 Area under the Receiver Operating Characteristic Curve

The area under the ROC curve (AUC) is a common summary index of the diagnostic accuracy of a binary biomarker. The AUC measures the ability of the marker to discriminate between the case and control groups (Pepe and Thompson, 2000; McIntosh and Pepe, 2002). By the definition of the AUC (the area under the ROC curve) and the fact that F and G are distribution functions of X and Y, respectively, the AUC can be expressed as

$$\int_0^1 R(t)dt = \int_0^1 (1-G(F^{-1}(1-t))dt = \int_{-\infty}^{\infty} (1-G(w))dF(w)$$

$$= 1 - \int_{-\infty}^{\infty} G(w)dF(w) = 1 - \Pr(Y \le X) = \Pr(Y > X).$$

Values of the AUC can range from 0.5, in the case of no differentiation between the case and control distributions, to 1, where the case and control distributions are perfectly separated.

Under binormal assumptions, where for the nondiseased population $X \sim N(\mu_1, \sigma_1^2)$ and for the diseased population $Y \sim N(\mu_2, \sigma_2^2)$, we can express the AUC (Wieand et al., 1989) as

$$A = \Pr(Y > X) = \Pr(Y - X > 0) = 1 - \Pr\left\{ \frac{(Y-X)-(\mu_2-\mu_1)}{\sqrt{\sigma_1^2+\sigma_2^2}} \le -\frac{\mu_2-\mu_1}{\sqrt{\sigma_1^2+\sigma_2^2}} \right\}$$

$$= 1 - \Phi\left(-\frac{\mu_2-\mu_1}{\sqrt{\sigma_1^2+\sigma_2^2}} \right) = \Phi\left(\frac{\mu_2-\mu_1}{\sqrt{\sigma_1^2+\sigma_2^2}} \right).$$

The index $A \ge 0.5$, when $\mu_2 \ge \mu_1$. By substituting MLEs for μ_i and σ_i^2, $i = 1,2$ into the above formula, the MLE of the AUC can be obtained directly. Given the estimator of the AUC under binormal distributional assumptions, one can easily construct large-sample confidence interval-based tests for the AUC using the delta method; see Kotz et al. (2003) for details. For nonnormal data a transformation of observations to normality may first be applied, e.g., the Box–Cox transformation (Box and Cox, 1964), prior to the parametric ROC approach being applied.

As we have seen in Chapter 7, a nonparametric estimator for the AUC can be obtained as

$$\hat{A} = \frac{1}{n_1 n_2} \sum_{i=1}^{n_1} \sum_{j=1}^{n_2} I(Y_j > X_i),$$

where $X_i, i=1,\ldots,n_1$ and $Y_j, j=1,\ldots,n_2$ are the observations for nondiseased and diseased populations, respectively (Zhou et al., 2002). It is equivalent to the well-known Mann–Whitney statistic, and the variance of this empirical estimator can be obtained using U-statistic theory (Serfling, 1980) as we have seen in Chapter 7. In Chapter 7, we have also discussed how to apply the EL method, where the resulting empirical likelihood ratio (ELR) statistic has the weighted χ_1^2 distribution. The EL method can be employed in a slightly different aspect using the approach by Qin and Zhou (2006) where the AUC is considered as the sample mean of *placement value*. Replacing the indicator function by a kernel function, one can also obtain a smoothed ROC curve (Zou et al., 1997). These techniques are explained in detail in Section 8.5.

8.4 Nonparametric Comparison of Two Receiver Operating Characteristic Curves

It is oftentimes of great importance for researchers to compare the discriminating ability of two biomarkers or even different diagnostic tests. If we use both diagnostic markers on the same n_1 controls and n_2 cases, we can represent the bivariate outcomes as $(X_{1j}, X_{2j})(j=1,\ldots,n_1)$ and $(Y_{1k}, Y_{2k})(k=1,\ldots,n_2)$, respectively. We denote the respective bivariate distributions as $F(x_1, x_2)$ and $G(y_1, y_2)$ and the marginal distributions as $F_i(x_i)$ and $G_i(y_i)$, $i=1,2$, respectively, and we assume that the n_1+n_2 bivariate vectors are mutually independent. Denote the sensitivity value on the ROC curve at specificity p by $S_i(p)$, $i=1,2$ (i.e., $S_i(p)=1-G_i\{F_i^{-1}(p)\}$), and define

$$\Delta = \int (S_1(p)-S_2(p))dW(p),$$

where W is a probability measure on the open unit interval. The parameter Δ allows one to compare sensitivities on a predefined range of specificities of clinical interest by adjusting the weight function W accordingly. When $W(p)$ is the uniform distribution on (0,1), the parameter Δ equals the difference of AUCs between two biomarkers. Wieand et al. (1989) considered a nonparametric estimate of Δ in the form of

$$\hat{\Delta} = \int (\hat{S}_1(p)-\hat{S}_2(p))dW(p),$$

where $\hat{S}_i(p)=1-\hat{G}_i(\hat{\xi}_{ip})$, $\hat{G}_i$ is the empirical distribution of G_i, and the sample quantile $\hat{\xi}_{ip}$ is the $[n_1 p]$-th order statistic among the n_1 values of X_i, where $[n_1p]$ is the smallest integer that equals or exceeds n_1p. When W is the uniform(0,1),

$$\hat{\Delta} = \int \{\hat{S}_2(p) - \hat{S}_1(p)\}dp = \frac{1}{n_1 n_2}\sum_k \sum_j \{I(Y_{2k} > X_{2j}) - I(Y_{1k} > X_{1j})\}. \quad (8.1)$$

Assume that W is a probability measure in $(0,1)$ and that there exists $\varepsilon > 0$ such that W has a bounded derivative in $(0,\varepsilon)$ and $(1-\varepsilon,1)$. Suppose further that $G_i(\xi_{ip})$, for $i = 1,2$, has continuous derivatives in $(0,1)$, which are monotone in $(0,\varepsilon)$ and $(1-\varepsilon,1)$. Define $s_i(p) = S_i'(p) = -G_i'(\xi_{ip})/F_i'(\xi_{ip})$ according to Wieand et al. (1989). Then, as $N = n_1 + n_2$ tends to ∞ with $n_1/N \to \lambda$, for $0 < \lambda < 1$, $N^{1/2}(\hat{\Delta} - \Delta)$ tends to a normal distribution with a generic form of the variance $\sigma^2 = \sigma_{11} - 2\sigma_{12} + \sigma_{22}$, where

$$\sigma_{ii} = \int_0^1 \int_0^1 \{(1-\lambda)^{-1} S_i(\max(p,q))(1 - S_i(\min(p,q)))$$
$$+ \lambda^{-1} s_i(p) s_i(q)(\min(p,q) - pq)\} dW(p) dW(q),$$

and

$$\sigma_{12} = (1-\lambda)^{-1} \int\int (G(\xi_{1p}, \xi_{2q})) - (1 - S_1(p))(1 - S_2(q)) dW(p) dW(q)$$
$$+ \lambda^{-1} \int\int (G(\xi_{1p}, \xi_{2q}) - pq) s_1(p) s_2(q) dW(p) dW(q).$$

Based on this asymptotic distribution of $\hat{\Delta}$, one can employ a nonparametric procedure for testing $H_0 : \Delta = 0$ versus $H_1 : \Delta > 0$. Wieand et al. (1989) showed that σ^2 is asymptotically equivalent to the variance formula provided by DeLong et al. (1988).

The expression (8.1) is comparing the nonparametric AUC estimates for two correlated biomarkers. As we have seen in Chapter 7, the relevant ELR statistic is obtained using the EL for the U-statistic. Also, the method by Qin and Zhou (2006) can be used, which is adapted to some extent in the following discussion with the best linear combinations (BLCs) of biomarkers.

8.5 Best Combinations Based on Values of Multiple Biomarkers

In practice, different biomarkers' levels are usually associated with disease in various magnitudes and in different directions. For example, low levels of high-density lipoprotein (HDL)-cholesterol and high levels of thiobarbuturic acid reacting substances (TBARS), biomarkers of oxidative stress and antioxidant status, are indicators of coronary heart disease (Schisterman et al., 2001). When multiple biomarkers are available, it is of great interest to seek a combination of biomarkers to improve diagnostic accuracy (Liu et al., 2011). Due to the simplicity in practical applications, we will attend the BLC of biomarkers, such that the combined score achieves the maximum AUC or the maximum treatment effect over all possible linear combinations. Consider a study with d continuous-scale biomarkers yielding measurements $\mathbf{X}_i = (X_{1i}, ..., X_{di})^T$, $i = 1, ..., n$, on n diseased patients, and measurements $\mathbf{Y}_j = (Y_{1j}, ..., Y_{dj})^T$, $j = 1, ..., m$, on m nondiseased patients, respectively. It is of interest to construct effective one-dimensional combined scores of biomarkers' measurements, that is, $X(\mathbf{a}) = \mathbf{a}^T\mathbf{X}$ and $Y(\mathbf{a}) = \mathbf{a}^T\mathbf{Y}$, such that the AUC based on these scores is maximized over all possible linear combinations of biomarkers. Define $A(\mathbf{a}) = \Pr(X(\mathbf{a}) > Y(\mathbf{a}))$; the statistical problem is to estimate the maximum AUC defined as $A = A(\mathbf{a}_0)$, where the vector $\mathbf{a}_0$ consists of the BLC coefficients satisfying $\mathbf{a}_0 = \arg\max_{\mathbf{a}} A(\mathbf{a})$.

In a parametric approach, assuming $\mathbf{X}_i \sim N(\mu_X, \Sigma_X)$, $i = 1, \ldots, n$, and $\mathbf{Y}_j \sim N(\mu_Y, \Sigma_Y)$, $j = 1, \ldots, m$, Su and Liu (1993) derived the BLC coefficients $\mathbf{a}_0 \propto \Sigma_C^{-1}\boldsymbol{\mu}$ and the corresponding optimal AUC as $\Phi(\omega^{1/2})$, where $\mu = \mu_X - \mu_Y$, $\Sigma_C = \Sigma_X + \Sigma_Y$, $\omega = \boldsymbol{\mu}^T\Sigma_C^{-1}\boldsymbol{\mu}$, and Φ is the standard normal cumulative distribution function. Based on Su and Liu's point estimator, we can derive the confidence interval estimation for the BLC-based AUC under multivariate normality assumptions (Reiser and Faraggi, 1997).

Chen et al. (2015) proposed using kernels to construct the EL-based confidence interval estimation for the BLC-based AUC, via construction of the ELR test statistic for testing the hypothesis $H_0 : A = A_0$ versus $H_1 : A \neq A_0$. In their approach they used the relationship (Qin and Zhou, 2006)

$$E_X\{1 - \bar{F}_Y(X)\} = Pr(X \geq Y),$$

where X and Y are the random variables corresponding to disease and nondiseased groups, respectively, and $\bar{F}_Y$ is the survival function of Y. The quantity $1 - \bar{F}_Y(X)$ is called placement value in Qin and Zhou (2006). Now, let k be a symmetric kernel function and define $K_h(x) = \int_{-\infty}^{x/h} k(u)du$, $v_i(\mathbf{a}) = m^{-1}\sum_{j=1}^{m} K_h(\mathbf{a}^T\mathbf{X}_i - \mathbf{a}^T\mathbf{Y}_j)$, $i = 1, ..., n$, where h is the bandwidth parameter. The value $v_i(\mathbf{a})$ provides the estimated survival function of $\mathbf{a}^T\mathbf{X}_i$ greater than $\mathbf{a}^T\mathbf{Y}_j$. Regarding the kernel estimation, we refer the reader to the textbook of Silverman (1986). Let $\mathbf{p} = (p_1, p_2, ..., p_n)^T$ be a probability weight vector, $\sum_{i=1}^{n} p_i = 1$ and $p_i \geq 0$ for all $i = 1, ..., n$. The EL for the BLC-based AUC evaluated at the true value A_0 of AUC can be defined as

$$L(A_0) = \sup\left\{\prod_{i=1}^{n} p_i : \sum_{i=1}^{n} p_i = 1, \sum_{i=1}^{n} p_i v_i(\hat{\mathbf{a}}_0) = A_0\right\},$$

where $\hat{\mathbf{a}}_0$ satisfies $\sum_{i=1}^{n} p_i \, \partial v_i(\mathbf{a})/\partial \mathbf{a} \,\big|_{\mathbf{a}=\hat{\mathbf{a}}_0} = \mathbf{0}$. One can show (using Lagrange multipliers) that

$$p_i = \frac{1}{n} \frac{1}{1+\lambda\left(v_i(\hat{\mathbf{a}}_0) - A_0\right)}, \; i = 1,\ldots,n,$$

where the Lagrange multiplier λ is the root of

$$\frac{1}{n} \sum_{i=1}^{n} \frac{v_i(\hat{\mathbf{a}}_0)}{1+\lambda\left(v_i(\hat{\mathbf{a}}_0) - A_0\right)} = A_0.$$

Under the alternative hypothesis, we have just the constraint $\sum_{i=1}^{n} p_i = 1$, and hence $L(A_0) = (1/n)^n$ at $p_i = 1/n$. Therefore, the empirical log-likelihood ratio test statistic is

$$l(A_0) = -2\log \mathrm{ELR}(A_0) = 2\sum_{i=1}^{n} \log(1+\lambda(v_i(\hat{\mathbf{a}}_0) - A_0)).$$

We define $\hat{\mathbf{a}}_K = \arg\max_{\mathbf{a}} A_{m,n}^{K}(\mathbf{a})$, where $A_{m,n}^{K}(\mathbf{a}) = n^{-1}\sum_{i=1}^{n} v_i(\mathbf{a})$. Under some general conditions (see Chen et al., 2015 for details), the asymptotic distribution of $l(A_0)$ under $H_0 : A = A_0$ is a scaled Chi-square distribution with one degree of freedom, that is,

$$\gamma(A_0) l(A_0) \xrightarrow{d} \chi_1^2, \text{ as } n, m \to \infty,$$

where

$$\gamma(A_0) = \frac{m\hat{\sigma}^2}{(m+n)s^2}, \hat{\sigma}^2 = n^{-1}\sum_{i=1}^{n}\Big(v_i(\hat{\mathbf{a}}_K) - n^{-1}\sum_{j=1}^{n} v_j(\hat{\mathbf{a}}_K)\Big)^2, s^2 = \frac{m\hat{\sigma}_{10}^2 + n\hat{\sigma}_{01}^2}{m+n},$$

$$\sigma_{10}^2 = Cov(K_h(\mathbf{a}_0{}^T\mathbf{X}_1 - \mathbf{a}_0{}^T\mathbf{Y}_1), K_h(\mathbf{a}_0{}^T\mathbf{X}_1 - \mathbf{a}_0{}^T\mathbf{Y}_2)),$$

$$\sigma_{01}^2 = Cov(K_h(\mathbf{a}_0{}^T\mathbf{X}_1 - \mathbf{a}_0{}^T\mathbf{Y}_1), K_h(\mathbf{a}_0{}^T\mathbf{X}_2 - \mathbf{a}_0{}^T\mathbf{Y}_1)),$$

and $\hat{\sigma}_{10}^2$ and $\hat{\sigma}_{01}^2$ are the corresponding estimates of σ_{10}^2 and σ_{01}^2. This result is similar to Qin and Zhou (2006). We refer to Chen et al. (2015) for the technical details of the proof.

Based on the asymptotic distribution of the statistic $l(A_0)$, the $100(1-\alpha)\%$ empirical likelihood-based confidence interval for the maximum AUC can be constructed as

$$R_\alpha = \left\{A_0 : \gamma(A_0) l(A_0) \le \chi_1^2(1-\alpha)\right\},$$

where $\chi_1^2(1-\alpha)$ is the $(1-\alpha)$-th quantile of the Chi-square distribution with 1 degree of freedom. The following R code for the EL-based confidence interval utilizes R package `emplik`. The dataset is randomly generated in the following code:

```
require(emplik)
require("mvtnorm")
sigma1=matrix(c(3,-0.1,0.9,-0.1,1.2,1.3,0.9,1.3,5),3,3)
sigma2=matrix(c(3,-1.2,2.5,-1.2,9,3.8,2.5,3.8,6),3,3)
data.x<-rmvnorm(30, matrix(c(0,0,0),3,1), sigma1)
data.y<-rmvnorm(30, matrix(c(0,0,0),3,1), sigma2)
```

The matrices `data.x` and `data.y` contain the datasets for the diseased and nondiseased groups, respectively, where rows correspond to observations and columns correspond to biomarkers.

```
n <- nrow(data.x)
m <- nrow(data.y)
h <- (m+n)^(-1/5) #define bandwidth used in Chen et al.(2015).
```

The following function produces linear combinations of the data:

```
combine<-function(data,lambda) data%*%as.vector(lambda)
```

The kernel functions are defined as

```
K.h <- function(x) pnorm (x/h,0,1)
k.h <- function(x) dnorm (x/h,0,1)/h
```

The following is the objective function $(mn)^{-1}\sum_i \sum_j K_h(\lambda^T \mathbf{X}_i - \lambda^T \mathbf{Y}_j)$ that we want to maximize by having the BLC:

```
find.lam.kernel <- function(lambda){
x.c <- combine(data.x,lambda)
y.c <- combine(data.y,lambda)
-mean(mapply(function(x) K.h(x-y.c),x.c))}
```

The following optimization provides λ estimate:

```
initial<-rep(1,ncol(data.x))          #arbitrary initial values
opt.kernel<- optim(initial,find.lam.kernel,method="BFGS")
A.kernel<- -opt.kernel$value                        #Estimate of AUC
A.kernel
[1] 0.564974
a.kernel<- opt.kernel$par                             #Estimate of λ
a.kernel
[1] -0.03135297 -1.12372221 3.19435174
```

Now, we have the BLCs based on the data as follows:

```
x.c<- combine(data.x,a.kernel)
y.c<- combine(data.y,a.kernel)
```

The function `CI.fun` produces the ELR test statistic.

```
xy.diff<- mapply(function(x) K.h(x-y.c),x.c)
vi<- apply(xy.diff,2,mean)
wj<- apply(xy.diff,1,mean)
S10<- sum((wj-mean(wj))^2)/(m-1)
S01<- sum((vi-mean(vi))^2)/(n-1)
S2<- (n*S01+m*S10)/(m+n)
alpha<-0.05; crit.val<-qchisq(1-alpha,df=1) #critical value
for 95% CI
  CI.fun<- function(AUC){
  ELR.A<- el.test(vi,AUC)
  ELR.A0<-ELR.A$`-2LLR`
  sigma2.hat<- mean((vi-AUC)^2)
  r<- m/(m+n)*sigma2.hat/S2
  ELR.A$`-2LLR`<-r*ELR.A0
  return(ELR.A)}
```

The function `findUL` from `emplik` package provides the confidence interval.

```
tmp=findUL(step=0.1,initStep=0,fun=CI.fun,MLE=A.kernel,
level=crit.val)
upper<- tmp$Up                                #CI's upper bound
lower<- tmp$Low                               #CI's lower bound
c(lower,upper)
[1] 0.4200584 0.6792192
```

8.6 Partial Area under the Receiver Operating Characteristic Curve

Recently, over-diagnosis of disease has become an increasingly important issue in the public health setting. A series of current studies warn against common medical screening practices in the general public as the practices may potentially over-diagnose a disease and may not deliver the promised benefit to the public (e.g., Loeb et al., 2014 on prostate cancer; Miller et al., 2014 on breast cancer). In this context, the partial area under the ROC curve (pAUC) investigating the ROC curve over the range of only high specificities (e.g., greater than 50%) is more appropriate than ever in the accurate evaluation of diagnostic tools, as opposed to the full area under the ROC curve (AUC) that examines the entire region of the curve. Higher specificity means a less expose to an unnecessary treatment for healthy individuals as a result of a lowered chance of misdiagnosing healthy individuals. This is particularly relevant in screening healthy populations for diseases, who have relatively low prevalence rates. High specificity will be achieved generally by setting up a stricter specificity cut point of a biomarker at the expense of lowered sensitivity rates. The pAUC (e.g., $\Pr\{Y > X > \theta\}$ for some quantile of X, θ) looks into the AUC on a limited range of specificity (or sensitivity) values (McClish, 1989; Huang et al., 2012). Dodd and Pepe (2003) proposed an estimator of the pAUC in the form of a U-statistic that incorporates the desirable range of specificity by using quantiles. In the estimate, it is necessary to estimate quantiles based on the sample, altering the covariance structures between the kernels in the U-statistic. Thus, a direct application of the common variance formula for a U-statistic (e.g., Sen, 1967) does not provide an accurate estimate of the true variance.

Herein, we first discuss the method to obtain the variance of the U-statistic estimator of the pAUC accurately. We extend the method to the case of two correlated biomarker comparisons. Then, we investigate an EL approach incorporating the proposed variance estimate, where the proposed variance estimate allows us to conveniently account for the correlations of the summand in constraints due to a *plug-in* method (Hjort et al., 2009) in the specification of the distribution of ELR statistic.

8.6.1 Alternative Expression of the pAUC Estimator for the Variance Estimation

Let X_i, $i = 1,\ldots,n_1$ be independent continuous random variables from group 1 with unknown distribution function $F(x) = \Pr\{X_i < x\}$, and let Y_i, $i = 1,\ldots,n_2$ be independent continuous random variables from group 2 with unknown distribution function $G(y) = \Pr\{Y_j < y\}$. Also, let $X_i \sim X$ and $Y_i \sim Y$. Assume that $\boldsymbol{\theta}_x = ({}^{p_1}\theta_x, {}^{p_2}\theta_x)^T$ is a vector of two true quantiles of the random variable X corresponding to the probabilities of p_1 and p_2 ($p_1 < p_2$). As the AUC of the ROC curve is $\int_0^1 \bar{G}\{\bar{F}^{-1}(t)\}dt = \Pr\{Y > X\}$, the two-sides truncated partial AUC, $P(\boldsymbol{\theta}_x)$ is expressed as $\int_{p_1}^{p_2} \bar{G}\{\bar{F}^{-1}(t)\}dt$ or

$$\Pr\{Y > X, {}^{p_1}\theta_x < X < {}^{p_2}\theta_x\} = \Pr\{Y > X > {}^{p_1}\theta_x\} - \Pr\{Y > X > {}^{p_2}\theta_x\}. \quad (8.2)$$

The corresponding U-statistic to estimate $P(\boldsymbol{\theta}_x)$ (Dodd and Pepe, 2003) is given as

$$\frac{1}{n}\left[\sum_{i=1}^{n_1}\sum_{j=1}^{n_2}\left\{I(Y_j > X_i)I(X_i > {}^{p_1}\theta_x) - I(Y_j > X_i)I(X_i > {}^{p_2}\theta_x)\right\}\right],$$

where $n = n_1 n_2$. In Definition (8.2), the pAUC is essentially a subtraction of two probabilities sharing the same structure. Hence, without loss of generality and for ease of notation, let us consider a simpler one-side truncated pAUC definition given as

$$P(\theta_x) \equiv \int_p^1 \bar{G}\{\bar{F}^{-1}(t)\}dt = \Pr\{Y > X > \theta_x\}, \tag{8.3}$$

where θ_x is the *p-th* quantile $(0 < p < 1)$ of the random variable X. Note that the quantity (8.3) has a practical interpretation as the true positive fraction (sensitivity) over a range of low false positive fraction (1-specificity) in an application to disease discrimination though a biomarker. The relevant U-statistic estimator of (8.3) is

$$\begin{aligned} P_n(\theta_x) &= \frac{1}{n}\sum\nolimits_{i=1}^{n_1}\sum\nolimits_{j=1}^{n_2} I(Y_j > X_i)I(X_i > \theta_x) \\ &\equiv \sum\nolimits_{i=1}^{n_1}\sum\nolimits_{j=1}^{n_2}\frac{1}{n}h(X_i, Y_j, \theta_x). \end{aligned} \tag{8.4}$$

The estimator $P_n(\theta_x)$ is a U-statistic with the degree of (1, 1), that is, in the summand, only one element from each group is included. Based on the theories of U-statistics (Lee, 1990), the exact variance has form

$$\mathrm{Var}(P_n(\theta_x)) = \frac{(n_2-1)\sigma_{10}^2 + (n_1-1)\sigma_{01}^2}{n_1 n_2} + \frac{\sigma_{11}^2}{n_1 n_2}, \tag{8.5}$$

where $\sigma_{10}^2 = \mathrm{Cov}(h(X_i, Y_j, \theta_x), h(X_i, Y_{j'}, \theta_x))$, $\sigma_{01}^2 = Cov(h(X_i, Y_j, \theta_x), h(X_{i'}, Y_j, \theta_x))$, and $\sigma_{11}^2 = \mathrm{Cov}(h(X_i, Y_j, \theta_x), h(X_i, Y_j, \theta_x))$ for $i \neq i'$ and $j \neq j'$ (see also Chapter 7). As, with known θ_x, $P_n(\theta_x)$ has a symmetric kernel with the degree of (1,1), the formula proposed by Sen (1967) can be directly applied as an estimate of the variance of the pAUC similar to the variance of AUC introduced in Chapter 7. Specifically, let

$$S_{10}^2 = \frac{1}{n_1 - 1}\sum_{i=1}^{n_1}\left(V_{10}(X_i) - P_n(\theta_x)\right)^2, \text{ and } S_{01}^2 = \frac{1}{n_2 - 1}\sum_{j=1}^{n_2}\left(V_{01}(Y_j) - P_n(\theta_x)\right)^2,$$

where $V_{10}(X_i) = \frac{1}{n_2}\sum_{j=1}^{n_2} h(X_i, Y_j, \theta_x)$ for $i = 1, \ldots, n_1$ and $V_{01}(Y_j) = \frac{1}{n_1}\sum_{i=1}^{n_1} h(X_i, Y_j, \theta_x)$ for $j = 1, \ldots, n_2$. Then, the estimator of (8.5) is given as

$$\hat{V}(P_n(\theta_x)) = \frac{n_1 + n_2}{n_1 n_2}\left(\frac{n_2 S_{10}^2 + n_1 S_{01}^2}{n_1 + n_2}\right). \tag{8.6}$$

The variance estimator (8.6) provides an accurate variance estimate when the value of θ_x is known. In practice, however, θ_x is unknown. Hence, let us consider the estimate of $P(\theta_x)$ given as

$$P_n(\tilde{\theta}_x) = \sum_{i=1}^{n_1} \sum_{j=1}^{n_2} \frac{1}{n} h(X_i, Y_j, \tilde{\theta}_x), \tag{8.7}$$

where $\tilde{\theta}_x$ is the *p-th* sample quantile of X. Due to the sample quantile, the statistic $P_n(\tilde{\theta}_x)$ in (8.7) does not keep the degree of $(1,1)$ strictly, and thus the variance formula (8.5) is no longer exact. To show differences of the variability of $P_n(\theta_x)$ and $P_n(\tilde{\theta}_x)$, Monte Carlo variances (5000 simulations per scenario) based on the various underlying distributions are shown in Table 8.1, where the values of θ_x are set to be the corresponding medians. The results in Table 8.1 show that the variance of $P_n(\tilde{\theta}_x)$ (simulated variance with an unknown quantile in the table) is generally much smaller than $P_n(\theta_x)$(simulated variance with a known quantile in the table). This fact may be somewhat counter-intuitive considered that additional sample estimate is incorporated into $P_n(\tilde{\theta}_x)$, whereas $P_n(\theta_x)$ uses the true θ_x.

To this end, Yu et al. (2016) developed an alternative expression of the kernel $h(X_i, Y_j, \tilde{\theta}_x)$ as a function of true quantile θ_x, which defines the relationship between $P_n(\tilde{\theta}_x)$ and $P_n(\theta_x)$. By expressing $h(X_i, Y_j, \tilde{\theta}_x)$ as a function of true quantile θ_x, the kernel will be in a form of a kernel with the degree of (1,1), enabling us to estimate the variance based on the typical variance estimator such as the one given in (8.6).

TABLE 8.1

Monte Carlo variances based on the median (0.5th quantile)

Underlying Distributions	Variance Method	Sample Sizes (n_1, n_2)						
		(20,20)	(20,30)	(30,30)	(30,50)	(50,50)	(50,100)	(100,100)
Normal(0,1) vs. Normal(1,2)	Var. w/ known quantile	0.006440	0.005651	0.004242	0.003399	0.002535	0.002065	0.001313
	Var. w/ sample quantile	0.002976	0.002122	0.001889	0.001376	0.001210	0.000732	0.000607
Gamma(1,2) vs. Gamma(3,1)	Var. w/ known quantile	0.011377	0.011053	0.007650	0.007835	0.004423	0.004528	0.002266
	Var. w/ sample quantile	0.000645	0.000527	0.000418	0.000333	0.000248	0.000181	0.000124
Lognormal(0,1) vs. Normal(5,2)	Var. w/ known quantile	0.010454	0.010333	0.006821	0.007053	0.004121	0.004040	0.002119
	Var. w/ sample quantile	0.002354	0.002130	0.001468	0.001381	0.000893	0.000838	0.000456

The following result shows a new expression of the kernel of $P_n(\tilde{\theta}_x)$.

Proposition 8.1

When n_1 and n_2 increase to ∞,

$$P_n(\tilde{\theta}_x) = \frac{1}{n}\sum_{i=1}^{n_1}\sum_{j=1}^{n_2} h^*(X_i, Y_j, \theta_x) + O(n_*^{-1/2}),$$

where $n_* = \min(n_1, n_2)$ and $h^*(X_i, Y_j, \theta_x)$ is given by

$$h^*(X_i, Y_j, \theta_x) = I(Y_j > X_i)I(X_i > \theta_x) - I(Y_j > \theta_x)\{I(X_i > \theta_x) - 1 + p\}.$$

The proof of Proposition 8.1 is shown in the Appendix. In an application of Proposition 8.1 for estimating the variance of $P_n(\tilde{\theta}_x)$, we use a simple implementation of Formula (8.6) as

$$\hat{V}(P_n(\tilde{\theta}_x)) = \frac{n_1 + n_2}{n_1 n_2}\left(\frac{n_2 S_{10}^{2\,*}(\tilde{\theta}_x) + n_1 S_{01}^{2\,*}(\tilde{\theta}_x)}{n_1 + n_2}\right), \tag{8.8}$$

where

$$S_{10}^{2\,*} = \frac{1}{n_1 - 1}\sum_{i=1}^{n_1}\left(V_{10}^{\,*}(X_i) - P_n(\tilde{\theta}_x)\right)^2, \text{ and } S_{01}^{2\,*} = \frac{1}{n_2 - 1}\sum_{j=1}^{n_2}\left(V_{01}^{\,*}(Y_j) - P_n(\tilde{\theta}_x)\right)^2$$

with

$$V_{10}^{\,*}(X_i) = \frac{1}{n_2}\sum_{j=1}^{n_2} h^*(X_i, Y_j, \tilde{\theta}_x) \text{ for } i = 1, \ldots, n_1$$

and

$$V_{01}^{\,*}(Y_j) = \frac{1}{n_1}\sum_{i=1}^{n_1} h^*(X_i, Y_j, \tilde{\theta}_x) \text{ for } j = 1, \ldots, n_2.$$

Now consider the estimator of the two-sides truncated pAUC, that is, Formula (8.7) with $h(X_i, Y_j, \tilde{\theta}_x)$ defined as $I(Y_j > X_i)I({}^{p_1}\tilde{\theta}_x < X < {}^{p_2}\tilde{\theta}_x)$, where ${}^{p_i}\tilde{\theta}_x$ is the sample p_i-*th* quantile. The same approach to prove Proposition 8.1 except using the vector $\boldsymbol{\theta}_x = ({}^{p_1}\theta_x, {}^{p_2}\theta_x)$ instead of θ_x gives rise to the expression of $h^*(X_i, Y_j, \boldsymbol{\theta}_x)$ given by

$$h^*(X_i, Y_j, \boldsymbol{\theta}_x) = h^*(X_i, Y_j, {}^{p_1}\theta_x) - h^*(X_i, Y_j, {}^{p_2}\theta_x). \tag{8.9}$$

Using Expression (8.9), the variance of the estimator of the two-sides pAUC is conveniently obtained by (8.8) in a similar manner to that of the estimator of the one-side pAUC. We obtain the test statistic to test the pAUC based on the variance estimate using the asymptotic normality of $P_n(\tilde{\theta}_x)$ (Dodd and Pepe, 2003; Qin et al. 2011). Yu et al. (2016) compared the performance of the proposed variance estimator and other existing methods (Cai and Dodd, 2008; He and Escobar, 2008; Qin et al., 2011; Adimari and Chiogna, 2012) through the simulation in settings of the various underlying distributions. The proposed method provides superior variance estimates throughout various underlying distributions compared with the other existing methods.

8.6.2 Comparison of Two Correlated pAUC Estimates

The results obtained above can be easily extended to the comparison between two correlated pAUCs. Suppose that individuals from population 1 provide independent observations $X_i = (X_{ai}, X_{bi})^T, i = 1, \ldots, n_1$, and individuals from population 2 provide independent observations $Y_i = (Y_{ai}, Y_{bi})^T, i = 1, \ldots, n_2$, where a and b indicate the first and second elements of the vectors. Let $X_i \sim X = (X_a, X_b)^T$, $Y_i \sim Y = (Y_a, Y_b)^T$, and

$$P(\theta_{x_k}) = \Pr\{Y_k > X_k, X_k > \theta_{x_k}\}, \; k = a, b, \tag{8.10}$$

where θ_{x_k} is the p-th quantile of variable X_k $(k = a, b)$ and thus $P(X_a > \theta_{x_a}) = P(X_b > \theta_{x_b})$.

We note that, for a slightly more general expression than (8.10), we can replace θ_{x_k} in (8.10) by ${}^{p_k}\theta_{x_k}$, p_k-th quantile for variable X_k, where p_a and p_b can be different probabilities.

To test the difference in the partial AUCs, the U-statistic $\hat{\delta}$ can be defined as

$$\hat{\delta}(\theta_{x_a}, \theta_{x_b}) = P_n(\theta_{x_a}) - P_n(\theta_{x_b}) = \sum_{i=1}^{n_1} \sum_{j=1}^{n_2} \left[\frac{1}{n} h(X_i, Y_j, \theta_{x_a}, \theta_{x_b}) \right],$$

where $h(X_i, Y_j, \theta_{x_a}, \theta_{x_b}) = h(X_{ai}, Y_{aj}, \theta_{x_a}) - h(X_{bi}, Y_{bj}, \theta_{x_b})$ based on Definition (8.4). Now, the direct application of Proposition 8.1 gives the following result:

Corollary 8.1

When n and n_1 increase to ∞,

$$\hat{\delta}(\tilde{\theta}_{x_a}, \tilde{\theta}_{x_b}) = \frac{1}{n} \sum_{i=1}^{n_1} \sum_{j=1}^{n_2} h^*(X_i, Y_j, \theta_{x_a}, \theta_{x_b}) + O(n_*^{-1/2}),$$

where $n_* = \min(n_1, n_2)$ and $h^*(X_i, Y_j, \theta_{x_a}, \theta_{x_b})$ is given by

$$h^*(X_i, Y_j, \theta_{x_a}, \theta_{x_b})$$
$$= \sum_{k=a,b} (-1)^{I(k=b)} \left[I(Y_{kj} > X_{ki}) I(X_{ki} > \theta_{x_k}) - I(Y_{kj} > \theta_x)\{I(X_{ki} > \theta_{x_k}) - 1 + p\} \right].$$

The variance of $\hat{\delta}(\tilde{\theta}_{x_a}, \tilde{\theta}_{x_b})$ may be obtained in a similar manner to that shown in DeLong et al. (1988). DeLong et al., 1988 extended Sen's variance estimator (8.6) to covariance estimates based on correlated variables. For detailed formula regarding two correlated AUC estimators, see Chapter 7. When we apply the variance formula, we replace $h(X_i, Y_j)$ by $h^*(X_i, Y_j, \tilde{\theta}_x)$, similar to (8.8).

8.6.3 An Empirical Likelihood Approach Based on the Proposed Variance Estimator

In Chapter 7, we showed that an ELR test based on a constraint in a form of a U-statistic has a weighted χ^2 distribution, where the weight is a function of the true variance of the U-statistic. Herein, we develop a test regarding the pAUC in the framework of the EL method as follows. Consider the null hypothesis for a pAUC value,

$$H_0: \ P(\theta_x) = p_0. \tag{8.11}$$

For the empirical constraint corresponding to (8.11), we have

$$\sum_{i=1}^{n_1} \sum_{j=1}^{n_2} w_{ij} h(X_i, Y_j, \boldsymbol{\theta}_x) = p_0, \tag{8.12}$$

where $\sum_{i=1}^{n_1} \sum_{j=1}^{n_2} w_{ij} = 1$ and $0 \le w_{ij} \le 1$. In the constraint (8.12), the summands are not independent, and a weight of each summand may not have a direct interpretation as a probability point mass, dissimilar to the common EL constraints based on independent summands. The corresponding ELR test does not have a common χ^2 distribution according to the result of the ELR test based on the general U-statistics as shown in Chapter 7 (Yuan et al., 2012; Yu et al., 2016).

We need to replace the unknown parameter (θ_x) by its sample estimate that is obtained without involving a maximization of the associated EL function. This type of approach is often referred as the *plug-in* approach (Hjort et al., 2009; Yu et al., 2011) in a more conventional EL framework. Following the plug-in approach concept, we replace unknown θ_x by $\tilde{\theta}_x$, which approximates Expression (8.12) as

$$\sum_{i=1}^{n_1} \sum_{j=1}^{n_2} w_{ij} h(X_i, Y_j, \tilde{\theta}_x) = p_0. \tag{8.13}$$

Under H_0, the corresponding EL is defined as

$$L_{\theta_0} = \max_{w_{ij}} \prod_{i=1}^{n_1} \prod_{j=1}^{n_2} w_{ij}, \tag{8.14}$$

where the maximization is subjected to $\sum_{i=1}^{n_1}\sum_{j=1}^{n_2} w_{ij} = 1,\ 0 \le w_{ij} \le 1$ and Constraint (8.13). To obtain L_{θ_0}, we maximize $\sum_{i=1}^{n_1}\sum_{j=1}^{n_2} \log w_{ij}$ by the method of the Lagrange multipliers. Then, we have

$$w_{ij} = \left\{ n(1 + \lambda(h(X_i, Y_j, \tilde{\theta}_x) - p_0)) \right\}^{-1}, i, j \in S, \tag{8.15}$$

where the Lagrange multiplier λ satisfies

$$\sum_{i=1}^{n_1} \sum_{j=1}^{n_2} \frac{h(X_i, Y_j, \tilde{\theta}_x) - p_0}{1 + \lambda(h(X_i, Y_j, \tilde{\theta}_x) - p_0)} = 0.$$

The EL function under H_1 is

$$L_1 = n^{-n}. \tag{8.16}$$

By (8.14) through (8.16), we obtain the ELR-type test statistic

$$R(p_0) = \prod_{i=1}^{n_1} \prod_{j=1}^{n_2} \left\{ 1 + \lambda(h(X_i, Y_j, \tilde{\theta}_x) - p_0) \right\}^{-1},$$

and the corresponding log-EL ratio test statistic is

$$l(p_0) = -2\log R(p_0) = 2\sum_{i=1}^{n_1} \sum_{j=1}^{n_2} \log(1 + \lambda(h(X_i, Y_j, \tilde{\theta}_x) - p_0)). \tag{8.17}$$

Let $V(P_n(\tilde{\theta}_x)) = \sigma^2\ (< \infty)$. Assume that $E_{F,G}\left|h(X_i, Y_j, \tilde{\theta}_x)\right|^{\alpha}$ exists up to some positive $\alpha\ (\ge 2)$ and p_0 is inside the convex hull of points given by the set $\{h(X_i, Y_j, \tilde{\theta}_x)$, for all i and j in the sample$\}$. Also, define $\lim_{n\to\infty} \sum_{i=1}^{n_1}\sum_{j=1}^{n_2} (h(X_i, Y_j, \tilde{\theta}_x) - p_0)^2/n = \eta^2$. Then, we can show the following result.

Proposition 8.2

Under H_0 at (8.11), $\gamma(p_0)l(p_0)$ converges in distribution to χ_1^2 distribution, where $\gamma(p_0) = \eta^2/[n_1 n_2 \sigma^2]$.

We provide the proof of Proposition 8.2 in the Appendix. To estimate σ^2, we use Formula (8.8), where p_0 is employed in place of $P_n(\tilde{\theta}_x)$ under H_0. Also, since

η^2 has a form of an expectation of the square of $h(X_i, Y_j, \tilde{\theta}_x) - p_0$, we use the sample variance of $h(X_i, Y_j, \tilde{\theta}_x)$ to estimate η^2.

The EL approach used above can be easily extended to the two correlated biomarkers problem mentioned in Section 8.6.2. Consider the following null hypothesis:

$$H_0 : P(\theta_{x_a}) - P(\theta_{x_b}) = \delta_0. \tag{8.18}$$

Often, $\delta_0 = 0$ indicating no difference between groups. Using the similar argument used in Chapter 7, the corresponding log-EL ratio test statistic is

$$l(\delta_0) = 2\sum_{i=1}^{n_1}\sum_{j=1}^{n_2} \log(1 + \lambda_2 (h(X_i, Y_j, \theta_{x_a}, \theta_{x_b}) - \delta_0)),$$

where λ_2 satisfies

$$\sum_{i=1}^{n_1}\sum_{j=1}^{n_2} \frac{h(X_i, Y_j, \theta_{x_a}, \theta_{x_b}) - \delta_0}{1 + \lambda_2 (h(X_i, Y_j, \theta_{x_a}, \theta_{x_b}) - \delta_0)} = 0.$$

Assume that $E_{F,G} \left| h(X_i, Y_j, \tilde{\theta}_{x_a}, \tilde{\theta}_{x_b}) \right|^\alpha$ exists up to some positive α (≥ 2), δ_0 is inside the convex hull of points given by the set of points $h(X_i, Y_j, \tilde{\theta}_{x_a}, \tilde{\theta}_{x_b})$ for all i and j in the sample, and we define $\lim_{n\to\infty} \sum_{i=1}^{n_1}\sum_{j=1}^{n_2} (h(X_i, Y_j, \tilde{\theta}_{x_a}, \tilde{\theta}_{x_b}) - \delta_0)^2 / n = \eta_2{}^2$. Also, let $V(\tilde{\delta}(\tilde{\theta}_{x_a}, \tilde{\theta}_{x_b})) = \sigma_2{}^2 (< \infty)$. Then, we have the following result.

Corollary 8.2

Under H_0 at (8.18), $\gamma(\delta_0) l(\delta_0)$ converges in distribution to a χ_1^2 distribution, where $\gamma(\delta_0) = \eta_2{}^2 / [n_1 n_2 \sigma_2{}^2]$.

The proof is omitted as it is similar to that of Proposition 8.2. The estimate of $\sigma_2{}^2$ is obtained in the same way as described below Corollary 8.1. We estimate $\eta_2{}^2$ using the sample variance of $h(X_i, Y_j, \tilde{\theta}_{x_a}, \tilde{\theta}_{x_b})$. The performance of the ELR-based tests and the normal distribution-based tests is compared using simulations (Yu et al., 2016). The normal distribution-based tests are constructed using the variance estimates explained in (8.8) and Corollary 8.1. When Forumla (8.8) is used, p_0 under H_0 is employed in place of $P_n(\tilde{\theta}_x)$ as

$$\hat{V}(p_0) = \frac{n_1 + n_2}{n_1 n_2} \left(\frac{n_2 S_{10}^{2\,*}(\tilde{\theta}_x) + n_1 S_{01}^{2\,*}(\tilde{\theta}_x)}{n_1 + n_2} \right),$$

where

$$S_{10}^{2\,*}(\tilde{\theta}_x) = \frac{1}{n_1 - 1} \sum_{i=1}^{n_1} \left(V_{10}{}^*(X_i) - p_0 \right)^2, \text{ and } S_{01}^{2\,*}(\tilde{\theta}_x) = \frac{1}{n_2 - 1} \sum_{j=1}^{n_2} \left(V_{01}{}^*(Y_j) - p_0 \right)^2$$

with

$$V_{10}^{*}(X_i) = \frac{1}{n_2}\sum_{j=1}^{n_2} h^{*}(X_i, Y_j, \tilde{\theta}_x), \text{ for } i = 1,\ldots, n_1$$

and

$$V_{01}^{*}(Y_j) = \frac{1}{n_1}\sum_{i=1}^{n_1} h^{*}(X_i, Y_j, \tilde{\theta}_x), \text{ for } j = 1,\ldots, n_2.$$

The test using $P_n(\tilde{\theta}_x)$ provides a slightly higher Type I error (TIE) rates than the test using p_0 in cases of the relatively small sample sizes, whereas the performance of the two tests will be similar when the sample sizes increase. Some TIE investigations for testing a pAUC are shown in Table 8.2. For the

TABLE 8.2

Monte Carlo Type I error rates of the truncated pAUC analysis (*Normal*: the Normal Approximation, EL: EL Method) with various underlying distributions for the pAUC with the 0.5th quantile, 0.9th quantile, and between the 0.5th and 0.9th quantiles. The target Type I error rate is 0.05

	Underlying Distributions	p_0	Method	Sample Sizes (n_1, n_2) (20,20)	(20,30)	(30,30)	(30,50)	(50,50)	(50,100)	(100,100)
0.5th	Normal (0,1) vs. Normal (0.5,2)	0.2224	EL	0.020	0.020	0.024	0.028	0.037	0.041	0.039
			Normal	0.020	0.021	0.027	0.030	0.038	0.042	0.042
	Lognormal (0,1) vs. Normal (0,3)	0.1137	EL	0.017	0.016	0.016	0.026	0.031	0.037	0.044
			Normal	0.032	0.031	0.032	0.038	0.044	0.043	0.048
	Gamma (2,0.5) vs. Gamma (5,1)	0.1851	EL	0.029	0.035	0.030	0.037	0.041	0.045	0.043
			Normal	0.035	0.041	0.039	0.044	0.044	0.050	0.045
0.9th	Normal (0,1) vs. Normal (0.5,2)	0.0270	EL	0.051	0.054	0.044	0.055	0.043	0.054	0.046
			Normal	0.023	0.040	0.041	0.049	0.044	0.052	0.049
	Lognormal (0,1) vs. Normal (0,3)	0.0046	EL	0.057	0.081	0.047	0.075	0.046	0.064	0.047
			Normal	0.133	0.088	0.109	0.104	0.085	0.092	0.075
	Gamma (2,0.5) vs. Gamma (5,1)	0.0045	EL	0.055	0.071	0.052	0.061	0.050	0.056	0.045
			Normal	0.137	0.091	0.115	0.082	0.090	0.087	0.072
(0.5th, 0.9th)	Normal (0,1) vs. Normal (0.5,2)	0.1954	EL	0.019	0.021	0.025	0.032	0.034	0.042	0.042
			Normal	0.023	0.025	0.030	0.033	0.035	0.043	0.044
	Lognormal (0,1) vs. Normal (0,3)	0.1091	EL	0.017	0.018	0.019	0.024	0.033	0.036	0.042
			Normal	0.032	0.034	0.037	0.039	0.045	0.044	0.051
	Gamma (2,0.5) vs. Gamma (5,1)	0.1805	EL	0.039	0.043	0.034	0.046	0.046	0.050	0.051
			Normal	0.045	0.046	0.043	0.059	0.054	0.053	0.054

pAUC with the median θ_x, the performance of the normal approximation and EL methods is comparable, where the two methods show slightly conservative TIE rates with relatively small sample sizes, whereas they show accurate TIE control with increasing sample size. However, for pAUC with 0.9th quantile θ_x, the EL method may have a better control of the TIE rate compared with the normal approximation. These results showcase that the EL approach has more robust TIE rate control than the normal approximation, especially with the cases of a higher quantile θ_x. The powers for all methods (not presented here) respond well for increasing sample sizes with a slightly larger power in the EL method when compared with the normal approximation. Simulation results of the TIE of the comparison of two correlated ROC curves by pAUCs are shown in Table 8.3. For normal, distributions used are

$$\begin{pmatrix} X \\ W \end{pmatrix} \sim N_2\left(\begin{pmatrix} 0 \\ 2 \end{pmatrix}, \begin{pmatrix} 1 & 1.35 \\ 1.35 & 2.25 \end{pmatrix}\right) \text{ versus } \begin{pmatrix} Y \\ Z \end{pmatrix} \sim N_2\left(\begin{pmatrix} \mu_Y \\ \mu_Z \end{pmatrix}, \begin{pmatrix} 0.25 & 0.45 \\ 0.45 & 1 \end{pmatrix}\right),$$

where μ_Y and μ_Z are calculated to obtain $p_0 = 0.008$ for 0.9th quantile and $p_0 = 0.2$ for the median. For lognormal, distributions used are

TABLE 8.3

Simulated Type I error rates of the comparison of correlated pAUC estimates with the various underlying distributions for the pAUC with the 0.5th quantile, 0.9th quantile, and between the 0.5th and 0.9th quantiles. The target Type I error rate is 0.05

			Sample Sizes (n_1, n_2)						
θ_x	Distributions	Method	(20,20)	(20,30)	(30,30)	(30,50)	(50,50)	(50,100)	(100,100)
0.5th	Same normal	EL	0.040	0.049	0.044	0.057	0.053	0.050	0.047
		Normal	0.040	0.049	0.044	0.057	0.053	0.050	0.047
	Different lognormal	EL	0.039	0.046	0.049	0.051	0.052	0.054	0.047
		Normal	0.039	0.045	0.049	0.051	0.051	0.054	0.047
0.9th	Same normal	EL	0.062	0.065	0.044	0.050	0.028	0.036	0.033
		Normal	0.029	0.038	0.019	0.030	0.020	0.030	0.029
	Different lognormal	EL	0.058	0.062	0.047	0.052	0.034	0.037	0.031
		Normal	0.028	0.036	0.022	0.034	0.025	0.029	0.027
(0.5th, 0.9th)	Same normal	EL	0.033	0.037	0.034	0.048	0.044	0.045	0.051
		Normal	0.028	0.035	0.031	0.046	0.043	0.045	0.050
	Different lognormal	EL	0.028	0.038	0.037	0.045	0.039	0.048	0.048
		Normal	0.023	0.034	0.035	0.044	0.039	0.047	0.047

$$\begin{pmatrix} \log X \\ \log W \end{pmatrix} \sim N_2\left(\begin{pmatrix} 0 \\ 2 \end{pmatrix}, \begin{pmatrix} 1 & 1.35 \\ 1.35 & 2.25 \end{pmatrix}\right) \text{ versus } \begin{pmatrix} \log Y \\ \log Z \end{pmatrix} \sim N_2\left(\begin{pmatrix} \mu_Y \\ \mu_Z \end{pmatrix}, \begin{pmatrix} 0.25 & 0.45 \\ 0.45 & 1 \end{pmatrix}\right),$$

where μ_Y and μ_Z are calculated to obtain $p_0 = 0.008$ for 0.9th quantile and $p_0 = 0.2$ for the median. Overall, the normal approximations and the EL method show a reasonable TIE rate control; however, the normal approximation is somewhat more conservative across the cases with the higher quantile θ_x. The power of the both methods responds well in general when sample sizes increase, although the EL method more frequently reaches a higher power than the normal approximations (results are not shown).

Example 8.1 An Example from DeLong et al. (1988)

We illustrate the application of the tests for pAUC comparison using a dataset provided in DeLong et al. (1988). In DeLong et al. (1988), the analytical goal is to evaluate the prognostic power of biomarkers such as Krebs–Goplerud (K–G) score (Krebs and Goplerud, 1983), total protein, and albumin on the surgical management of bowel obstruction for the ovarian cancer patients, where the successful outcome is a survival of more than 2 months. The Krebs–Goplerud (K–G) score is a rank-based assessment tool using several risk factors (e.g., patients' age, tumor spread and etc.), whereas the other two biomarkers under investigation indicate patients' nutritional status. DeLong et al. compared the AUCs of those biomarkers based on the entire region of specificity and concluded no significant differences in prognostic powers of the biomarkers. A close examination of the ROCs of the biomarkers reveals an interesting fact (Figure 8.2). Although there is no evidence that one biomarker is better than the other based on the overall AUCs, it appears that the ROCs of albumin and the K–G score cross one another around a specificity of 0.5. That is, for the area of high specificity (shaded area in Figure 8.2), albumin may have better sensitivity than the K–G score. Note that Figure 8.2 is obtained using the K–G score and albumin based on 12 successes and 37 failures. The dataset is available in the user guide in SAS Institute Inc (2009). The dataset is provided in the R-code example in the following.

Thus, we carried out the tests for pAUCs with the median for specificity higher than 0.5 using the proposed method. This area of specificities is meaningful as it indicates that the biomarker has a correct diagnostic power greater than 50% (or making decision by flipping a coin among the nondiseased group). For tied values of successes (say, Y_{kj}) and failures (say, X_{ki}), the value of 0.5 is assigned to calculate $I(Y_{kj} > X_{ki})$ and the variances are estimated accordingly. The estimated pAUCs for the K–G score and albumin are 0.169 and 0.271, respectively. The p-values for the tests based on the normal approximation and the EL method are 0.2300 and 0.2331, respectively, indicating they are not significantly different with the given dataset at the conventional significance level, 0.05. For comparison, the tests based on the entire region of specificity produce the p-values of 0.9102 and 0.9103 for the tests based on the normal approximation and EL method, respectively. This result demonstrates that using the pAUC may elicit a different conclusion than the consideration of the whole AUC regarding the comparison of the prognostic power of the biomarkers. The R-code to produce the result is as follows. For the EL method, optimization can be carried out using `optim` function in R in a similar way to Yu et al. (2015). Herein, we carry out optimization using `el.test` from `emplik` package.

The data are provided as

```
#K-G score for success (x) and failure (y) groups
x<-c(2,3,7,8,4,4,6,6,4,6,8,5)
y<-c(9,7,7,6,5,6,7,7,6,7,6,7,6,6,5,
5,7,9,8,8,7,7,6,7,7,6,6,7,8,7,5)
#Albumin for success (w) and failure (z) groups
w<-c(3.0,2.9,0.9,4.2,3.0,2.5,4.0,3.3,2.8,2.8,3.6,1.7)
z<-c(3.2,3.8,4.1,2.3,3.8,3.1,3.2,3.7,3.3,3.2,3.7,3.6,4.1,
2.6,3.3,2.1,3.7,3.9,3.2,4.3,4.5,4.3,4.2,3.6,1.6,3.8,3.5,
3.7,4.3,3.5,4.0)
```

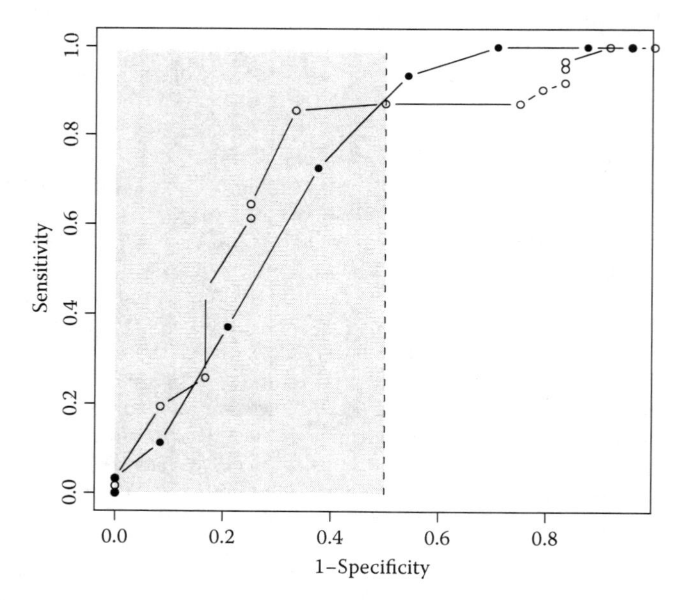

FIGURE 8.2
The ROC curves for K–G score (bullets) and albumin (circles). The shaded part corresponds to specificity greater than 0.5.

The following code is to compare the two correlated biomarkers using the test based on the normal approximation:

```
n1<-length(x);n2<-length(y);n<-n1+n2
m<-n1*n2
```

In the following codes, pauc_xy and pauc_wz contain the pAUCs.

```
probforQ<-0.5;
medx<-quantile(x,probforQ);
medw<-quantile(w,probforQ) #sample medians
#kernels of sample pAUC for K-G
indicator_xy1=matrix(data=NA, n1, n2)
for ( a in 1:n1) {for ( b in 1:n2) {
indicator_xy1[a,b]=as.numeric(x[a]<y[b])*
as.numeric(x[a]>medx)
}}
indicator_xy2=matrix(data=NA, n1, n2) #kernels in
Collorary 8.6.1
for ( p in 1:n1) {for ( q in 1:n2) {
         indicator_xy2 [p,q] = as.numeric(x[p]<y[q])*
as.numeric(x[p]>medx)-
         (as.numeric(x[p]>medx)-(1-probforQ))*
as.numeric(y[q]>medx)
}}
indicators_vxy1=c(indicator_xy1) #To vectorize the
matrix data
indicators_vxy2=c(indicator_xy2)
# kernels for sample pAUC for albumin
indicator_wz1=matrix(data=NA, n1, n2)
for ( a in 1:n1) {for ( b in 1:n2) {
         indicator_wz1[a,b]=
as.numeric(w[a]<z[b])*as.numeric(w[a]>medw)
}}
indicator_wz2=matrix(data=NA, n1, n2) #kernels in
Collorary 8.6.1
for ( p in 1:n1) {for ( q in 1:n2) {
         indicator_wz2[p,q]=as.
numeric(w[p]<z[q])*as.numeric(w[p]>medw)-
         (as.numeric(w[p]>medw)-(1-probforQ))*
as.numeric(z[q]>medw)
}}
indicators_vwz1=c(indicator_wz1) #To vectorize the
matrix data
indicators_vwz2=c(indicator_wz2)
#centerval has the kernel, i.e.,h(Xi,Yj,θxa,θxb).
centerval<-indicators_vxy1-indicators_vwz1
```

The following is to calculate the variance v and the test statistic norm:

```
pauc_xy<-mean(indicators_vxy1);
pauc_wz<-mean(indicators_vwz1)
v10_x=apply(indicator_xy2,1,mean);v01_y=apply(
indicator_xy2,2,mean)
v10_w=apply(indicator_wz2,1,mean);v01_z=apply(
indicator_wz2,2,mean)
s10_12=sum((v10_x-pauc_xy)*(v10_w-pauc_wz))/(n1-1)
s10_11=sum((v10_x-pauc_xy)^2)/(n1-1)
s10_22=sum((v10_w-pauc_wz)^2)/(n1-1)
s01_12=sum((v01_y-pauc_xy)*(v01_z-pauc_wz))/(n2-1)
s01_11=sum((v01_y-pauc_xy)^2)/(n2-1)
s01_22=sum((v01_z-pauc_wz)^2)/(n2-1)
s=matrix(c(s10_11,s10_12,s10_12,s10_22),nrow=2,ncol=2,
byrow=T)/n1+matrix(c(s01_11,s01_12,s01_12,s01_22),nrow=2,
ncol=2,byrow=T)/n2
v=matrix(c(1,-1),nrow=1) %*% s %*%
t(matrix(c(1,-1),nrow=1))
normtest <-(pauc _xy-pauc_wz)^2/v
normtest
[1,] 1.440682
#p-value for the normal-based test
1-pchisq(normtest, 1)
[1,] 0.230029
```

The following codes are to carry out the EL test to compare two pAUCs:

```
inilamval<-sum(centerval)*m/sum(centerval^2)
#0 is the null value, i.e., no differences between pAUCs
outval <-el.test(centerval, 0, inilamval)
lr<- outval$`-2LLR`
var_phi<-var(centerval)
eltest=lr*(var_phi/(v*m))
[1,] 1.422098
pvalue_el=1-pchisq(eltest,1) #p-value provided by the EL test.
[1,] 1.440682
```

8.7 Concluding Remarks

We showed EL applications to ROC curve analysis including the BLCs of biomarkers based on ROC curve and pAUC. In application of EL method, we used two techniques: placement value technique (Qin and Zhou, 2006; Chen et al., 2015) and an application of EL for U-statistics (Chapter 7). For the pAUC, we also used the concept of the plug-in estimator that alters the variance of statistics when it is used. An EL statistic for the pAUC with the plug-in estimator was developed by incorporating an appropriate weight. We showed that the EL tests may have a better testing performance compared to the tests based on the normal approximation, especially in controlling the TIE rates. Overall, the results presented in this chapter demonstrate that the tests based on EL methods have workable properties and may be conveniently applied for the analysis relevant to ROC curves.

Appendix

Let us define $G_n(\tilde{\theta}_x)$ as

$$G_n(\tilde{\theta}_x) = [P_n(\tilde{\theta}_x) - P_n(\theta_x)] - [P(\tilde{\theta}_x) - P(\theta_x)],$$

where $P(\tilde{\theta}_x) = \Pr\{Y > X > \tilde{\theta}_x\}$, $P_n(\theta_x)$, $P_n(\tilde{\theta}_x)$, and $P(\theta_x)$ are defined previously. Let $\{a_{n_1} : n_1 = 1, 2, \ldots\}$ be a sequence of positive constants such that

$$a_{n_1} \sim (\log n_1)/{n_1}^{1/2} \quad \text{as} \quad n_1 \to \infty.$$

Let $I_{n_1} = (\theta_x - a_{n_1}, \theta_x + a_{n_1})$, and

$$H_{n,n_1} = \sup\{ | G_n(\tilde{\theta}_x) | : \tilde{\theta}_x \text{ in } I_{n_1} \}. \tag{A.8.1}$$

Then, we can show the following new result using the outline of reasonings from Bahadur (1966).

Lemma 8.1

$H_{n,n_1,1} = O({n_1}^{-1/2})$ as $n_1, n_2 \to \infty$.

Proof

Let $\{b_{n_1} : n_1 = 1, 2, \ldots\}$ be a sequence of positive integers such that $b_{n_1} \sim {n_1}^{1/4}$ as $n_1 \to \infty$.

For any integer r, let $\eta_{r,n_1} = \theta_x + a_{n_1} {b_{n_1}}^{-1} r$ and an interval $J_{r,n_1} = [\eta_{r,n_1}, \eta_{r+1,n_1}]$.

Let $\alpha_{r,n_1} = P(\eta_{r,n_1}) - P(\eta_{r+1,n_1})$. Since $P_n(\eta)$ and $P(\eta)$ are nonincreasing functions of a real number η, for $\tilde{\theta}_x$ in J_{r,n_1} for any integer r, we have

$$\begin{aligned} G_n(\tilde{\theta}_x) &\le P_n(\eta_{r,n_1}) - P_n(\theta_x) - P(\eta_{r+1,n_1}) + P(\theta_x) \\ &= P_n(\eta_{r,n_1}) - P_n(\theta_x) - P(\eta_{r,n_1}) + P(\theta_x) - P(\eta_{r+1,n_1}) + P(\eta_{r,n_1}) \\ &= G_n(\eta_{r,n_1}) + \alpha_{r,n_1}, \end{aligned}$$

where $G_n(\eta_{r+1,n}) \geq 0$ and $\alpha_{r,n_1} \geq 0$. Similarly

$$\begin{aligned} G_n(\tilde{\theta}_x) &\geq P_n(\eta_{r+1,n_1}) - P_n(\theta_x) - P(\eta_{r,n_1}) + P(\theta_x) \\ &= P_n(\eta_{r+1,n_1}) - P_n(\theta_x) - P(\eta_{r+1,n_1}) + P(\theta_x) - P(\eta_{r,n_1}) + P(\eta_{r+1,n_1}) \\ &= G_n(\eta_{r+1,n_1}) - \alpha_{r,n_1}, \end{aligned}$$

where $G_n(\eta_{r+1,n}) \leq 0$. Thus, by Definition (A.8.1),

$$\begin{aligned} H_{n,n_1} &\leq \max\{|G_n(\eta_{r,n_1})|: -b_{n_1} \leq r \leq b_{n_1}\} + \max\{|\alpha_{r,n_1}|: -b_{n_1} \leq r \leq b_{n_1} - 1\} \\ &\equiv \max\{|G_n(\eta_{r,n_1})|: -b_{n_1} \leq r \leq b_{n_1}\} + \beta_{n_1}. \end{aligned} \tag{A.8.2}$$

Note, when r increases, $G_n(\eta_{r,n_1})$ decreases. Since $\eta_{r+1,n_1} - \eta_{r,n_1} = a_{n_1} b_{n_1}^{-1}$ for each r, $|\eta_{r,n_1} - \theta_x| \leq a_n$ for $|r| \leq b_{n_1}$ and $P(.)$ is sufficiently smooth in a fixed neighborhood of θ_x,

$$\beta_{n_1} = O(n_1^{-3/4} \log n_1).$$

Now consider

$$\begin{aligned} |G_n(\eta_{r,n_1})| &= |\{P_n(\eta_{r,n_1}) - P(\eta_{r,n_1})\} - \{P_n(\theta_x) - P(\theta_x)\}| \\ &\leq |P_n(\eta_{r,n_1}) - P(\eta_{r,n_1})| + |P_n(\theta_x) - P(\theta_x)| \\ &= O(n^{-1/2}), \end{aligned}$$

where $O(n^{-1/2})$ is achieved by the property of general U-statistics (Hoeffding, 1948), where $n = n_1 n_2$. Note that $O(n^{-1/2})$ is a slower convergence than $O(n^{-3/4} \log n)$ when n increases sufficiently. Thus, when both n and n_1 increase, the right-hand side of Inequality (A.8.2) is $O(n_1^{-1/2})$.

Proof of Proposition 8.1

We can express $P(\tilde{\theta}_x)$ in the form

$$P_n(\tilde{\theta}_x) - P(\theta_x) = G_n(\tilde{\theta}_x) - 2P(\theta_x) + P_n(\theta_x) + P(\tilde{\theta}_x), \tag{A.8.3}$$

where $G_n(\tilde{\theta}_x)$ in the right-hand side of (A.8.3) is $O(n_1^{-1/2})$ by Lemma 8.1. Thus, (A.8.3) becomes

$$P_n(\tilde{\theta}_x) - P(\theta_x) = P_n(\theta_x) - P(\tilde{\theta}_x) + 2\{P(\tilde{\theta}_x) - P(\theta_x)\} + O(n_1^{-1/2}). \tag{A.8.4}$$

Now, by applying the Taylor expansion on the smooth function P, we have

$$P(\tilde{\theta}_x) - P(\theta_x) = (\tilde{\theta}_x - \theta_x)P'(\theta_x) + O(n_1^{-1/2}), \tag{A.8.5}$$

where $P'(\theta_x)$ is the derivative of $P(\theta_x)$ with respect to θ_x. Using (A.8.5), (A.8.4) becomes

$$\begin{aligned} P_n(\tilde{\theta}_x) - P(\theta_x) &= P_n(\theta_x) - [P(\theta_x) + (\tilde{\theta}_x - \theta_x)^T P'(\theta_x)] + 2(\tilde{\theta}_x - \theta_x)^T P'(\theta_x) + O(n_1^{-1/2}) \\ &= [P_n(\theta_x) - P(\theta_x)] + (\tilde{\theta}_x - \theta_x)^T P'(\theta_x) + O(n_1^{-1/2}). \end{aligned} \tag{A.8.6}$$

We note that

$$P(\theta_x) = \Pr(Y > X > \theta_x) = \int_{\theta_x}^{\infty} \left[\int_{\theta_x}^{y} f(x)dx \right] g(y)dy, \tag{A.8.7}$$

and

$$\frac{\partial}{\partial \theta_x} \int_{\theta_x}^{\infty} \left[\int_{\theta_x}^{y} f(x)dx \right] g(y)dy = -f(\theta_x)[1 - G(\theta_x)]. \tag{A.8.8}$$

Using the Bahadur (1966)'s representation, Equations (A.8.6) through (A.8.8), we have

$$\begin{aligned} P_n(\tilde{\theta}_x) &= \frac{1}{n} \sum_{i=1}^{n_1} \sum_{j=1}^{n_2} I(Y_j > X_i) I(X_i > \theta_x) \\ &\quad - f(\theta_x)[1 - G(\theta_x)] \frac{\sum_{i=1}^{n_1} I(X_i > \theta_x) - n_1(1-p)}{n_1 f(\theta_x)} + O(n_1^{-1/2}). \end{aligned} \tag{A.8.9}$$

Based on the $\sqrt{n_2}$ rate convergence of the empirical distribution function

$$\hat{G}(z) = \frac{\sum_{j=1}^{n_2} I(Y_j \le z)}{n_2}$$

to $G(z)$ and using the relationship

$$\sum_{i=1}^{n_1} I(X_i > z) - n_1(1-p) = \sum_{i=1}^{n_1} \{ I(X_i > z) - (1-p) \},$$

We have that (A.8.9) gives the desired expression.

Proof of Proposition 8.2

The proof is similar to that of Proposition 7.2, thus we only explain deviating parts. We first check the asymptotic properties regarding the convergence of $P_n(\tilde{\theta}_x)$ as follows. By Lemma 8.1, we have

$$[P_n(\tilde{\theta}_x) - P_n(\theta_x)] - [P(\tilde{\theta}_x) - P(\theta_x)] = O(n_*^{-1/2}) \text{ or}$$

$$-[P_n(\tilde{\theta}_x) - P_n(\theta_x)] + [P(\tilde{\theta}_x) - P(\theta_x)] = O(n_*^{-1/2}).$$

By (A.8.5) and the convergence of the sample quantile to the true quantile, we have $P(\tilde{\theta}_x) - P(\theta_x) = O(n_1^{-1/2})$. Thus, $\left|P_n(\tilde{\theta}_x) - P_n(\theta_x)\right| = O(n_*^{-1/2})$. This indicates that $P_n(\tilde{\theta}_x)$ has an asymptotic property of $P_n(\theta_x)$ with a difference of a multiplicative constant. Now, following the proof of Proposition 7.2, the EL ratio test statistic (8.17) can be expressed as

$$-2\log R(p_0) = \frac{(P_n(\tilde{\theta}_x) - p_0)^2 \cdot (n_1 n_2)^2}{\sum_{i=1}^{n_1} \sum_{j=1}^{n_2} (\psi_{ij}^c)^2} + o_p(1),$$

where $\psi_{ij}^c = h(X_i, Y_j, \tilde{\theta}_x) - p_0$. By the fact that the variance of $P_n(\tilde{\theta}_x)$ is bounded and Slutsky's theorem, we conclude with

$$-2\log R(\theta_0) \frac{\eta^2}{n_1 n_2 \sigma^2} \xrightarrow{d} \chi_1^2.$$

9

Various Topics

9.1 Introduction

The statistical methodology has been continuously developed to tackle various data analytical issues. Since the empirical likelihood (EL) was introduced, many novel uses of the EL methods are found in the literature. Incorporating the EL concept into existing statistical methods may give rise to improvement in inference over parametric approaches as shapes of rejection areas and confidence regions reflect the characteristic of observed data. In this chapter, we will present several interesting topics that have been discussed in the EL literature. Mainly, we concentrate our discussions on regression methods, censored data analysis, missing data, and survey sampling. We will try to provide some details in terms of describing analytical issues and building the EL constraints and relevant inferential results. This overview will demonstrate that the EL methodology has a flexibility to be applied to various topics of interest as far as users can formulate a statistical question in a form of the estimating equations (i.e., constraints). Having said that, we note that this overview is supplementary and not intended to provide thorough technical details such as proofs of asymptotic results for the subjects. Rather, we attempt to outline some of the usages of the EL method that may be of interest for many users.

9.2 Various Regression Approaches

9.2.1 General Framework

Regression models are one major area that the EL method has been actively employed (Chen and Van Keilegom, 2009; Wu and Ying, 2001). Consider the pairs of observations consisted of the vector of covariates and the response value (X_i, Y_i), $i = 1,...,n$ from n independent subjects. A typical parametric regression model is

$$Y_i = m(X_i, \beta) + \varepsilon_i,\ i = 1,...,n,$$

where $m(X,\beta)$ is the known regression function with the p-dimensional coefficient vector β and $\varepsilon_i \sim (0, \sigma^2(X_i))$ with $\text{Var}(\varepsilon_i \mid X_i) = \sigma^2(X_i)$. For the linear regression, we have $m(X,\beta) = X^T\beta$ and for the generalized linear model $m(X,\beta) = G(X^T\beta)$ using the link function G. The least squares regression estimator of β is obtained by minimizing

$$\sum\nolimits_{i=1}^{n} \{Y_i - m(X_i,\beta)\}^2,$$

and this is achieved by solving

$$\sum\nolimits_{i=1}^{n} \frac{\partial m(X_i,\beta)}{\partial \beta} \{Y_i - m(X_i,\beta)\} = 0 \tag{9.1}$$

with respect to β.

The EL function is $\prod_{i=1}^{n} p_i$ that is maximized given the empirical constraint related to (9.1),

$$\sum\nolimits_{i=1}^{n} p_i \frac{\partial m(X_i,\beta)}{\partial \beta} \{Y_i - m(X_i,\beta)\} = 0.$$

If the convex hull made of vectors $\left(\frac{\partial m(X_i,\beta)}{\partial \beta_1}\{Y_i - m(X_i,\beta)\},\ldots,\frac{\partial m(X_i,\beta)}{\partial \beta_p}\{Y_i - m(X_i,\beta)\}\right)$, $i = 1,\ldots,n$ contains 0, then we obtain p_i's applying the Lagrange multiplier method using a function,

$$\sum\nolimits_{i=1}^{n} \log p_i + \lambda_0\left(\sum\nolimits_{i=1}^{n} p_i - 1\right) + \lambda_1^T\left(\sum\nolimits_{i=1}^{n} p_i \frac{\partial m(X_i,\beta)}{\partial \beta}\{Y_i - m(X_i,\beta)\}\right).$$

Using similar calculations to the previous chapters (e.g., Chapter 5), we can show $\lambda_0 = -n$ and p_i's have the form

$$p_i = \frac{1}{n} \frac{1}{1 + \lambda^T \frac{\partial m(X_i,\beta)}{\partial \beta}\{Y_i - m(X_i,\beta)\}},$$

where $\lambda = -n\lambda_1$ satisfying

$$\sum\nolimits_{i=1}^{n} \frac{\frac{\partial m(X_i,\beta)}{\partial \beta}\{Y_i - m(X_i,\beta)\}}{1 + \lambda^T \frac{\partial m(X_i,\beta)}{\partial \beta}\{Y_i - m(X_i,\beta)\}} = 0. \tag{9.2}$$

Without the empirical constraint, the maximum EL estimator (MELE) $\tilde{\beta}$ satisfies (9.2) without λ and thus the maximum of the EL is achieved with $p_i = 1/n$. Subsequently, –2log-EL ratio (ELR) statistic to test $H_0 : \beta = \beta_0$ is

$$R(\beta_0) = 2\sum_{i=1}^{n} \log\left\{1 + \lambda^T \frac{\partial m(X_i, \beta)}{\partial \beta}\{Y_i - m(X_i, \beta)\}\right\}\Bigg]_{\beta=\beta_0}.$$

Under H_0, $R(\beta_0)$ has asymptotically a χ_p^2 distribution. The EL confidence region with the confidence level $1-\alpha$ is

$$\{\beta : R(\beta) \le \chi_{p,1-\alpha}^2\}. \tag{9.3}$$

The regression function $m(X_i) = E(Y_i \mid X_i)$ can incorporate some nonparametric techniques such as the kernel smooth method, splines, orthogonal series, and wavelets method (Chen and Van Keilegom, 2009). For example, consider d-dimensional covariate X. Using a d-dimensional kernel function $K_h(t)$ with the bandwidth h and the Nadaraya–Watson estimator (Nadaraya, 1964; Watson, 1964), the regression model can be expressed as

$$Y_i = m(X_i) + e_i,$$

where $E(e_i \mid X_i) = 0$, $\mathrm{Var}(e_i \mid X_i = x) = \sigma^2(x)$, and $m(x)$ is estimated by a kernel estimator

$$\frac{\sum_{i=1}^n K_h(x - X_i)Y_i}{\sum_{i=1}^n K_h(x - X_i)}.$$

This kernel estimator is obtained by minimizing the weighted sum of squares $\sum_{i=1}^n K_h(x - X_i)\{Y_i - m(x)\}^2$, which leads to

$$\sum_{i=1}^{n} K_h(x - X_i)\{Y_i - m(x)\} = 0.$$

Under the null hypothesis $H_0 : m(x) = \theta(x)$, the EL function $\prod_{i=1}^n p_i$ is maximized given the constraint

$$\sum_{i=1}^{n} p_i K_h(x - X_i)\{Y_i - \theta(x)\} = 0,$$

along with $\sum_{i=1}^n p_i = 1$. Under the alternative hypothesis, $p_i = 1/n$. The resulting −2 log ELR statistic has a χ_1^2 distribution, when $n^{2/(4+d)h^2} \to 0$ using the approach of undersmoothing (Chen and Van Keilegom, 2009). The confidence interval is estimated in the manner of (9.3) that does not require an explicit variance estimator of estimate of β.

A similar approach is possible given more complicated models, for example, and

$$Y_i = g(\beta^T X_i) + \theta^T Z_i + \varepsilon_i,$$

where Y_i, X_i, and Z_i are the response, p-, and q-dimensional explanatory variables, respectively, $\|\beta\| = 1$, $g(\cdot)$ is an unknown univariate link function, and

$E(\varepsilon_i \mid X_i, Z_i) = 0$ (Wang and Jing, 2003; Zhu and Xue, 2006). In the context of (9.1), the relevant constraint, in this case, is

$$\sum_{i=1}^{n} p_i \xi_i(\beta, \theta) = 0, \tag{9.4}$$

where $\xi_i(\beta,\theta) = \{Y_i - g(\beta^T X_i) - \theta^T Z_i\}(g'(\beta^T X_i) X_i^T J_\beta, Z_i^T)^T$ and J_β is the Jacobian matrix of the vector β with the constraint $\|\beta\| = 1$. The EL approach may be carried out based on Contstraint (9.4); however, g and its derivative g' should be estimated. Wang and Jing (2003) used the Nadaraya–Watson kernel estimator for the estimation of g. Zhu and Xue (2006) used the estimator based on a local linear smoother (Fan and Gijbels, 1996), which provides the definition of g and g' simultaneously. Specifically, g and g' can be estimated by

$$\hat{g}(t;\beta,\theta) = \sum_{i=1}^{n} \frac{U_{ni}(t;\beta)}{\sum_{j=1}^{n} U_{nj}(t;\beta)} \left\{ Y_i - \theta^T Z_i \right\},$$

$$\hat{g}'(t;\beta,\theta) = \sum_{i=1}^{n} \frac{\tilde{U}_{ni}(t;\beta)}{\sum_{j=1}^{n} U_{nj}(t;\beta)} \left\{ Y_i - \theta^T Z_i \right\},$$

where $U_{ni}(t;\beta) = K_h(\beta^T X_i - t)\{S_{n,2}(t;\beta) - (\beta^T X_i - t) S_{n,1}(t,\beta)\}$, $\tilde{U}_{ni}(t;\beta) = K_h(\beta^T X_i - t)\{(\beta^T X_i - t) S_{n,0}(t,\beta) - S_{n,1}(t;\beta)\}$, and $S_{n,l}(t,\beta) = \frac{1}{n}\sum_{i=1}^{n} (\beta^T X_i - t)^l K_h(\beta^T X_i - t)$, $l = 0,1,2$. Now, the replacement of g and g' by $\hat{g}$ and $\hat{g}'$ (plug-in estimator) gives rise to −2log-ELR statistic to have a distribution of a sum of weighted independent χ_1^2 random variables asymptotically. In order to make the asymptotic distribution available in a closed form, a conditional centering of $\xi_i(\beta,\theta)$ is considered, that is,

$$\hat{\eta}_i(\beta,\theta) = \{Y_i - \hat{g}(\beta^T X_i) - \theta^T Z_i\}$$

$$\left(\hat{g}'(\beta^T X_i)(X_i - \hat{\mu}_1(\beta^T X_i;\beta))^T J_\beta, (Z_i - \hat{\mu}_2(\beta^T X_i;\beta))^T \right)^T,$$

where

$$\hat{\mu}_1(t;\beta) = \sum_{i=1}^{n} \frac{U_{ni}(t;\beta)}{\sum_{j=1}^{n} U_{nj}(t;\beta)} X_i$$

and

$$\hat{\mu}_2(t;\beta) = \sum_{i=1}^{n} \frac{U_{ni}(t;\beta)}{\sum_{j=1}^{n} U_{nj}(t;\beta)} Z_i.$$

The sample variance using $\hat{\eta}_i(\beta,\theta)$ is asymptotically an unbiased variance estimator of $\xi_i(\beta,\theta)$. Also, using β and θ under H_o, the sample mean using $\hat{\eta}_i(\beta,\theta)$ converges to 0. These facts allow −2log-ELR based on $\hat{\eta}_i(\beta,\theta)$ converges to χ_{p+q}^2 distribution.

9.2.2 Analyzing Longitudinal Data

Wang et al. (2010) considered the EL method for the regression model with longitudinal data,

$$Y_i = X_i \beta + e_i, \ i = 1,\ldots,n,$$

where n is the number of experimental units, Y_i is the m_i-dimensional repeated observations, X_i is the $m_i \times q$ matrix of covariates, β is the q-dimensional regression coefficient.

Following the usual generalized least squares estimation, Wang et al. (2010) defined $Z_i(\beta) = V_i^{-1}(Y_i - X_i\beta)$ with $V_i = \text{cov}(Y_i \mid X_i)$, and the estimating equation was constructed as $\sum_{i=1}^{n}\sum_{j=1}^{m_i} p_{ij}\ X_{ij}\hat{z}_{ij}(\beta) = 0$, where X_{ij}^T and z_{ij} are j-th row of X_i and j-th element of $\hat{Z}_i(\beta) = \hat{V}_i^{-1}(Y_i - X_i\beta)$, respectively. In the analysis, $\hat{V}_i$ is calculated based on the nonparametric sample variance matrix obtained from the residuals of a generalized estimating equation fit with working independence assumption or the maximum likelihood estimator based on a certain correlation structure assumption. It is proven that the resulting distribution of –2log-ELR statistic to test β is asymptotically a sum of the weighted independent χ_1^2 distributed random variables. The weights are eigenvalues of $\Sigma_2^{-1}\Sigma_1$, where Σ_1 and Σ_2 can be considered as the asymptotic variance of $N^{-1/2}\sum_{i=1}^{n}\left\{\sum_{j=1}^{m_i} X_{ij}z_{ij}(\beta)\right\}$ and the convergence of $N^{-1}\sum_{i=1}^{n}\sum_{j=1}^{m_i}(X_{ij}\hat{z}_{ij}(\beta))(X_{ij}\hat{z}_{ij}(\beta))^T$, respectively ($N$: total sample size). Wang et al. (2010) also provided an experiment-wise EL approach (i.e., p_i is used instead of p_{ij}) and inference for a linear combination of parameters as well.

9.2.3 Application to the Longitudinal Partial Linear Regression Model

Consider a data triplet (Y_{ij}, x_{ij}, t_{ij}), $i = 1,\ldots,k$, $j = 1,\ldots,n_i$, where i indicates an independent subject, j indicates the repeated observation, Y_{ij} is the response, x_{ij} is the p-dimensional covariate, and t_{ij} is the observed time. Based on the semiparametric longitudinal model evaluated in Zeger and Diggle (1994),

$$Y_{ij} = x_{ij}^T\beta + g(t_{ij}) + e_i(t_{ij}) + \varepsilon_{ij},$$

where $g(\cdot)$ is an arbitrary smooth function, $e_1(t),\ldots,e_k(t)$ are independent mean-zero processes, ε_{ij} is the independent error, You et al. (2006) implemented the EL approach for estimating β. The basic idea is to use the relationship $\sum_{i=1}^{k}\sum_{j=1}^{n_i}(Y_{ij} - x_{ij}{}^T\beta - \hat{g}(x_{ij},\beta)) = 0$, where $\hat{g}(x_{ij},\beta)$ is the estimate of $g(x_{ij},\beta)$ given the value of β. In order to obtain $\hat{g}(x_{ij},\beta)$, using the relationship $Y_{ij} - x_{ij}{}^T\beta = g(t_{ij}) + e_i(t_{ij}) + \varepsilon_{ij}$ and linearly approximating $g(t) \simeq a + b(t - t_{ij})$, the following local least square function is minimized with respect to a and b.

$$\sum_{i=1}^{k}\sum_{j=1}^{n_i}\{Y_{ij} - x_{ij}^T\beta - a - b(t_{ij} - t)\}^2 K_h(t_{ij} - t),$$

where $K_h(\cdot)$ is a kernel function with a bandwidth h. You et al. (2006) utilized available formulas to estimate a and b (Chiou and Müller, 1999) and were able to express the summand of the estimating equation in a form of $Y_{ij} - x_{ij}^T\beta - \hat{g}(x_{ij}, \beta) = \hat{Y}_{ij} - \hat{x}_{ij}^T\beta$ and subsequently, the empirical estimating equation has a form of $\sum_{i=1}^{k}\sum_{j=1}^{n_i} p_{ij}(\hat{Y}_{ij} - \hat{x}_{ij}^T\beta) = 0$. It is shown that the resulting −2log-ELR statistic has asymptotically a χ_p^2 distribution under the null hypothesis for β.

9.2.4 Empirical Likelihood Approach for Marginal Likelihood Functions

Qin and Zhang (2005) discussed an EL approach for the marginal likelihood function that is constructed as a result of incomplete information of the subjects' membership in terms of treatment received or genotypes. Their approach is centered on the exponential-tilt model that defines two different density functions ($f(x)$, $g(x)$) from two different populations as

$$f(x)/g(x) = \exp(\alpha + \beta x), \tag{9.5}$$

for some appropriate parameters α and β (β and x can be extended to vectors). Qin and Zhang (2005) noted that Model (9.5) is equivalent to the logistic regression model.

Consider observable pairs (X_{1i}, X_{2i}), $i = 1,\ldots,n$, where X_{1i} and X_{2i} are independent and have density functions $g(x)$ and $f(x)$, respectively. Then the likelihood function is

$$\prod_{i=1}^{n} g(x_{1i})f(x_{2j}). \tag{9.6}$$

Now, suppose that we observe n pairs of (Y_{1i}, Y_{2i}), but we do not know which one has the density $f(x)$ or $g(x)$. In that case, a marginal likelihood function can be formed as

$$\prod_{i=1}^{n} \{f(y_{1i})g(y_{2i}) + f(y_{2i})g(y_{1i})\}.$$

Applying the exponential-tilt model and letting $g(x_{ji}) = p_{ji}$, Qin and Zhang (2005) obtained the marginal log-likelihood function

$$l_M(\alpha, \beta) = \sum_{i=1}^{n} \log\{\exp(\alpha + \beta y_{1i}) + \exp(\alpha + \beta y_{2i})\} + \sum_{i=1}^{n}\sum_{j=1}^{2} \log p_{ji}. \tag{9.7}$$

The probability mass p_{ji} is obtained using the typical EL procedure with the constraint

$$\sum_{i=1}^{n}\sum_{j=1}^{2} p_{ji}\exp(\alpha + \beta y_{ji}) = 1, \tag{9.8}$$

which is based on the relationship $f(x)/g(x) = \exp(\alpha + \beta x)$ and $g(x_{ji}) = p_{ji}$. Using the Lagrange multiplier argument, we have $p_{ji} = (2n)^{-1}\{1 + \gamma(\exp(\alpha + \beta y_{ji}) - 1)\} - 1$, where γ satisfies

$$\sum_{i=1}^{n}\sum_{j=1}^{2}\frac{\exp(\alpha+\beta y_{ji})-1}{1+\gamma\{\exp(\alpha+\beta y_{ji})-1\}}=0.$$

The full log-likelihood corresponding to (9.6) is

$$l_F(\alpha,\beta)=\sum_{i=1}^{n}(\alpha+\beta x_{2i})+\sum_{i=1}^{n}\sum_{j=1}^{2}\log p_{ji}. \tag{9.9}$$

Consider $X_{1i} \sim Y_{1j}$ and $X_{2i} \sim Y_{2j}$. This condition yields

$$\begin{aligned}P(X_{1i}=y_{1i},X_{2i}=y_{2i}\mid Y_{1i}=y_{1i},Y_{2i}=y_{2i}) &= \frac{P(X_{1i}=y_{1i},X_{2i}=y_{2i},Y_{1i}=y_{1i},Y_{2i}=y_{2i})}{P(Y_{1i}=y_{1i},Y_{2i}=y_{2i})}\\ &= \frac{P(X_{1i}=y_{1i},X_{2i}=y_{2i})}{P(Y_{1i}=y_{1i},Y_{2i}=y_{2i})}\\ &= \frac{g(y_{1i})f(y_{2i})}{g(y_{1i})f(y_{2i})+g(y_{2i})f(y_{1i})}\\ &= \frac{\exp(\alpha+\beta y_{2i})}{\exp(\alpha+\beta y_{2i})+\exp(\alpha+\beta y_{1i})}.\end{aligned}$$

This implys that the conditional log-likelihood function is

$$l_C(\alpha,\beta)=\sum_{i=1}^{n}\beta y_{2i}-\sum_{i=1}^{n}\log\{\exp(\beta y_{1i})+\exp(\beta y_{2i})\}. \tag{9.10}$$

Notice the relationships of (9.7), (9.9), and (9.10), we obtain that

$$l_C(\alpha,\beta)=l_F(\alpha,\beta)-l_M(\alpha,\beta).$$

This relationship can be also understood by

$$\mathrm{P}_r(X_{1i}=y_{1i},X_{2i}=y_{2i}\mid Y_{1i}=y_{1i},Y_{2i}=y_{2i})=\frac{P_r(X_{1i}=y_{1i},X_{2i}=y_{2i})}{P_r(Y_{1i}=y_{1i},Y_{2i}=y_{2i})}.$$

Qin and Zhang (2005) commented that a conditional likelihood is commonly used to eliminate nuisance parameters, in this case α and $g(\cdot)$ as demonstrated in (9.10).

For the marginal log-likelihood function, Qin and Zhang (2005) indicated the fact

$$E\left\{\frac{\partial l_M(\alpha_0,\beta_0)}{\partial\alpha_0}\right\}=0,\ \ E\left\{\frac{\partial l_M(\alpha_0,\beta_0)}{\partial\beta_0}\right\}=0,$$

where α_0 and β_0 are the true values of α and β. Define $\hat{\alpha}$ and $\hat{\beta}$ to be the maximum likelihood estimators based on the marginal log-likelihood function (9.7). Then it is shown that

$$\begin{pmatrix} \hat{\alpha}-\alpha_0 \\ \hat{\beta}-\beta_0 \end{pmatrix} = \frac{1}{n} S^{-1} \begin{pmatrix} \partial l_M(\alpha_0,\beta_0)/\partial\alpha_0 \\ \partial l_M(\alpha_0,\beta_0)/\partial\beta_0 \end{pmatrix} + o_p(n^{-1/2}), \tag{9.11}$$

where nS is the converged matrix of the negative of the second derivatives of $\partial l_M(\alpha_0,\beta_0)$ similar to the observed information matrix. Equation (9.11) leads to

$$\sqrt{n}\begin{pmatrix} \hat{\alpha}-\alpha_0 \\ \hat{\beta}-\beta_0 \end{pmatrix} \to N_2(0,\Sigma),$$

where $\Sigma = S^{-1}BS^{-1}$. Note B is the variance matrix of

$$1/\sqrt{n}\begin{pmatrix} \partial l_M(\alpha_0,\beta_0)/\partial\alpha_0 \\ \partial l_M(\alpha_0,\beta_0)/\partial\beta_0 \end{pmatrix}.$$

Further, it is shown the −2log-likelihood ratio statistic based on the marginal likelihood function to test $\beta = \beta_0$ has a χ_1^2 distribution asymptotically.

The construction of the marginal likelihood function may require careful considerations. In this context, see the following examples:

- Consider some old clinical trial data where the identity of membership (i.e., case and control) is lost, whereas it is known that there are r controls with the density function $g(x)$ and $n-r$ cases with the density function $f(x)$. The marginal likelihood function has the form

$$\sum_{i\in\Psi}\prod_{k=1}^{r} g(x_{ik})\prod_{k=r+1}^{n} f(x_{ik}),$$

where Ψ is $n!/\{r!(n-r)!\}$ permutations of the membership. Using the semiparametric likelihood function expression similar to (9.7) and Constraint (9.8), Qin and Zhang (2005) showed that

$$l_M(\alpha,\beta) = (n-r)\alpha + \log\left\{\sum_{\Psi}\exp\left(\sum_{k=r+1}^{n}\beta^T x_{ik}\right)\right\}$$

$$-\sum_{i=1}^{n}\log\{1+\tfrac{n-r}{r}\exp(\alpha+\beta^T x_i)\}.$$

- Suppose that there are two genotypes for n subjects (D_i, $i=1,\ldots,n$) that take a value of 0 or 1. Its phenotype is expressed as X_i, $i=1,\ldots,n$. The genotype is not known. Among n subjects, there are $n-m$ subjects that have parents' known genotype information $(D_{i,F}, D_{i,M})$ and m subjects that do not have those. The marginal likelihood function consists of three parts *penetrance* $f(x_i \mid D_i)$, *population frequency* $P(D_i)$, and *transmission probability of genotype* $P(D_i \mid D_{i,F}, D_{i,M})$ in the form

$$\sum_{D_1=0,1,\ldots,D_n=0,1} \left\{ \prod_{i=1}^{m} P(D_i) \prod_{i=m+1}^{n} P(D_i \mid D_{i,F}, D_{i,M}) \prod_{i=1}^{n} f(x_i \mid D_i) \right\}. \qquad (9.12)$$

The density function $f(x_i \mid D_i)$ is a general density as a function of D_i and can be expressed as $f(x_i \mid D_i) = \exp\{D_i(\alpha + \beta^T x_i)\} g(x_i)$, where $g(x_i)$ is the baseline density and replaced by p_i. With Constraint (9.8) and the marginal likelihood function (9.12), we have the marginal log-likelihood function as

$$l_M(\alpha,\beta) = \log\left[\sum_{D_1,\ldots,D_n} \left\{ \prod_{i=1}^{m} P(D_i) \prod_{i=m+1}^{n} P(D_i|D_{i,F}, D_{i,M}) \prod_{i=1}^{n} \exp(D_i(\alpha+\beta^T x_i)) \right\} \right]$$
$$-\sum_{i=1}^{n} \log[1+\tau\{\exp(\alpha+\beta^T x_i)-1\}],$$

where τ is the Lagrange multiplier satisfying Constraint (9.8).

9.2.5 Empirical Likelihood in the Linear Regression Framework with Surrogate Covariates

In a linear model, the covariates of interest may not be exactly observed or too expensive to be observed. For example, lab analysis of biohazardous specimens (e.g., saliva) can be much more costly than data collection through questionnaire in smoking prevention projects (Wang and Rao, 2002a). Wang and Rao (2002a) discussed an EL approach for linear models where covariates consist of surrogate covariates presenting errors and independent validation covariates. Consider the linear model

$$Y = X^T \beta + \varepsilon, \qquad (9.13)$$

where Y is a response variable, X is a d-dimensional covariate, and ε is a random error.

Let $\tilde{X}$ be the surrogate variables and X be the true variables. Available data are the primary data $(Y_i, \tilde{X}_i)$, $i = 1,\ldots,N$ and the independent validation data $(X_i, \tilde{X}_i)$, $i = N+1,\ldots,N+n$. Let $u(\tilde{X}) = E(X \mid \tilde{X})$. Then the linear model can be written as

$$Y = u(\tilde{X})^T \beta + \eta,$$

where $\eta = \varepsilon + X^T\beta - u(\tilde{X})^T\beta$. Also define $Z_i(\beta) = u(\tilde{X}_i)\{Y_i - u(\tilde{X}_i)^T\beta\}$, then $E(Z_i(\beta)) = 0$ if β is the true parameter. Thus, the EL ratio is

$$\prod_{i=1}^{N} p_i N^{-N},$$

where the product of p_i is maximized subject to

$$\sum_{i=1}^{N} p_i = 1, \; \sum_{i=1}^{N} p_i Z_i(\beta) = 0. \tag{9.14}$$

If β is the true parameter, -2 log-ELR statistic has asymptotically a χ_d^2 distribution. The fact that $u(\tilde{X}_i)$ needs to be estimated gives rise to the EL statistic to be a different distribution. Similar to a nonparametric regression, $u(\tilde{X}_i)$ can be estimated as

$$\hat{u}(\tilde{x}) = \left\{\sum_{j=N+1}^{N+n} X_j K\left(\frac{\tilde{x}-\tilde{X}_j}{h_n}\right)\right\} \Big/ \left\{\sum_{j=N+1}^{N+n} K\left(\frac{\tilde{x}-\tilde{X}_j}{h_n}\right)\right\}, \tag{9.15}$$

where $K(\cdot)$ and h_n are the kernel function and bandwidth, respectively, that are functions of the sample size. In order to prevent too small value of (9.15), Wang and Rao (2002a) used a truncated version of the estimation, that is,

$$\tilde{u}(\tilde{x}) = \frac{\hat{u}(\tilde{x})\hat{f}_n(\tilde{x})}{\tilde{f}_n(\tilde{x})},$$

where $\hat{f}(\tilde{x})$ is a kernel density estimation at $\tilde{x}$ and $\tilde{f}(\tilde{x}) = \max\{\hat{f}(\tilde{x}), b_n\}$ with some positive constant b_n (b_n is a sequence that converges to 0 with increasing sample size, see also (9.35). Let $\tilde{Z}_i(\beta) = Z_i(\beta)|_{u(\tilde{x}_i)=\tilde{u}(\tilde{x}_i)}$, and we replace $Z_i(\beta)$ by $\tilde{Z}_i(\beta)$ in Constraint (9.14). Using the Taylor expansion, -2log-ELR statistic can be approximated as

$$\hat{l}(\beta) \simeq \left\{\frac{1}{\sqrt{N}}\sum_{i=1}^{N} \tilde{Z}_i(\beta)\right\}^T \left\{\frac{1}{N}\sum_{i=1}^{N} \tilde{Z}_i(\beta)\,\tilde{Z}_i(\beta)^T\right\}^{-1} \left\{\frac{1}{\sqrt{N}}\sum_{i=1}^{N} \tilde{Z}_i(\beta)\right\}. \tag{9.16}$$

Suppose $\sum_{i=1}^{N} \tilde{Z}_i(\beta)\,\tilde{Z}_i(\beta)^T/N \to V_0(\beta)$ in probability and $V(\beta)$ is the true variance of $\sum_{i=1}^{N} \tilde{Z}_i(\beta)/\sqrt{N}$. The value $V(\beta)$ consists of the variance of the original linear model (9.13) and the variance caused by modeling $E(X \mid \tilde{X})$. Consequently, $V(\beta)$ is estimated based on the primary data for the former and the validation data for the latter. The estimators of $V_0(\beta)$ and $V(\beta)$ can be obtained accordingly. To make that (9.16) have asymptotically a χ^2 distribution, $V(\beta)$ needs to be incorporated into (9.16) and this leads to the result that $\hat{l}(\beta)$ converges to $\sum_{i=1}^{d} w_i\, \chi_{1,i}^2$ where $\chi_{1,i}^2$ indicates independent random variables with a χ_1^2 distribution and w_i values are eigenvalues of $V_0^{-1}(\beta)\, V(\beta)$.

For an alternative approximation of the distribution of the ELR test, the distribution of the sum of weighted χ_1^2 distributions can be approximated by a χ_d^2 distribution by multiplying an appropriate weight, that is, $\rho \sum_{i=1}^{d} w_i\, \chi_{1,i}^2$ will have a χ_d^2 distribution where $\rho = d/tr\{V_0^{-1}(\beta)\, V(\beta)\}$ (Rao and Scott, 1981;

Wang and Rao, 2002a). Based on a simulation study, the aforementioned proposed methods by Wang and Rao (2002a) perform better than a method based on a normal approximation of the least square estimator of β in terms of coverage accuracy and average length of the confidence interval.

With relatively small sample sizes, the coverage rate of the confidence intervals based on the EL approach introduced above may be somewhat lower than the target confidence level according to the simulations carried out by Wang and Rao (2002a). They introduce the partially smoothed bootstrap EL that may give a improved coverage rate than the methods without bootstrapping. Suppose that the empirical distributions of the primary data and validation data are denoted by μ_n and v_n, respectively. The bootstrap data are selected using the empirical distributions as $(\tilde{X}_1^*, Y_1^*),\ldots,(\tilde{X}_M^*, Y_M^*)$ for the primary data and $(\tilde{X}_{M+1}^*, X_{M+1}^*),\ldots,(\tilde{X}_{M+m}^*, X_{M+m}^*)$ for the validation data. We note that M and m can be any sufficiently large numbers and not necessarily match with N and n (Wang and Rao, 2002a). Now, the validation data are smoothed in a manner of $\tilde{X}_{M+i}^{**} = \tilde{X}_{M+i}^* + h_n \xi_{M+i}$, $i = 1,\ldots,m$, where h_n is the bandwidth previously defined and ξ_{M+i} indicates the random variable with the density $K(\cdot)$. This smoothing method gives higher weights to the points closer to the bootstrap data. Based on those *partially* smoothed bootstrap data, -2log-ELR statistic (say, $\hat{l}^{**}(\hat{\beta})$) is obtained. The distribution of $\hat{l}^{**}(\hat{\beta})$ is obtained using the Monte Carlo simulation and $(1-\alpha)$-*th* quantile (say, $\hat{c}_\alpha^{**}$) is calculated. Wang and Rao proposed to obtain the confidence interval of β satisfying $\{\tilde{\beta} : \hat{l}(\tilde{\beta}) \le \hat{c}_\alpha^{**}\}$. Through the simulations, it is shown that the partially smoothed bootstrap EL approach provides somewhat conservative confidence intervals with relatively small sample sizes unlike the *simple* bootstrap EL or the normal approximation that has much lower coverage rates than the target confidence level.

9.3 Empirical Likelihood Based on Censored Data

9.3.1 Testing the Hazard Function

Suppose that $X_1,\ldots,X_n$ are independent identically distributed (i.i.d.) non-negative random variables with the distribution function F, and $C_1,\ldots,C_n$ are i.i.d. censoring times with the distribution function G. We assume right censoring unless otherwise specified. Let $T_i = \min(X_i, C_i)$ and $\delta_i = I(X_i \le C_i)$ be the observation and indicator that the observed value is X_i, respectively. The likelihood function based on (T_i, δ_i) is (Pan and Zhou, 2002)

$$L(F) = \prod_{i=1}^{n} [\Delta F(t_i)]^{\delta_i} [1 - F(t_i)]^{1-\delta_i}, \tag{9.17}$$

where $\Delta F(X_i) = F(X_i) - F(X_i -)$. Using the relationship between the hazard $\Delta\Lambda(t)$ and the distribution function

$$\Delta\Lambda(t) = \frac{\Delta F(t)}{1 - F(t-)} \quad \text{and} \quad 1 - F(t) = \prod_{s \le t} (1 - \Delta\Lambda(s)),$$

the likelihood function (9.17) can be written as

$$\prod_{i=1}^{n} [\Delta\Lambda(t)]^{\delta_i} [1 - F(t_i -)]^{\delta_i} [1 - F(t_i)]^{1-\delta_i}$$

$$= \prod_{i=1}^{n} [\Delta\Lambda(t_i)]^{\delta_i} \left[\prod_{j:t_j < t_i} (1 - \Delta\Lambda(t_j))\right]^{\delta_i} \left[\prod_{j:t_j \le t_i} (1 - \Delta\Lambda(t_j))\right]^{1-\delta_i}. \tag{9.18}$$

Pan and Zhou (2002) proposed to use a simpler form of the likelihood than (9.18) in the form

$$\prod_{i=1}^{n} [\Delta\Lambda(t_i)]^{\delta_i} \exp(-\Lambda(t_i)), \tag{9.19}$$

where the cumulative hazard function $\Lambda(t_i) = \sum_{j:t_j \le t_i} \Delta\Lambda(t_j)$. A constraint to be tested is

$$\int g(t) d\Lambda(t) = \theta, \tag{9.20}$$

where $g(t)$ is a function satisfying some moment conditions at true parameters. Without loss of generality, let $T_1 < \ldots < T_n$ without tied values. Let $w_i = \Delta\Lambda(t_i)$ $(0 < w_i \le 1)$. If the last observation is failed at $\max\{t_i, i=1,\ldots,n\}$, then

$$\Delta\Lambda(\max t_i) = \frac{\Delta F(\max t_i)}{1 - F(\max t_i -)} = 1,$$

which motivates Pan and Zhou (2002) to use $w_n = 1$. If the observation is censored, $w_n = 0$. Thus, the empirical constraint based on (9.20) is

$$\sum_{i=1}^{n-1} \delta_i g(t_i) w_i + g(t_n)\delta_n = \theta.$$

The log EL using (9.19) can be presented as

$$l(\theta) = \sum_{i=1}^{n} \delta_i \log w_i - \sum_{i=1}^{n} \Lambda(t_i), \tag{9.21}$$

using the definition $\Lambda(t_i) = \sum_{j:t_j \le t_i} \Delta\Lambda(t_j)$ and $w_i = \Delta\Lambda(t_i)$. The target function for the Lagrange multiplier method can be presented as

$$G = \sum_{i=1}^{n} \delta_i \log w_i - \sum_{i=1}^{n} \sum_{j=1}^{i} w_j + n\lambda \left[\theta - \sum_{i=1}^{n-1} \delta_i g(t_i) w_i - g(t_n)\delta_n\right]. \tag{9.22}$$

Notice in (9.22) that δ_i is not considered for the cumulative hazard function in $\sum_{i=1}^{n}\sum_{j=1}^{i} w_j$. Also, a restriction such as $\sum_{i=1}^{n} w_i = 1$ is not used as $\sum_{i=1}^{n} w_i$ is considered to be the estimator of the cumulative hazard function. The ELR statistic to test $H_0 : \theta = \theta_0$ has the form

$$R(\theta_0) = \frac{\max l(\theta_0)}{\max l(\theta_1)},$$

where $l(\theta_1)$ by (9.21) is maximized without the constraint of H_0, which leads to $w_i = \delta_i/(n-i+1)$. Pan and Zhou (2002) showed $-2\log R(\theta_0)$ has asymptotically a χ_1^2 distribution.

9.3.2 Estimating the Quantile Function

Assume the data setting presented in Section 9.3.1. Li et al. (1996) considered an EL method to obtain the confidence interval for a quantile function. Using the likelihood function (9.17), the likelihood ratio is constructed in a form

$$R(p,t) = \frac{\sup\{L(F) : F(t) = p \text{ and } F \in \Theta\}}{\sup\{L(F) : F \in \Theta\}},$$

where p is the probability corresponding to a quantile and Θ is the space of all distribution functions on $[0,\infty)$.

The ordered uncensored survival times are denoted by $0 < V_1 < \ldots < V_k < \infty$ and let $r_j = \sum_{i=1}^{n} I(T_i \geq V_j)$. Applying the Lagrange method, one can show (Li et al., 1996)

$$-2\log R(p,t) = -2\sum\nolimits_{j:V_j \leq t}\left\{(r_j - 1)\log\left(1 + \frac{\lambda_n(t)}{r_j - 1}\right) - r_j \log\left(1 + \frac{\lambda_n(t)}{r_j}\right)\right\}$$

where $\lambda_n(t)$ satisfies

$$\prod\nolimits_{j:V_j \leq t}\left(1 - \frac{1}{r_j + \lambda_n(t)}\right) = 1 - p.$$

Suppose that the true distribution functions of X_i and C_i are F_0 and G_0. Assume that $\mathrm{U}(t)$ is defined as a Gaussian process with mean 0 and the covariance function $Cov\{\mathrm{U}(s),\mathrm{U}(t)\} = \sigma^2(\min\{s,t\})$, where

$$\sigma^2(s) = \int_0^s \frac{dF_0(u)}{[1 - F_0(u)][1 - F_0(u-)][1 - G_0(u-)]}.$$

Based on the asymptotic distribution of the Kaplan–Meier estimator, Li et al. (1996) showed that

$$-2\log R(p,t) \xrightarrow{d} \left[\frac{U(F_0^{-1}(p))}{\sigma(F_0^{-1}(p))}\right]^2.$$

Subsequently, the confidence interval is given as

$$\{t : -2\log R(p,t) \le -2\log r\},$$

where $-2\log r$ corresponds to a quantile of χ_1^2 distribution. The lower bound and upper bound of the confidence interval are searched among the values of $V_1,\ldots,V_k$, that is, the lower bound is the first value satisfying $-2\log R(p,V_j) \le -2\log r$ and the upper bound is the first subsequent value satisfying $-2\log R(p,V_j) > -2\log r$. It is shown that the corresponding coverage rates are close to the nominal value except cases under heavy censoring and small sample sizes.

9.3.3 Testing the Mean Survival Time

Assume the data setting presented in Section 9.3.1. Zhou (2005) computed an ELR statistic, where the log-EL function is expressed as

$$l = \sum_{i=1}^{n}\left[\delta_i \log p_i + (1-\delta_i)\log\left(\sum_{j:t_j>t_i} p_j\right)\right], \tag{9.23}$$

where $p_i = \Delta F(t_i) = F(t_i) - F(t_i-)$, which directly corresponds to a *probability* rather than the hazard. This is the direct application of the likelihood function (9.17). The null hypothesis is given as $H_0 : E(g(X)) = \mu$. The constraint under H_0 is therefore

$$\sum_{i=1}^{n} p_i = 1, \quad \sum_{i=1}^{n} p_i g(t_i) = \mu.$$

Notice that, for these constraints, δ_i is not considered; however, Zhou (2005) mentioned that the maximization of (9.23) will force $p_i = 0$ for censored observations. Zhou also mentioned that obtaining the solution for p_i is not easy. He discussed a possible approach with a more general censoring mechanism such as left censoring or interval censoring. Let $A_i = [L_i, R_i]$, $i = 1,\ldots,n$, where L_i and R_i are appropriate numbers to provide information of true X_i. For example, $X_i \in [2,3]$ (interval censoring), $L_i = 2$, and $R_i = 3$. If $X_i \in [-\infty, 3]$ (left censoring), $L_i = -\infty$ and $R_i = 3$. If $X_i = 3$ (not censored), $L_i = 3$ and $R_i = 3$. Let the collection of endpoints of intervals A_i's be $\{L_i, 1 \le i \le n\}$ and $\{R_i, 1 \le i \le n\}$. Now, we construct a set of disjoint intervals $[q_i, p_i], i = 1,\ldots,m$, where $q_i \in \{L_i, 1 \le i \le n\}$, $p_i \in \{R_i, 1 \le i \le n\}$, and $q_1 \le p_1 < q_2 \le p_2 < \ldots < q_m \le p_m$ (Turnbull, 1976). The EL is

$$\prod_{i=1}^{n} \sum_{j=1}^{m} \alpha_{ij} s_j, \tag{9.24}$$

where $\alpha_{ij} = 1$ if $[q_j, p_j] \in A_i$, 0 otherwise, and $\sum_{i=1}^{m} s_i = 1,\ s_i \geq 0$. Note that $\sum_{j=1}^{m} \alpha_{ij} s_j$ estimates $P_r(X \in A_i)$ This definition gives rise to

$$\hat{P}(X \in [q_l, p_l]) = \frac{\sum_{i=1}^{n} (\alpha_{il} s_l / \sum_{k=1}^{m} \alpha_{ik} s_k)}{\sum_{i=1}^{n} \sum_{j=1}^{m} (\alpha_{ij} s_j / \sum_{k=1}^{m} \alpha_{ik} s_k)} \equiv \pi_l(s).$$

Under the null hypothesis, (9.24) is maximized given the estimating equation

$$\sum_{i=1}^{m} s_i\, g(t_i) = \mu.$$

The target function for the Lagrange multiplier method is

$$\sum_{i=1}^{n} \log\left(\sum_{j=1}^{m} \alpha_{ij} s_j\right) - \gamma\left(\sum_{j=1}^{m} s_j - 1\right) - \lambda\left(\sum_{j=1}^{m} s_j g(t_j) - \mu\right). \tag{9.25}$$

The partial derivative of Equation (9.25) with respect to s_j is

$$d_j(s) = \sum_{i=1}^{n} \frac{\alpha_{ij}}{\sum_{k=1}^{m} \alpha_{ik} s_k} - \gamma - \lambda(g(t_j) - \mu), \tag{9.26}$$

where we can show that γ is 0. Zhou (2005) argued that solving $d_j(s) = 0$ for s_j is equivalent to solving the following *self-consistent* equation

$$s_j = \left\{1 + \frac{d_j(s)}{n + \lambda(g(t_j) - \mu)}\right\} s_j, \tag{9.27}$$

where λ is the solution of

$$0 = \sum_{l=1}^{m} \frac{(g(t_l) - \mu) \sum_{i=1}^{n} \left(\alpha_{il}\, s_l / \sum_{k=1}^{m} \alpha_{ik} s_k\right)}{\sum_{i=1}^{n} \sum_{j=1}^{m} \left(\alpha_{ij} s_j / \sum_{k=1}^{m} \alpha_{ik} s_k\right) + \lambda(g(t_l) - \mu)}. \tag{9.28}$$

It can be shown $\sum_{i=1}^{n} \sum_{j=1}^{m} (\alpha_{ij} s_j / \sum_{k=1}^{m} \alpha_{ik} s_k) = n$. We note that the equation such as (9.28) can be obtained if the log EL has the form $\sum_{i=1}^{m} \left[\sum_{i'=1}^{n} (\alpha_{i'i} s_i / \sum_{k=1}^{m} \alpha_{i'k} s_k)\right] \log s_i$, where $\sum_{i'=1}^{n} (\alpha_{i'i} s_i / \sum_{k=1}^{m} \alpha_{i'k} s_k)$ could be interpreted as an estimate of the expectation of the frequencies that the events happen in $[q_i, p_i]$ (see Equation (3.1) in Turnbull, 1976). The self-consistent Equation (9.27) is based on Equation (3.9) in Turnbull (1976), where $d_j(s)$ is infinitesimal difference of the log-likelihood function with respect to s_j much like the derivative of the log-likelihood function. Zhou (2005) provided (9.27) replacing $d_j(s)$ in Turnbull (1976) by

$$d_j(s) = \sum_{i=1}^{n} \frac{\alpha_{ij}}{\sum_{k=1}^{m} \alpha_{ik} s_k} - \lambda(g(t_j) - \mu).$$

Also, n in Turnbull (1976) is replaced by $n + \lambda(g(t_j) - \mu)$, which could be analogous to the replacement of $d_j(s)$. The value of s_j is obtained iteratively using (9.27). The Kaplan–Meyer estimator can be used for the initial s. The EL under the alternative hypothesis is obtained simply applying Turnbull's (1976) approach. The R function `el.cen.EM()` in `emplik` package is available for the EL approach proposed by Zhou (2005).

9.3.4 Mean Quality-Adjusted Lifetime with Censored Data

Quality-adjusted lifetime (QAL) is a measure combining patient's quality of life and survival time and has used to evaluate treatment effects for many chronic diseases (Zhao and Tian, 2001). For i-th individual ($i = 1,\dots,n$), QAL is defined as

$$Q_i = \int_0^{T_i} q\{V_i(t)\}dt,$$

where T_i is the time to an event of interest (not censoring), $V_i(t)$ is any health-related event at time t, and $q(\cdot)$ is a known utility function evaluating $V_i(t)$.

Zhao and Wang (2008) discussed the regression model of QAL in the form

$$E(Q_i \mid Z_i) = g(\beta, Z_i),$$

where Z_i is the $(p+1)$-dimensional covariate vector, β is the parameter vector, $g(\cdot)$ is an appropriate function for the generalized linear regression model.

Let $\Delta_i = I(T_i \le C_i)$ with the censoring time C_i. With the presence of censoring, an estimating equation has the form

$$\sum_{i=1}^{n} \frac{\Delta_i}{\hat{K}(T_i)} h(Z_i)\{Q_i - g(\beta, Z_i)\} = 0,$$

where $\hat{K}(T_i)$ is the Kaplan–Meier estimator and $h(Z_i)$ is a modified $(p+1)$-dimensional function based on an efficient estimating equation (Robins et al., 1992). We note that Zhao and Wang (2008) also provided a more efficient estimating equation, too. The EL procedure can be carried out based on the empirical constraint related to the estimating equation as

$$\sum_{i=1}^{n} p_i \frac{\Delta_i}{\hat{K}(T_i)} h(Z_i)\{Q_i - g(\beta, Z_i)\} = 0,$$

where p_i is the empirical probability mass. It is argued that the resulting −2 log-ELR ratio statistic has the distribution of a sum of the weighted independent χ_1^2 random variables. EL methods were shown to outperform the normal approximation methods in terms of the coverage probability (CP).

9.3.5 Regression Approach for the Censored Data

Applications of EL for regression on censored data can be carried out in the similar framework of EL for the regression without censored data (Zhou and Liang, 2005). For example, consider the accelerated failure model

$$Y_i = \beta^T X_i + \varepsilon_i, i = 1, \ldots, n,$$

where Y_i is the log of the survival time, X_i is the covariate vector, and ε_i is an error term with an unspecified distribution.

The EL can be obtained using observations in the form $e_i(b) = \tilde{y}_i - b^T x_i$ (Zhou and Li, 2008), where $\tilde{y}_i$ is observed minimum of Y_i and censoring time. The likelihood function is constructed similar to (9.17). The survival function $1-F$ at (9.17) can be estimated as $\prod_{j:\, e_j(b)>e_i(b)} m[i,j]$, where $m[i,j] = \Delta\hat{S}_{KM}(e_j(b))/\hat{S}_{KM}(e_i(b)) \cdot I(e_j(b) > e_i(b))$ with the Kaplan–Meier estimator, $\hat{S}_{KM}(t)$, and the jump at $e_j(b)$, $\Delta\hat{S}_{KM}(e_j)$. Note that $m[i,i]$ is defined to be 1. The quantity $m[i,j]$ can be interpreted as an estimate of the probability of $e_j(b)$ given that the observation is greater than $e_i(b)$. Now, in the manner of the Buckley-James estimating equation (Ritov, 1990), the coefficient b can be obtained to satisfy

$$0 = \frac{1}{n}\sum_{i=1}^{n}\left\{\delta_i\, x_i\, e_i(b) + (1-\delta_i)\, x_i \sum_{j:e_j(b)>e_i(b)} e_j(b)\, m[i,j]\right\}, \tag{9.29}$$

where δ_i is the indicator that the observed data is the time to event (not censored). Similarity between the estimating equations (9.1) and (9.29) is easily observable. Let $w_j = \sum_{k=1}^{n} m[k,j]/n = \sum_{k\le j} m[k,j]/n$, an estimate of $\Delta\hat{S}_{KM}(e_j(b))$ owing to the definition of $m[i,j]$. The expression (9.29) can be rewritten as the summation of weighted $e_i(b)$ as

$$0 = \sum_{i=1}^{n} \delta_i\, e_i(b) \frac{\sum_{k=1}^{n} m[k,i] x_k}{n w_i} \Delta\hat{S}_{KM}(e_i(b)).$$

Replacing $\Delta\hat{S}_{KM}(e_i(b))$ by p_i, the EL constraint is

$$0 = \sum_{i=1}^{n} \delta_i\, e_i(b) \frac{\sum_{k=1}^{n} m[k,i] x_k}{n w_i} p_i.$$

The corresponding EL is

$$EL(F) = \prod_{i=1}^{n} p_i^{\delta_i} \left[1 - \sum_{e_j \le e_i} p_j \right]^{1-\delta_i}.$$

Zhou and Li (2008) showed

$$-2\log\{\sup_F EL(F)/EL(\hat{S}_{KM})\} \xrightarrow{d} \chi_1^2,$$

where $\hat{S}_{KM}$ is the Kaplan–Meier estimator of $\tilde{y}_i$ without the model assumption. The asymptotic distribution has the degrees of freedom 1 as it is based on the right-censored scalar observation $e_i(b)$.

An EL approach to semiparametric regression such as the Cox proportional regression is possible. Consider a linear transformation model (Chen et al., 2002; Lu and Liang, 2006),

$$H(T) = -\beta^T Z + \varepsilon,$$

where H is a monotone increasing function, T is the survival time, Z and β are p-dimensional covariate and parameter, ε is the error term with the known distribution.

Let T_i, $\tilde{T}_i$, δ_i, C_i, Z_i, $i = 1,\ldots,n$ be the independently observed survival time and $\min(T_i, C_i)$, $I(T_i \le C_i)$, the censoring time and covariate, respectively. Say $T_i \sim T$, $\delta_i \sim \delta$, and $C_i \sim C$. Define at-risk process $Y(t) = I(\tilde{T} \ge t)$ and the individual counting process $N(t) = \delta I(\tilde{T} \le t)$. A martingale process is defined by $M(t) = N(t) - \int_0^t Y(s) d\Lambda\{\beta^T Z + H(s)\}$, where Λ is the cumulative hazard function of ε. The estimating equations for the solution $(\hat{\beta}, \hat{H})$ are

$$\sum_{i=1}^{n} \int_0^\infty Z_i[dN_i(t) - Y_i(t) d\Lambda\{\beta^T Z_i + H(t)\}] = 0, \tag{9.30}$$

$$\sum_{i=1}^{n} [dN_i(t) - Y_i(t) d\Lambda\{\beta^T Z_i + H(t)\}] = 0, \tag{9.31}$$

where $H(0) = -\infty$ and subscript i indicates individual observation. Chen et al. (2002) explained that the Cox proportional hazard model is a special case of solutions of (9.30) in the following way. Let $\lambda(t) = \Lambda(t) = \exp(t)$, then $d\Lambda\{\beta^T Z_i + H(t)\} = d[\exp\{\beta^T Z_i + H(t)\}]$. Now, we have $d[\exp\{H(t)\}] = \sum_{i=1}^{n} dN_i(t) / \sum_{j=1}^{n} \{Y_j(t)\exp(\beta^T Z_j)\}$ from (9.31), and plugging it to (9.30), we have

$$\sum_{i=1}^{n} \int_0^\infty \left\{ Z_i - \frac{\sum_{j=1}^{n} Z_j Y_j(t) \exp(\beta^T Z_j)}{\sum_{j=1}^{n} Y_j(t) \exp(\beta^T Z_j)} \right\} dN_i(t) = 0,$$

which is the score function of the Cox proportional hazard model. The difference between a failure time t_l and t_l- ($l=1,\ldots,k$; k is the number of failures) at (9.31) gives rise to

$$1-\sum_{i=1}^{n} Y_i(t_l)[\Lambda\{\beta^T Z_i + H(t_l)\} - \Lambda\{\beta^T Z_i + H(t_l-)\}] = 0, l = 1,\ldots,k.$$

Starting with some initial value of $\hat{\beta}$, $\hat{H}(t_l)$ can be computed. Then $\hat{H}(t_l)$ is used to obtain the updated $\hat{\beta}$ via (9.30). This procedure will be repeated until predetermined convergence criteria are met. Lu and Liang (2006) employed the EL for linear-transformed models to test the parameter β_0. For the EL constraint under the null hypothesis value β, Equation (9.30) becomes

$$\sum_{i=1}^{n} p_i \int_0^{\infty} Z_i[dN_i(t) - Y_i(t)d\Lambda\{\beta^T Z_i + H(t)\}] = 0, \tag{9.32}$$

with the probability point mass p_i. The typical procedure of the EL can be carried out with known $H(t)$. In that case, the limiting distribution of the −2log-ELR test statistic is a χ_p^2 distribution. When $H(t)$ is estimated and plugged in (9.32), the limiting distribution is the distribution of a sum of p independent weighted χ_1^2 random variables, where the weights are the eigenvalues of a matrix as the function of the variances of $\int_0^{\infty} Z_i[dN_i(t) - Y_i(t)d\Lambda\{\beta^T Z_i + H(t)\}]$ and $\int_0^{\infty} Z_i[dN_i(t) - Y_i(t)d\Lambda\{\beta^T Z_i + \hat{H}(t)\}]$ with the estimator $\hat{H}(t)$.

9.4 Empirical Likelihood with Missing Data

9.4.1 Fully Observed Data Case

Commonly, missing mechanisms have three categories, missing completely at random (MCAR) where missing data are independent of other observed or unobserved data, missing at random (MAR) where missing data depend on only observed observation, and nonignorable missing where missingness is associated with unobserved data (Little and Rubin, 2014). Unless the missing data happen with the mechanism of MCAR, the data analysis completely ignoring the individuals with missing data would give rise to biased parameter estimates (Qin et al., 2009).

Suppose that responses can be missing in a regression setting. Independent observations are denoted by (X_i, Y_i, δ_i), $i=1,\ldots,n$, where $Y_i \sim Y$, $X_i \sim X$, and $\delta_i \sim \delta$ are the univariate response, d-dimensional covariate, and missing indicator of response (1 if observed, 0 if missing), respectively. The regression model is given by $Y_i = m(X_i, \beta) + \varepsilon_i$, where β is the parameter vector and ε_i represents random error with $E(\varepsilon_i \mid X_i, Y_i) = 0$. MAR is ofter described using the probability

$$P_r(\delta_i = 1 \mid Y_i, X_i) = P_r(\delta_i = 1 \mid X_i).$$

Under MAR, the full likelihood is

$$\begin{aligned} L &= \prod_{i=1}^{n} f(X_i, Y_i, \delta_i = 1) \prod_{i=1}^{n} f(X_i, \delta_i = 0) \\ &= \prod_{i=1}^{n} f(X_i, Y_i) P(\delta_i = 1 \mid X_i, Y_i) \prod_{i=1}^{n} f(X_i) P(\delta_i = 0 \mid X_i) \\ &= \prod_{i=1}^{n} w(X_i, \theta)^{\delta_i} \{1 - w(X_i, \theta)\}^{1-\delta_i} \prod_{i=1}^{n} f(X_i, Y_i)^{\delta_i} f(X_i)^{1-\delta_i}, \end{aligned} \tag{9.33}$$

where $w(X_i, \theta) = P(\delta_i = 1 \mid X_i)$ with the relevant missing propensity parameter θ associated with X_i and $f(\cdot)$ indicates the density function associated with the variables inside the parenthesis.

The likelihood function (9.33) indicates that θ can be estimated separately based on the maximization of the first product. If the regression parameter β is estimated using the only completely observed data, the EL is obtained in the form

$$L_C = \max \prod_{i=1}^{n} p_i^{\delta_i},$$

subject to

$$\sum_{i=1}^{n} p_i \delta_i = 1 \text{ and } \sum_{i=1}^{n} p_i \delta_i \frac{\partial m(X_i, \beta)}{\partial \beta} \{Y_i - m(X_i, \beta)\} = 0.$$

Note that this approach does not fully take advantage of the concept of MAR. Some approaches based on MAR are considered in the following section.

9.4.2 Using Imputation

Assume the data setting stated in Section 9.4.1. Suppose we want to test $E(Y)$ and consider that the relationship $E(Y \mid X = x) = m(x)$ is true. Let $\tilde{Y}_i = \delta_i Y_i + (1 - \delta_i) m(X_i)$. Then, $E(Y_i) = E(\tilde{Y}_i)$ (Wang and Rao, 2002b). In a framework of a nonparametric regression, $m(x)$ can be estimated as

$$\hat{m}_n(x) = \frac{\sum_{i=1}^{n} \delta_i Y_i K((x - X_i)/h_n)}{\sum_{i=1}^{n} \delta_i K((x - X_i)/h_n)}, \tag{9.34}$$

where K and h_n are a kernel function and a bandwidth as a function of the sample size. Wang and Rao (2002b) proposed to use the truncated version of (9.34) preventing the cases that the denominator of (9.34) is too small, that is

$$\hat{m}_{b_n}(x) = \frac{\hat{m}_n(x)\hat{g}_n(x)}{\hat{g}_{b_n}(x)}, \tag{9.35}$$

where

$$\hat{g}_n(x) = (nh_n^d)^{-1}\sum_{i=1}^n \delta_i K\left(\frac{x - X_i}{h_n}\right), \ \hat{g}_{b_n}(x) = \max\{\hat{g}_n(x), b_n\},$$

and b_n is a sequence that converges to 0 with increasing sample size. Also let $m_{b_n}(x)$ be Equation (9.35) based on the true target values of estimators $\hat{m}_n(x)$, $\hat{g}_n(x)$, and $\hat{g}_{b_n}(x)$. Now, $\tilde{Y}_i$ is estimated by $\hat{Y}_i = \delta_i Y_i + (1-\delta_i)\hat{m}_{b_n}(X_i)$. The corresponding EL is obtained using the constraints

$$\sum_{i=1}^n p_i = 1, \ \sum_{i=1}^n p_i \hat{Y}_i = \theta,$$

where $\theta = E(Y_i)$. The ELR has the form

$$R_\theta = 2\sum_{i=1}^n \log(1 + \lambda(\hat{Y}_i - \theta)), \tag{9.36}$$

where λ satisfies

$$\frac{1}{n}\sum_{i=1}^n \frac{\hat{Y}_i - \theta}{1 + \lambda(\hat{Y}_i - \theta)} = 0.$$

Since Y_i values are imputed, Equation (9.36) does not follow a χ^2 distribution. Wang and Rao (2002b) showed that the ELR has a weighted χ_1^2 distribution with the true parameter θ as

$$R_\theta \xrightarrow{d} \frac{V(\theta)}{\tilde{V}(\theta)}\chi_1^2, \tag{9.37}$$

where

$$\begin{aligned} V(\theta) &= E(\sigma^2(X)/P(X)) + V(m(X)), \\ \tilde{V}(\theta) &= E(\sigma^2(X)P(X)) + V(m(X)), \end{aligned} \tag{9.38}$$

with $\sigma^2(X) = V(Y \mid X)$ and $P_r(X) = P_r(\delta = 1 \mid X)$. $V(\theta)$ and $\tilde{V}(\theta)$ in (9.37) indicate the variance of $\sum_{i=1}^n \hat{Y}_i/\sqrt{n}$ and the converging value (in probability) of $\sum_{i=1}^n (\hat{Y}_i - \theta)^2/n$, respectively. The variance of $\sum_{i=1}^n \hat{Y}_i/\sqrt{n}$ is obtained first by representing $\sum_{i=1}^n \hat{Y}_i/\sqrt{n}$ as

$$\frac{1}{\sqrt{n}}\sum_{i=1}^n (\hat{Y}_i - \theta) = \sqrt{n}(R_n + S_n + T_n + U_n),$$

where

$$R_n = n^{-1}\sum_{i=1}^{n}(m(X_i)-\theta),\ S_n = n^{-1}\sum_{i=1}^{n}\delta_i(Y_i - m(X_i)),$$

$$T_n = n^{-1}\sum_{i=1}^{n}(1-\delta_i)(\hat{m}_{b_n}(X_i)-m_{b_n}(X_i)),\ \text{and}$$

$$U_n = -n^{-1}\sum_{i=1}^{n}(1-\delta_i)(m(X_i)-m_{b_n}(X_i)).$$

It is shown that T_n and U_n converge to 0 in probability, and R_n and S_n as the sample means of independent observations lead to $V(\theta)$ in (9.38). We note that $\sum_{i=1}^{n}(\hat{Y}_i-\theta)^2/n$, the sample variance, is not an accurate estimator of $V(\hat{Y}_i)$ as $\hat{Y}_i$'s are not independent observations. Using the typical approach to obtain the approximation of R_θ (Wang and Rao, 2002b), we have

$$R_\theta = \left[\frac{1}{\sqrt{n}}\sum_{i=1}^{n}(\hat{Y}_i-\theta)\right]^2/\tilde{V}(\theta)+o_p(1). \tag{9.39}$$

Typically in the approximation of the ELR statistic such as (9.39), $\tilde{V}(\theta)$ is a variance estimator giving rise to R_θ to have χ_1^2 distribution approximation; however, the approximation is not true in this case leading to the result (9.37).

9.4.3 Incorporating Missing Probabilities

Instead of imputing missing response, the likelihood can be constructed based on fully observed data with missing probability incorporated (Qin and Zhang, 2007). Assume the data setting presented in Section 9.4.1. Consider the likelihood function shown in (9.33). For notational convenience, let $(x_i, y_i), i = 1,\ldots,n_1$, indicate fully observed data and $(x_i, y_i), i = n_1+1,\ldots,n$ indicate that the response y_i's are missing. Then, the conditional likelihood function is given by

$$L_C = \prod_{i=1}^{n_1}\frac{w(x_i,\theta)f(x_i,y_i)}{\iint w(x_i,\theta)f(x_i,y_i)dxdy} \equiv \prod_{i=1}^{n_1}\frac{w(x_i,\theta)p_i}{\eta}, \tag{9.40}$$

where p_i, $i = 1,\ldots,n_1$ are empirical probability mass and θ is estimated by the binomial likelihood based on

$$L_B = \prod_{i=1}^{n} w(x_i,\theta)^{\delta_i}\{1-w(x_i,\theta)\}^{1-\delta_i}.$$

In Qin and Zhang (2007), it is of interest to estimate the average treatment effect or

$$\mu = E(Y) = \int y\ f(x,y)\,dx\,dy.$$

The value η can be estimated by $\hat{\eta} = \sum_{i=1}^{n} w(x_i, \hat{\theta})$, where $\hat{\theta}$ is the estimate of θ. Some additional constraint using fully observed x_i's can be existed. For example, we have the expectation $E(Y \mid X = x) = a(x)$, where $a(x)$ is an arbitrary function of x. Let $\hat{a} = \sum_{i=1}^{n} a(x_i)/n$. The conditional EL (9.40) is maximized subject to

$$\sum_{i=1}^{n_1} p_i = 1,\ \sum_{i=1}^{n_1} p_i\{w(x_i, \hat{\theta}) - \hat{\eta}\} = 0,\ \sum_{i=1}^{n_1} p_i\{a(x_i) - \hat{a}\} = 0. \tag{9.41}$$

The value of p_i has the form

$$p_i = \frac{1}{n_1} \frac{\hat{\eta}\ w^{-1}(x_i, \hat{\theta})}{1 + \pi^T r(x_i, \hat{\theta}, \hat{\eta}, \hat{a})},\ i = 1, \ldots, n_1,$$

where $\pi^T = (\hat{\eta}\lambda_1 - 1, \hat{\theta}\lambda_2)$ with the Lagrange multipliers λ_1 and λ_2, and $r(x, \theta, \eta, a)^T = (1 - \eta w^{-1}(x, \theta),\ w^{-1}(x, \theta)\{a(x) - a\})$. The estimator of $E(Y)$ is given by

$$\hat{\mu}_{\text{EL}} = \sum_{i=1}^{n_1} p_i y_i = \frac{1}{n_1} \sum_{i=1}^{n} \frac{\hat{\eta}\ w^{-1}(x_i, \hat{\theta})}{1 + \pi^T r(x_i, \hat{\theta}, \hat{\eta}, \hat{a})} \delta_i y_i$$

Qin and Zhang showed that $\hat{\mu}_{\text{EL}}$ has a variance with a size asymptotically equivalent to that of the estimator proposed by Robins et al. (1995) achieving the semiparametric lower bound asymptotically. Unlike the estimator proposed by Robin et al., $\hat{\mu}_{\text{EL}}$ does not require specifying the model for $E(Y \mid X = x) = \mu(x)$ at the coefficient level for the third expression in constraints (9.41). Due to the fact

$$\hat{\mu}_{\text{EL}} = \sum_{i=1}^{n_1} p_i y_i = \sum_{i=1}^{n_1} p_i (y_i - \mu(x_i)) + \sum_{i=1}^{n_1} p_i \mu(x_i)$$
$$\xrightarrow{p} E\{c\ (y_i - \mu(x_i))\} + E\{\mu(x_i)\},$$

where c is a function of $w(x_i, \theta)$ (Qin and Zhang, 2007), and misspecification of $w(x_i, \theta)$ would not affect the consistency of $\hat{\mu}_{\text{EL}}$ as $E\{y_i - \mu(x_i)\} \xrightarrow{p} 0$. A confidence interval for μ can be obtained using the bootstrap method (say, hybrid EL). First, obtain B bootstrap samples from the data (x_i, y_i, δ_i), $i = 1, \ldots, n$, then $\hat{\mu}_{\text{EL}}$ is repeatedly calculated using each bootstrap sample (say, $\hat{\mu}_{\text{EL}}^*$). The confidence interval will be obtained using standard bootstrap confidence interval methods based on generated $\hat{\mu}_{\text{EL}}^*$. It is shown that these hybrid EL confidence intervals have better coverage probabilities than the bootstrap percentile confidence intervals, whereas the average length of the hybrid EL method is longer than that of the bootstrap percentile confidence intervals.

9.4.4 Missing Covariates

Consider a partition of a vector of d-dimensional covariates $X_i^T = (X_i^{(1)T}, X_i^{(2)T})$, where $X_i^{(1)}$ represents missing covariates. In this case, MAR is interpreted as

$$P(\delta_i = 1 \mid X_i, Y_i) = P(\delta_i = 1 \mid X_i^{(2)}, Y_i) = w_2(X_i^{(2)}, Y_i; \hat{\theta}),$$

where δ_i is 1 if $X_i^{(1)}$ is missing, or otherwise 0, and $\hat{\theta}$ is the binary likelihood estimator similar to (9.33). Unlike the case with missing responses, the model approach would not be possible. Chen and Van Keilegom (2009) discussed incorporating inverse-probability-weighting in the constraint of the EL in the manner

$$\sum_{i=1}^{n} p_i = 1, \; \sum_{i=1}^{n} p_i \delta_i w_2^{-1}(X_i^{(2)}, Y_i; \hat{\theta}) \frac{\partial m(X_i, \beta)}{\partial \beta} \{Y_i - m(X_i, \beta)\} = 0.$$

The resulting –2log-ELR has the form

$$2\sum_{i=1}^{n} \log(1 + \lambda^T Z_i(\beta, \hat{\theta})),$$

where $Z_i = \delta_i w_2^{-1}(X_i^{(2)}, Y_i; \hat{\theta})(\partial m(X_i, \beta)/\partial \beta)\{Y_i - m(X_i, \beta)\}$. Chen and Van Keilegom noted that the asymptotic distribution of the statistic above is a distribution of a sum of weighted independent χ_1^2 random variables due to using $\hat{\theta}$, the estimator of θ.

9.5 Empirical Likelihood in Survey Sampling

9.5.1 Pseudo-Empirical Log-Likelihood Approach

In survey sampling, a sample is selected from a finite population (say, U whose size is N). Typically, the sample is selected without replacement and the probability to select a sampling unit may not be equally likely (unequal probability sampling).

Consider nonstratified sampling. The EL function can be constructed reflecting different inclusion probabilities in a manner of the Horvitz–Thompson (HT) estimation (Yates and Grundy, 1953). Specifically, Chen and Sitter (1999) proposed a pseudo-empirical log-likelihood (PELL) function, for a sample s ($\subset U$, the population index set), given by

$$\hat{l}_{\mathrm{HT}} = \sum_{i \in s} d_i \log(p_i),$$

where $d_i = \pi_i^{-1}$, the design weight, and π_i is the inclusion probability for unit i. Note that the finite population correction is not incorporated assuming the sampling fraction is small. Maximizing $\hat{l}_{\mathrm{HT}}$ subject to $\sum_{i \in s} p_i = 1$ results in $p_i = \tilde{d}_i = d_i / \sum_{j \in s} d_j$, which corresponds to the Hajek estimator (Wu and Rao, 2006).

Wu and Rao (2006) used the PELL function, for a sample of size n, defined by

$$l_{ns} = n \sum_{i \in s} \tilde{d}_i \log(p_i). \tag{9.42}$$

If $\tilde{d}_i$ values are equal, Equation (9.42) is reduced to usual EL with a sample with equal probability sampling. Let $\theta_0 = N^{-1} \sum_{i=1}^{N} g(y_i)$ indicate a population mean of interest with the data transformation $g(y_i)$. Without additional constraints, the peudo-MELE (maximum EL estimator, Chapter 2) of the population mean is

$$\hat{\theta}_H = \sum_{i \in s} \tilde{d}_i \, g(y_i). \tag{9.43}$$

If $g(y_i) = y_i$, θ_0 is the population mean (say, the corresponding estimator is $\hat{\bar{y}}_H$) and if $g(y_i) = I(y_i \le t)$, θ_0 is the distribution function (let the corresponding estimator be $\hat{F}_H(t)$). An improved estimator (Wu and Rao, 2006) is developed incorporating auxiliary information

$$\sum_{i \in s} p_i, \quad \sum_{i \in s} p_i z_i = \bar{z}, \tag{9.44}$$

where a size measure $z_i \propto \pi_i$ (i.e., first-order inclusion probability) and $\bar{z}$ is the known population mean of z_i. The second constraint indicates additional information of the population mean of the size measure z_i, for example, $\sum_{i \in s} p_i \pi_i = n/N$. Consider $\sum_{i \in s} p_i y_i$, an estimator of the population mean. Maximization with the additional constraint provides an improved pseudo-MELE (say, $\hat{\bar{y}}_E$) and is asymptotically equivalent to a generalized regression estimator $\hat{\bar{y}}_{\mathrm{GR}} = \hat{\bar{y}}_H + \hat{B}(\bar{z} - \hat{\bar{z}}_H)$, where $\hat{\bar{y}}_H$ and $\hat{\bar{z}}_H$ are the estimators (9.43) using z_i and $g(y_i)$, respectively, and $\hat{B} = \sum_{i \in s} \tilde{d}_i \, (z_i - \hat{\bar{z}}_H) y_i / \sum_{i \in s} \tilde{d}_i \, (z_i - \hat{\bar{z}}_H)^2$, a weighted estimator of the population regression coefficient. In the case that y_i and z_i are closely related and $z_i \propto \pi_i$, $\hat{\bar{y}}_E$ may provide a shorter confidence interval than that based on $\hat{\bar{y}}_H$ (Wu and Rao, 2006). We note that the auxiliary information can have a more general form

$$\sum_{i \in s} p_i x_i = \bar{x},$$

where x_i is an auxiliary variable (possibly a vector) related to y_i and $\bar{x}$ is the known population mean of x_i. Again, the resulting estimator is asymptotically equivalent to a generalized regression estimator.

Consider the PELL ratio

$$r_{ns}(\theta) = -2\{l_{ns}(\theta) - l_{ns}(\theta^C)\},$$

where $l_{ns}(\theta)$ is the maximized l_{ns} in (9.42) subject to

$$\sum_{i \in s} p_i = 1, \quad \sum_{i \in s} p_i g(y_i) = \theta,$$

and $l_{ns}(\theta^C)$ is maximized l_{ns} without the constraint $\sum_{i \in s} p_i g(y_i) = \theta$, that is, $l_{ns}(\theta^C) = n \sum_{i \in s} \tilde{d}_i \log(\tilde{d}_i)$. Now, consider the design effect (deff) associated with $\hat{\bar{y}}_H$ defined by

$$\text{deff}_H = V_p(\hat{\bar{y}}_H)/(S_y^2/n),$$

where S_y^2 is the population variance (notice $V(\hat{\bar{y}}_H) = S_y^2/n$ under simple random sampling) and $V_p(\cdot)$ is the variance under a certain survey design. Note that the estimator $\hat{\bar{y}}_H$ reflects a certain survey design using $\tilde{d}_i$. For $\theta = \bar{y}$, under some regularity conditions, it is shown (Wu and Rao, 2006) that

$$r_{ns}(\theta)/\text{deff}_H \xrightarrow{d} \chi_1^2. \tag{9.45}$$

In (9.45), a different value of deff_H will be used if $g(y_i)$ is of interest instead of y_i. Let $\tilde{l}_{ns}(\theta)$ indicate $l_{ns}(\theta)$ maximized with auxiliary information, that is, subjected to

$$\sum_{i \in s} p_i = 1, \quad \sum_{i \in s} p_i x_i = \bar{x}, \quad \sum_{i \in s} p_i y_i = \theta. \tag{9.46}$$

As discussed earlier, the corresponding estimator of the population mean of y_i is asymptotically equivalent to the generalized regression estimator. Specifically, the generalized regression estimator is

$$\hat{\bar{y}}_{\text{GR}} = \hat{\bar{y}}_H + B(\bar{x} - \hat{\bar{x}}_H), \tag{9.47}$$

where $B = \{N^{-1}\sum_{i=1}^N (x_i - \bar{x})^2\}^{-1}\{N^{-1}\sum_{i=1}^N (x_i - \bar{x})(y_i - \bar{y})\}$. The corresponding design effect is

$$\text{deff}_{\text{GR}} = V_p(\hat{\bar{y}}_{\text{GR}})/(S_r^2/n), \tag{9.48}$$

where S_r^2/n is $V(\hat{\bar{y}}_{\text{GR}})$ under simple random sampling. Let $\tilde{l}_{ns}(\theta^C)$ be $l_{ns}(\theta)$ with Constraints (9.46) lacking $\sum_{i \in s} p_i y_i = \theta$. Then, under $\theta = \bar{y}$, Wu and Rao (2006) showed

$$\tilde{r}_{ns}(\theta)/\text{deff}_{\text{GR}} \xrightarrow{d} \chi_1^2,$$

where $\tilde{r}_{ns}(\theta) = -2\{\tilde{l}_{ns}(\theta) - \tilde{l}_{ns}(\theta^C)\}$. The design effects need to be estimated from sample. For example, the Sen–Yates–Grundy type of estimator of $V_p(\hat{\bar{y}}_H)$ is proposed to be used as

$$v(\hat{\bar{y}}_H) = \frac{1}{\hat{N}^2}\sum_{i\in s}\sum_{j>i}\frac{\pi_i\pi_j - \pi_{ij}}{\pi_{ij}}\left(\frac{e_i}{\pi_i} - \frac{e_j}{\pi_j}\right)^2, \tag{9.49}$$

with $\hat{N} = \sum_{i\in s} d_i$, $e_i = y_i - \hat{\bar{y}}_H$ and the second-order inclusion probability π_{ij} (Wu and Rao, 2006). Also, the unbiased estimator of S_y^2 is expressed as

$$\hat{s}_y^2 = \frac{1}{N(N-1)}\sum_{i\in s}\sum_{j>i}\frac{(y_i - y_j)^2}{\pi_{ij}}. \tag{9.50}$$

The design effect (9.48) is similarly obtained by replacing e_i in (9.49) and y_i in (9.50) by $r_i = y_i - \hat{\bar{y}}_H - \hat{B}(x_i - \bar{x})$.

Now, let us consider stratified sampling with L strata. From each stratum h, the sample s_h is selected with sample size n_h $(h = 1,\ldots,L)$. The population size of the stratum h is N_h. Also, let $w_h = N_h/N$ be the known stratum weight where N_h is the size of population stratum h. The pseudo-PELL (Wu and Rao, 2006) is given by

$$l_{st} = n\sum_{h=1}^{L} w_h \sum_{i\in s_h}\tilde{d}_{hi}\log(p_{hi}),$$

where subscript h indicates the membership to the stratum h and $\tilde{d}_{hi} = d_{hi}/\sum_{j\in s_h} d_{hj}$. With the constraint

$$\sum_{i\in s_h} p_{hi} = 1,\ h = 1,\ldots,L, \tag{9.51}$$

we have $p_{hi} = \tilde{d}_{hi}$. The pseudo-MELE of the parameter $\theta_0 = N^{-1}\sum_{h=1}^{L}\sum_{i=1}^{N_h} g(y_{hi}) = \sum_{h=1}^{L} w_h\theta_h$ is given by $\hat{\theta}_{st_H} = \sum_{h=1}^{L} w_h\hat{\theta}_{H_h}$ where $\hat{\theta}_{H_h}$ is the $\hat{\theta}_H$ for the stratum h. Similar discussions can be given for pseudo-MELEs incorporating auxiliary information. For example, if the population mean regarding x_{hi} is known to be $\bar{x}$, the constraints for stratified sampling corresponding to Equation (9.44) are

$$\sum_{i\in s_h} p_{hi} = 1,\ h = 1,\ldots,L,\ \sum_{h=1}^{L} w_h \sum_{i\in s_h} p_{hi}x_{hi} = \bar{x}.$$

The PELL ratio can be similarly developed to the cases without stratification. Consider the PELL ratio

$$\tilde{r}_{st}(\theta) = -2\{\tilde{l}_{st}(\theta) - \tilde{l}_{st}(\theta^C)\},$$

where $\tilde{l}_{st}(\theta^C)$ is maximized l_{st} subject to Constraint (9.51) and $l_{st}(\theta)$ is maximized l_{st} subject to

$$\sum_{i\in s_h} p_{hi} = 1,\ h = 1,\ldots,L,\ \sum_{h=1}^{L} w_h \sum_{i\in s_h} p_{hi}\, x_{hi} = \bar{x},\ \sum_{h=1}^{L} w_h \sum_{i\in s_h} p_{hi}\, y_{hi} = \theta.$$

Let us define the design effect

$$\text{deff}_{st\ \text{GR}} = \sum_{h=1}^{L} w_h^2\, V_p\left(\sum_{i\in s_h} \tilde{d}_{hi}\, r_{hi}\right) / \, (S_r^2/n),$$

where $r_{hi} = (y_{hi} - \bar{y}) - B(x_{hi} - \bar{x})$ with B in (9.47) and $S_r^2 = (N-1)^{-1}\sum_{h=1}^{L}\sum_{i=1}^{N_h} r_{hi}^2$. With some regularity conditions and under $\theta = \bar{y}$, Wu and Rao (2006) showed

$$\tilde{r}_{st}(\theta)/\text{deff}_{st\ \text{GR}} \xrightarrow{d} \chi_1^2.$$

The case without the auxiliary information can be handled similarly, where the design effect will be obtained letting $B = 0$.

It is shown that the confidence interval based on the EL approach provides in general improved coverage rate based on longer average lengths than the confidence intervals based on the normal approximation. Wu and Rao (2006) noted that pseudo-ELR confidence intervals of the distribution function $F(t)$ at t can be obtained by replacing y_i by $I(y_i < t)$; however, the auxiliary information would not improve efficiency of estimation due to low correlation between $I(y_i < t)$ and x_i.

9.5.2 Many Zero Values Problem in Survey Sampling

Consider that one is interested in monitoring the amount of excessive claims in accounting practice. Among randomly selected claims, most of them are legitimate (thus, zero of excessive claim) but a few may be excessive (Kvanli et al., 1998; Chen et al., 2003). Data sets such as this one give rise to analytical challenges because of many zeros (Takeshi, 1984; Tobin, 1958). The data distribution is skewed to right but the log transformation may not be possible because of many zeros and gives distortion of estimates if arbitrary small number is added to zeros (e.g., Yu et al., 2014a). Normal approximation-based approach to the analysis of zero-inflated data would not perform satisfactorily unless appropriate mixture distributions are assumed for the data analysis. Chen et al. (2003) investigated an EL approach to the data with many zeros in the context of survey sampling. The nonparametric approach can be preferable as minimal assumptions are required compared to parametric approaches.

As the starting point, the mixture model is considered as

$$f(y;\mu,\theta,r) = r\, f_1(y;\mu,\theta) I(y \neq 0) + (1-r) I(y = 0), \tag{9.52}$$

where f and f_1 denote the distribution of Y, the random variable of the data of interest, and the distribution of Y that is not 0 and its mean is μ, respectively. Also, r is the fixed rate of zero data and θ is a nuisance parameter. This setting gives rise to that the number of zeros in the sample size of n to be fixed (say, that is, k). The hypothesis of interest is $H_0 : \tau = r\mu$. The τ is the unconditional mean of Y. Unlike the parametric approach (e.g., Kvanli et al., 1998), the EL approach can be performed by letting $f_1(y_i; \mu, \theta)$ in Equation (9.52) be p_i and using constraints (Chen et al., 2003)

$$\sum_{i=1}^{n-k} p_i = 1, \quad \sum_{i=1}^{n-k} p_i y_i = \mu.$$

In fact, Chen et al. (2003) noted that the resulting ELR statistic is same as the ELR without the model assumption such as (9.52), thus the standard EL method to test the mean can be applied directly.

The EL approach can be easily extended for survey sampling. For example, consider a population with two strata and simple random sampling within strata (Chen et al., 2003). We noted that Chen et al. (2003) incorporated w_h, the weight for stratum h into the constraint not the EL, thus strictly speaking the method is not conventional PELL. The log-EL is given by

$$l_{st} = \sum_{h=1}^{2} \sum_{i \in s_h} \log(p_{hi}),$$

subject to

$$\sum_{i \in s_h} p_{hi} = 1, \ h = 1, 2, \ \sum_{h=1}^{2} w_h \sum_{i=1}^{n_h} p_{hi} y_{hi} = \tau.$$

The EL l_{st} under the alternative hypothesis results in $p_{hi} = 1/n_h$. Under the null hypothesis $H_0 : \tau = \sum_{h=1,2} w_h E(y_{hi})$ and with some regularity conditions, Chen et al. (2003) showed that the ELR statistic has asymptotically a χ_1^2 distribution. In Chen et al. (2003), Monte Carlo studies show generally favorable results of the EL approach for various underlying distributions.

References

Adimari, G., & Chiogna, M. (2012). Jackknife empirical likelihood based confidence intervals for partial areas under ROC curves. *Statistica Sinica, 22*, 1457–1477.

Altman, N., & Leger, C. (1995). Bandwidth selection for kernel distribution function estimation. *Journal of Statistical Planning and Inference, 46*(2), 195–214.

Arvesen, J. N. (1969). Jackknifing U-statistics. *The Annals of Mathematical Statistics, 40*(6), 2076–2100.

Austin, P. C., Mamdani, M. M., Juurlink, D. N., & Hux, J. E. (2006). Testing multiple statistical hypotheses resulted in spurious associations: A study of astrological signs and health. *Journal of Clinical Epidemiology, 59*(9), 964–969.

Azzalini, A. (1981). A note on the estimation of a distribution function and quantiles by a kernel method. *Biometrika, 68*(1), 326–328.

Baggerly, K. A. (1998). Empirical likelihood as a goodness-of-fit measure. *Biometrika, 85*(3), 535–547.

Bahadur, R. R. (1966). A note on quantiles in large samples. *The Annals of Mathematical Statistics, 37*(3), 577–580.

Bamber, D. (1975). The area above the ordinal dominance graph and the area below the receiver operating characteristic graph. *Journal of Mathematical Psychology, 12*(4), 387–415.

Barndorff-Nielsen, O. E., & Cox, D. R. (1989). *Asymptotic techniques; for use in statistics* (No. 04; QA276, B31.). London: Chapman and Hall.

Barton, W. H., & Zhou, M. (2012). emplik2: Empirical-likelihood test (two-sample, censored data). R package version 1.10.

Berger, J. O. (2010). *Statistical decision theory and Bayesian analysis*. New York, NY: Springer Science & Business Media.

Bleistein, N., & Handelsman, R. A. (2010). *Asymptotic expansions of integrals*. New York, NY: Courier Corporation.

Boucai, L., & Surks, M. I. (2009). Reference limits of serum TSH and free T4 are significantly influenced by race and age in an urban outpatient medical practice. *Clinical Endocrinology, 70*(5), 788–793.

Box, G. E., & Cox, D. R. (1964). An analysis of transformations. *Journal of the Royal Statistical Society. Series B (Methodological), 26*, 211–252.

Brandt, P. (2014). MSBVAR: Markov-Switching, Bayesian, vector autoregression models. *R package version 0.9-1.*

Bravo, F. (2003). Second-order power comparisons for a class of nonparametric likelihood-based tests. *Biometrika, 90*(4), 881–890.

Broemeling, L. D. (2007). *Bayesian biostatistics and diagnostic medicine*. Boca Raton, FL: CRC Press.

Brunner, E., & Munzel, U. (2000). The nonparametric Behrens-Fisher problem: Asymptotic theory and a small-sample approximation. *Biometrical Journal, 42*(1), 17–25.

Buckley, J., & James, I. (1979). Linear regression with censored data. *Biometrika, 66*(3), 429–436.

Cai, T., & Dodd, L. E. (2008). Regression analysis for the partial area under the ROC curve. *Statistica Sinica, 18,* 817–836.
Carlin, B. P., & Louis, T. A. (2000). *Bayes and empirical Bayes methods for data analysis.* Boca Raton, FL: Chapman & Hall/CRC Press.
Carlin, B. P., & Louis, T. A. (2008). *Bayesian methods for data analysis.* Boca Raton, FL: CRC Press.
Castorina, R., Bradman, A., Fenster, L., Barr, D. B., Bravo, R., Vedar, M. G., ... Eskenazi, B. (2010). Comparison of current-use pesticide and other toxicant urinary metabolite levels among pregnant women in the CHAMACOS cohort and NHANES. *Environmental Health Perspectives, 118*(6), 856.
Chang, I. H., & Mukerjee, R. (2008). Bayesian and frequentist confidence intervals arising from empirical-type likelihoods. *Biometrika, 95*(1), 139–147.
Chen, H., & Chen, J. (2000). Bahadur representations of the empirical likelihood quantile processes. *Journal of Nonparametric Statistics, 12*(5), 645–660.
Chen, J., Chen, S. Y., & Rao, J. N. K. (2003). Empirical likelihood confidence intervals for the mean of a population containing many zero values. *Canadian Journal of Statistics, 31*(1), 53–68.
Chen, J., & Lazar, N. A. (2010). Quantile estimation for discrete data via empirical likelihood. *Journal of Nonparametric Statistics, 22*(2), 237–255.
Chen, J., & Qin, J. (1993). Empirical likelihood estimation for finite populations and the effective usage of auxiliary information. *Biometrika, 80*(1), 107–116.
Chen, J., & Sitter, R. R. (1999). A pseudo empirical likelihood approach to the effective use of auxiliary information in complex surveys. *Statistica Sinica, 9,* 385–406.
Chen, J., Variyath, A. M., & Abraham, B. (2008). Adjusted empirical likelihood and its properties. *Journal of Computational and Graphical Statistics, 17*(2), 426–443.
Chen, K., Jin, Z., & Ying, Z. (2002). Semiparametric analysis of transformation models with censored data. *Biometrika, 89*(3), 659–668.
Chen, L. (1995). Testing the mean of skewed distributions. *Journal of the American Statistical Association, 90*(430), 767–772.
Chen, M. H., & Shao, Q. M. (1999). Monte Carlo estimation of Bayesian credible and HPD intervals. *Journal of Computational and Graphical Statistics, 8*(1), 69–92.
Chen, S. X. (1994). Comparing empirical likelihood and bootstrap hypothesis tests. *Journal of Multivariate Analysis, 51*(2), 277–293.
Chen, S. X., & Hall, P. (1993). Smoothed empirical likelihood confidence intervals for quantiles. *The Annals of Statistics, 21,* 1166–1181.
Chen, S. X., & Van Keilegom, I. (2009). A review on empirical likelihood methods for regression. *Test, 18*(3), 415–447.
Chen, X., Vexler, A., & Markatou, M. (2015). Empirical likelihood ratio confidence interval estimation of best linear combinations of biomarkers. *Computational Statistics & Data Analysis, 82,* 186–198.
Chib, S., Shin, M., & Simoni, A. (2018). Bayesian estimation and comparison of moment condition models. *Journal of the American Statistical Association.* In Press. doi: 10.1080/01621459.2017.1358172.
Chiou, J. M., & Muller, H. G. (1999). Nonparametric quasi-likelihood. *Annals of Statistics, 27,* 36–64.
Choi, K., & Marden, J. (1997). An approach to multivariate rank tests in multivariate analysis of variance. *Journal of the American Statistical Association, 92*(440), 1581–1590.

Claeskens, G., & Hjort, N. L. (2004). Goodness of fit via non-parametric likelihood ratios. *Scandinavian Journal of Statistics, 31*(4), 487–513.

Claeskens, G., Jing, B. Y., Peng, L., & Zhou, W. (2003). Empirical likelihood confidence regions for comparison distributions and ROC curves. *Canadian Journal of Statistics, 31*(2), 173–190.

Consonni, G., & Veronese, P. (1992). Conjugate priors for exponential families having quadratic variance functions. *Journal of the American Statistical Association, 87*(420), 1123–1127.

Crawley, M. J. (2012). *The R book*. Chichester: John Wiley & Sons.

Cressie, N., & Read, T. R. (1984). Multinomial goodness-of-fit tests. *Journal of the Royal Statistical Society. Series B (Methodological), 46*, 440–464.

Daniels, M. J., & Hogan, J. W. (2008). *Missing data in longitudinal studies: Strategies for Bayesian modeling and sensitivity analysis*. Boca Raton, FL: CRC Press.

DasGupta, A. (2008). *Asymptotic theory of statistics and probability*. New York, NY: Springer Science & Business Media.

David, H. A., & Nagaraja, H. N. (2003). *Order statistics*. New York, NY: John Wiley & Sons.

DeLong, E. R., DeLong, D. M., & Clarke-Pearson, D. L. (1988). Comparing the areas under two or more correlated receiver operating characteristic curves: A nonparametric approach. *Biometrics, 44*, 837–845.

DiCiccio, T., Hall, P., & Romano, J. (1988). *Bartlett adjustment for empirical likelihood*. Stanford University, Department of Statistics, Technical report.

DiCiccio, T., Hall, P., & Romano, J. (1991). Empirical likelihood is Bartlett-correctable. *The Annals of Statistics, 19*, 1053–1061.

DiCiccio, T. J., Kass, R. E., Raftery, A., & Wasserman, L. (1997). Computing Bayes factors by combining simulation and asymptotic approximations. *Journal of the American Statistical Association, 92*(439), 903–915.

Dodd, L. E., & Pepe, M. S. (2003). Partial AUC estimation and regression. *Biometrics, 59*(3), 614–623.

Dupont, H., Chalhoub, V., Plantefève, G., De Vaumas, C., Kermarrec, N., Paugam-Burtz, C., & Mantz, J. (2004). Variation of infected cell count in bronchoalveolar lavage and timing of ventilator-associated pneumonia. *Intensive Care Medicine, 30*(8), 1557–1563.

Efron, B., & Morris, C. (1972). Limiting the risk of Bayes and empirical Bayes estimators—Part II: The empirical Bayes case. *Journal of the American Statistical Association, 67*(337), 130–139.

Einmahl, J. H., & McKeague, I. W. (2003). Empirical likelihood based hypothesis testing. *Bernoulli, 9*, 267–290.

Erkanli, A. (1994). Laplace approximations for posterior expectations when the mode occurs at the boundary of the parameter space. *Journal of the American Statistical Association, 89*(425), 250–258.

Evans, M., & Swartz, T. (1995). Methods for approximating integrals in statistics with special emphasis on Bayesian integration problems. *Statistical Science, 10*, 254–272.

Fan, J., Farmen, M., & Gijbels, I. (1998). Local maximum likelihood estimation and inference. *Journal of the Royal Statistical Society: Series B (Statistical Methodology), 60*(3), 591–608.

Fan, J., & Gijbels, I. (1996). *Local polynomial modelling and its applications: Monographs on statistics and applied probability 66* (Vol. 66). Boca Raton, FL: CRC Press.

Fan, J., Zhang, C., & Zhang, J. (2001). Generalized likelihood ratio statistics and Wilks phenomenon. *Annals of Statistics, 29,* 153–193.

Fang, K. T., & Mukerjee, R. (2006). Empirical-type likelihoods allowing posterior credible sets with frequentist validity: Higher-order asymptotics. *Biometrika, 93*(3), 723–733.

Fanous, A. A., Natarajan, S. K., Jowdy, P. K., Dumont, T. M., Mokin, M., Yu, J., ... Snyder, K. V. (2015). High-risk factors in symptomatic patients undergoing carotid artery stenting with distal protection: Buffalo Risk Assessment Scale (BRASS). *Neurosurgery, 77*(4), 531–543.

Fernholz, L. T. (1991). Almost sure convergence of smoothed empirical distribution functions. *Scandinavian Journal of Statistics,* 255–262.

Fleiss, J. L. (1989). A critique of recent research on the two-treatment crossover design. *Controlled Clinical Trials, 10*(3), 237–243.

Fraser, D. A. S. (1954). Completeness of order statistics. *Canadian Journal of Mathematics, 6,* 42–45.

Freedman, D. A. (2009). *Statistical models: Theory and practice.* New York, NY: Cambridge University Press.

Freeman, P. R. (1989). The performance of the two-stage analysis of two-treatment, two-period crossover trials. *Statistics in Medicine, 8*(12), 1421–1432.

Freidlin, B., & Gastwirth, J. L. (2000). Should the median test be retired from general use? *The American Statistician, 54*(3), 161–164.

Freiman, J. A., Chalmers, T. C., Smith Jr, H., & Kuebler, R. R. (1978). The importance of beta, the type II error and sample size in the design and interpretation of the randomized control trial: Survey of 71 negative trials. *New England Journal of Medicine, 299*(13), 690–694.

Gehan, E. A. (1965). A generalized Wilcoxon test for comparing arbitrarily singly-censored samples. *Biometrika, 52*(1–2), 203–224.

Gelman, A., Carlin, J. B., Stern, H. S., Dunson, D. B., Vehtari, A., & Rubin, D. B. (2013). *Bayesian data analysis.* Boca Raton, FL: CRC Press.

Ghalanos, A., & Theussl, S. (2012). Rsolnp: General non-linear optimization using augmented Lagrange multiplier method. *R package version, 1.*

Ghosh, M. (1995). Inconsistent maximum likelihood estimators for the Rasch model. *Statistics & Probability Letters, 23*(2), 165–170.

Gini, C. (1912). Variabilità e mutabilità. Contributi allo studio dele relazioni e delle distribuzioni statistiche. *Studi Economico-Giuridici della Università di Cagliari.*

Greenwood, J. A., Landwehr, J. M., Matalas, N. C., & Wallis, J. R. (1979). Probability weighted moments: Definition and relation to parameters of several distributions expressable in inverse form. *Water Resources Research, 15*(5), 1049–1054.

Grizzle, J. E. (1965). The two-period change-over design and its use in clinical trials. *Biometrics, 21,* 467–480.

Gurevich, G., & Vexler, A. (2010). Retrospective change point detection: From parametric to distribution free policies. *Communications in Statistics—Simulation and Computation®, 39*(5), 899–920.

Gurevich, G., & Vexler, A. (2011). A two-sample empirical likelihood ratio test based on samples entropy. *Statistics and Computing, 21*(4), 657–670.

Guzman, D. S. M., Drazenovich, T. L., KuKanich, B., Olsen, G. H., Willits, N. H., & Paul-Murphy, J. R. (2014). Evaluation of thermal antinociceptive effects and pharmacokinetics after intramuscular administration of butorphanol tartrate to American kestrels (Falco sparverius). *American Journal of Veterinary Research, 75*(1), 11–18.

Hall, P. (1983). Inverting an Edgeworth expansion. *The Annals of Statistics, 11*(2), 569–576.
Hall, P. (2013). *The bootstrap and Edgeworth expansion*. Springer Science & Business Media.
Hall, P., & La Scala, B. (1990). Methodology and algorithms of empirical likelihood. *International Statistical Review/Revue Internationale de Statistique, 58*, 109–127.
Hall, P., & Owen, A. B. (1993). Empirical likelihood confidence bands in density estimation. *Journal of Computational and Graphical Statistics, 2*(3), 273–289.
He, D., Wang, M., Chen, X., Gao, Z., He, H., Zhau, H. E., ... Nan, X. (2004). Ethnic differences in distribution of serum prostate-specific antigen: A study in a healthy Chinese male population. *Urology, 63*(4), 722–726.
He, Y., & Escobar, M. (2008). Nonparametric statistical inference method for partial areas under receiver operating characteristic curves, with application to genomic studies. *Statistics in Medicine, 27*(25), 5291–5308.
Hjort, N. L., McKeague, I. W., & Van Keilegom, I. (2009). Extending the scope of empirical likelihood. *The Annals of Statistics, 37*, 1079–1111.
Hoeffding, W. (1948). A class of statistics with asymptotically normal distribution. *The annals of mathematical statistics*, 293–325.
Hosking, J. R. (1990). L-moments: Analysis and estimation of distributions using linear combinations of order statistics. *Journal of the Royal Statistical Society. Series B (Methodological), 52*, 105–124.
Hosking, J. R. M., Wallis, J. R., & Wood, E. F. (1985a). An appraisal of the regional flood frequency procedure in the UK Flood Studies Report. *Hydrological Sciences Journal, 30*(1), 85–109.
Hosking, J. R. M., Wallis, J. R., & Wood, E. F. (1985b). Estimation of the generalized extreme-value distribution by the method of probability-weighted moments. *Technometrics, 27*(3), 251–261.
Hsieh, F., & Turnbull, B. W. (1996). Nonparametric and semiparametric estimation of the receiver operating characteristic curve. *The Annals of Statistics, 24*(1), 25–40.
Huang, X., Qin, G., Yuan, Y., & Zhou, X. H. (2012). Confidence intervals for the difference between two partial AUCs. *Australian & New Zealand Journal of Statistics, 54*(1), 63–79.
Huang, Y., & Ke, B. S. (2014). Influence analysis on crossover design experiment in bioequivalence studies. *Pharmaceutical Statistics, 13*(2), 110–118.
Hutson, A. D. (2007). An "exact" two-group median test with an extension to censored data. *Nonparametric Statistics, 19*(2), 103–112.
Hyndman, R. J., & Yao, Q. (2002). Nonparametric estimation and symmetry tests for conditional density functions. *Journal of Nonparametric Statistics, 14*(3), 259–278.
James, W., & Stein, C. (1961). Estimation with quadratic loss. In *Proceedings of the fourth Berkeley symposium on mathematical statistics and probability* (Vol. 1, No. 1961, pp. 361–379). Berkeley: University of California Press.
Jing, B. Y. (1995). Two-sample empirical likelihood method. *Statistics & Probability Letters, 24*(4), 315–319.
Jing, B. Y., Yuan, J., & Zhou, W. (2009). Jackknife empirical likelihood. *Journal of the American Statistical Association, 104*(487), 1224–1232.
Johnson, R. A. (1970). Asymptotic expansions associated with posterior distributions. *The Annals of Mathematical Statistics, 41*(3), 851–864.
Johnson, R. A., & Wichern, D. W. (2002). *Applied multivariate statistical analysis*. Upper Saddle River, NJ: Prentice-Hall.

Jung, J. W., & Koch, G. G. (1999). Multivariate non-parametric methods for Mann–Whitney statistics to analyse cross-over studies with two treatment sequences. *Statistics in Medicine, 18*(8), 989–1017.

Kang, L., Vexler, A., Tian, L., Cooney, M., & Louis, G. M. B. (2010). Empirical and parametric likelihood interval estimation for populations with many zero values: Application for assessing environmental chemical concentrations and reproductive health. *Epidemiology, 21*(4), S58–S63.

Kass, R. E., & Vaidyanathan, S. K. (1992). Approximate Bayes factors and orthogonal parameters, with application to testing equality of two binomial proportions. *Journal of the Royal Statistical Society. Series B (Methodological), 54,* 129–144.

Katz, R. W., Parlange, M. B., & Naveau, P. (2002). Statistics of extremes in hydrology. *Advances in Water Resources, 25*(8), 1287–1304.

Kenward, M. G., & Jones, B. (1987). The analysis of data from 2 × 2 cross-over trials with baseline measurements. *Statistics in Medicine, 6*(8), 911–926.

Koenig, S. M., & Truwit, J. D. (2006). Ventilator-associated pneumonia: Diagnosis, treatment, and prevention. *Clinical Microbiology Reviews, 19*(4), 637–657.

Kotz, S., Lumelskii, Y., & Pensky, M. (2003). *The stress-strength model and its generalizations: Theory and applications.* Singapore: World Scientific.

Krebs, H. B., & Goplerud, D. R. (1983). Surgical management of bowel obstruction in advanced ovarian carcinoma. *Obstetrics & Gynecology, 61*(3), 327–330.

Kvanli, A. H., Shen, Y. K., & Deng, L. Y. (1998). Construction of confidence intervals for the IVIean of a population containing many zero values. *Journal of Business & Economic Statistics, 16*(3), 362–368.

Landwehr, J. M., Matalas, N. C., & Wallis, J. R. (1979). Probability weighted moments compared with some traditional techniques in estimating Gumbel parameters and quantiles. *Water Resources Research, 15*(5), 1055–1064.

Lazar, N., & Mykland, P. A. (1998). An evaluation of the power and conditionality properties of empirical likelihood. *Biometrika, 85*(3), 523–534.

Lazar, N. A. (2003). Bayesian empirical likelihood. *Biometrika, 90*(2), 319–326.

Lee, E. T., Desu, M. M., & Gehan, E. A. (1975). A Monte Carlo study of the power of some two-sample tests. *Biometrika, 62*(2), 425–432.

Lee, J. (1990). *U-statistics: Theory and practice.* New York, NY: Marcel Dekker.

Lehmann, E. L., & Romano, J. P. (2005). *Testing statistical hypotheses.* New York, NY: Springer Science & Business Media.

Letón, E., & Zuluaga, P. (2005). Relationships among tests for censored data. *Biometrical Journal, 47*(3), 377–387.

Li, G., Hollander, M., McKeague, I. W., & Yang, J. (1996). Nonparametric likelihood ratio confidence bands for quantile functions from incomplete survival data. *The Annals of Statistics, 24*(2), 628–640.

Li, G., & Wang, Q. H. (2003). Empirical likelihood regression analysis for right censored data. *Statistica Sinica, 13,* 51–68.

Lieberman, O. (1994). A Laplace approximation to the moments of a ratio of quadratic forms. *Biometrika, 81*(4), 681–690.

Limpert, E., Stahel, W. A., & Abbt, M. (2001). Log-normal Distributions across the Sciences: Keys and Clues: On the charms of statistics, and how mechanical models resembling gambling machines offer a link to a handy way to characterize log-normal distributions, which can provide deeper insight into variability and probability—normal or log-normal: That is the question. *AIBS Bulletin, 51*(5), 341–352.

Little, R. J., & Rubin, D. B. (2014). *Statistical analysis with missing data*. Hoboken, NJ: John Wiley & Sons.
Liu, C., Liu, A., & Halabi, S. (2011). A min–max combination of biomarkers to improve diagnostic accuracy. *Statistics in Medicine, 30*(16), 2005–2014.
Liu, Y., Zou, C., & Zhang, R. (2008). Empirical likelihood for the two-sample mean problem. *Statistics & Probability Letters, 78*(5), 548–556.
Lloyd, C. J. (1998). Using smoothed receiver operating characteristic curves to summarize and compare diagnostic systems. *Journal of the American Statistical Association, 93*(444), 1356–1364.
Loeb, S., Bjurlin, M. A., Nicholson, J., Tammela, T. L., Penson, D. F., Carter, H. B., … Etzioni, R. (2014). Overdiagnosis and overtreatment of prostate cancer. *European Urology, 65*(6), 1046–1055.
Loewen, G. M., Tracy, E., Blanchard, F., Tan, D., Yu, J., Raza, S., Matsui, S. I., & Baumann, H. (2005). Transformation of human bronchial epithelial cells alters responsiveness to inflammatory cytokines. *BMC Cancer, 5*(1), 145.
Lopez, E. M. M., Keilegom, I. V., & Veraverbeke, N. (2009). Empirical likelihood for non-smooth criterion functions. *Scandinavian Journal of Statistics, 36*(3), 413–432.
Lorenz, M. O. (1905). Methods of measuring the concentration of wealth. *Publications of the American Statistical Association, 9*(70), 209–219.
Lu, W., & Liang, Y. (2006). Empirical likelihood inference for linear transformation models. *Journal of multivariate analysis, 97*(7), 1586–1599.
Ma, S., & Huang, J. (2005). Regularized ROC method for disease classification and biomarker selection with microarray data. *Bioinformatics, 21*(24), 4356–4362.
Ma, S., & Huang, J. (2007). Combining multiple markers for classification using ROC. *Biometrics, 63*(3), 751–757.
Mann, H. B., & Whitney, D. R. (1947). On a test of whether one of two random variables is stochastically larger than the other. *The Annals of Mathematical Statistics, 18*, 50–60.
McClish, D. K. (1989). Analyzing a portion of the ROC curve. *Medical Decision Making, 9*(3), 190–195.
McIntosh, M. W., & Pepe, M. S. (2002). Combining several screening tests: Optimality of the risk score. *Biometrics, 58*(3), 657–664.
Metz, C. E., Herman, B. A., & Shen, J. H. (1998). Maximum likelihood estimation of receiver operating characteristic (ROC) curves from continuously-distributed data. *Statistics in medicine, 17*(9), 1033–1053.
Miecznikowski, J. C., Vexler, A., & Shepherd, L. A. (2013). dbEmpLikeGOF: An R package for nonparametric likelihood-ratio tests for goodness-of-fit and two-sample comparisons based on sample entropy. *Journal of Statistical Software, 54*(3), 1–19.
Milán-Segovia, R. C., Vigna-Pérez, M., Romero-Méndez, M. C., Medellín-Garibay, S. E., Vargas-Morales, J. M., Magaña-Aquino, M., & Romano-Moreno, S. (2014). Relative bioavailability of isoniazid in a fixed-dose combination product in healthy Mexican subjects. *The International Journal of Tuberculosis and Lung Disease, 18*(1), 49–54.
Miller, A. B., Wall, C., Baines, C. J., Sun, P., To, T., & Narod, S. A. (2014). Twenty five year follow-up for breast cancer incidence and mortality of the Canadian National Breast Screening Study: Randomised screening trial. *BMJ, 348*, g366.
Miyata, Y. (2004). Fully exponential Laplace approximations using asymptotic modes. *Journal of the American Statistical Association, 99*(468), 1037–1049.
Monahan, J. F., & Boos, D. D. (1992). Proper likelihoods for Bayesian analysis. *Biometrika, 79*(2), 271–278.

Mood, A. M. (1954). On the asymptotic efficiency of certain nonparametric two-sample tests. *The Annals of Mathematical Statistics, 25*(3), 514–522.

Mukerjee, R. (1994). Comparison of tests in their original forms. *Sankhyā: The Indian Journal of Statistics, Series A, 56*, 118–127.

Nadaraya, E. A. (1964). Some new estimates for distribution functions. *Theory of Probability & Its Applications, 9*(3), 497–500.

Nature Environment Research Council. (1975). *Flood studies report, I, hydrological studies.* London: Natural Environment Research Council.

Newton, M. A., & Raftery, A. E. (1994). Approximate Bayesian inference by the weighted likelihood bootstrap (with discussion). *Journal of the Royal Statistical Society Series B, 56*, 1–48.

Neyman, J., & Pearson, E. S. (1928). On the use and interpretation of certain test criteria for purposes of statistical inference: Part I. *Biometrika, 20A*, 175–240.

Neyman, J., & Pearson, E. S. (1933). The testing of statistical hypotheses in relation to probabilities a priori. In *Mathematical Proceedings of the Cambridge Philosophical Society* (Vol. 29, No. 4, pp. 492–510). Cambridge: Cambridge University Press.

Neyman, J., & Pearson, E. S. (1936). Sufficient statistics and uniformly most powerful tests of statistical hypotheses. *Statistical Research Memorandum, 1*, 113–137.

Neyman, J., & Pearson, E. S. (1938). *Contributions to the theory of testing statistical hypotheses.* Printed in Great Britain by W. Lewis, MA, at the University Press.

Neyman, J., & Pearson, E. S. (1992). On the problem of the most efficient tests of statistical hypotheses. In S. Kotz & N. Johnson (Eds.), *Breakthroughs in statistics* (pp. 73–108). New York, NY: Springer.

Oremek, G. M., & Seiffert, U. B. (1996). Physical activity releases prostate-specific antigen (PSA) from the prostate gland into blood and increases serum PSA concentrations. *Clinical Chemistry, 42*(5), 691–695.

Owen, A. (1990). Empirical likelihood ratio confidence regions. *The Annals of Statistics, 18*, 90–120.

Owen, A. (1991). Empirical likelihood for linear models. *The Annals of Statistics, 19*, 1725–1747.

Owen, A. B. (1988). Empirical likelihood ratio confidence intervals for a single functional. *Biometrika, 75*(2), 237–249.

Owen, A. B. (2001). *Empirical likelihood.* John Wiley & Sons.

Pan, X. R., & Zhou, M. (2002). Empirical likelihood ratio in terms of cumulative hazard function for censored data. *Journal of Multivariate Analysis, 80*(1), 166–188.

Peng, L., & Qi, Y. (2006). Confidence regions for high quantiles of a heavy tailed distribution. *The Annals of Statistics, 34*, 1964–1986.

Pepe, M. S. (1997). A regression modelling framework for receiver operating characteristic curves in medical diagnostic testing. *Biometrika, 84*(3), 595–608.

Pepe, M. S. (2003). *The statistical evaluation of medical tests for classification and prediction.* New York, NY: Oxford University Press.

Pepe, M. S., Cai, T., & Longton, G. (2006). Combining predictors for classification using the area under the receiver operating characteristic curve. *Biometrics, 62*(1), 221–229.

Pepe, M. S., & Thompson, M. L. (2000). Combining diagnostic test results to increase accuracy. *Biostatistics, 1*(2), 123–140.

Polson, N. G. (1991). A representation of the posterior mean for a location model. *Biometrika, 78*(2), 426–430.

Qin, G., Jin, X., & Zhou, X. H. (2011). Non-parametric interval estimation for the partial area under the ROC curve. *Canadian Journal of Statistics, 39*(1), 17–33.

Qin, G., & Jing, B. Y. (2001). Empirical likelihood for censored linear regression. *Scandinavian Journal of Statistics, 28*(4), 661–673.

Qin, G., & Zhou, X. H. (2006). Empirical likelihood inference for the area under the ROC curve. *Biometrics, 62*(2), 613–622.

Qin, J. (2000). Miscellanea. Combining parametric and empirical likelihoods. *Biometrika, 87*(2), 484–490.

Qin, J., & Lawless, J. (1994). Empirical likelihood and general estimating equations. *The Annals of Statistics, 22*, 300–325.

Qin, J., & Leung, D. H. (2005). A semiparametric two-component "compound" mixture model and its application to estimating malaria attributable fractions. *Biometrics, 61*(2), 456–464.

Qin, J., & Wong, A. (1996). Empirical likelihood in a semi-parametric model. *Scandinavian Journal of Statistics, 23*, 209–219.

Qin, J., & Zhang, B. (2005). Marginal likelihood, conditional likelihood and empirical likelihood: Connections and applications. *Biometrika, 92*(2), 251–270.

Qin, J., & Zhang, B. (2007). Empirical-likelihood-based inference in missing response problems and its application in observational studies. *Journal of the Royal Statistical Society: Series B (Statistical Methodology), 69*(1), 101–122.

Qin, J., Zhang, B., & Leung, D. H. (2009). Empirical likelihood in missing data problems. *Journal of the American Statistical Association, 104*(488), 1492–1503.

Qin, Y., Rao, J. N. K., & Wu, C. (2010). Empirical likelihood confidence intervals for the Gini measure of income inequality. *Economic Modelling, 27*(6), 1429–1435.

R Development Core Team. (2014). *R: A language and environment for statistical computing.* Vienna: R Foundation for Statistical Computing.

Rao, J. N., & Scott, A. J. (1981). The analysis of categorical data from complex sample surveys: Chi-squared tests for goodness of fit and independence in two-way tables. *Journal of the American Statistical Association, 76*(374), 221–230.

Reiser, B., & Faraggi, D. (1997). Confidence intervals for the generalized ROC criterion. *Biometrics, 53*, 644–652.

Rimm, E. B., Stampfer, M. J., Ascherio, A., Giovannucci, E., Colditz, G. A., & Willett, W. C. (1993). Vitamin E consumption and the risk of coronary heart disease in men. *New England Journal of Medicine, 328*(20), 1450–1456.

Ritov, Y. (1990). Estimation in a linear regression model with censored data. *The Annals of Statistics, 18*, 303–328.

Robins, J. M., & Rotnitzky, A. (1992). Recovery of information and adjustment for dependent censoring using surrogate markers. In N. Jewell, K. Dietz, & V. Farewell (Eds.), *AIDS epidemiology* (pp. 297–331). Boston, MA: Birkhäuser.

Robins, J. M., Rotnitzky, A., & Zhao, L. P. (1995). Analysis of semiparametric regression models for repeated outcomes in the presence of missing data. *Journal of the American Statistical Association, 90*(429), 106–121.

Rosbach, J. T., Vonk, M., Duijm, F., Van Ginkel, J. T., Gehring, U., & Brunekreef, B. (2013). A ventilation intervention study in classrooms to improve indoor air quality: The FRESH study. *Environmental Health, 12*(1), 110.

SAS Institute Inc. (2009). *SAS/STAT 9.2 user's guide* (2nd ed.). Cary, NC: SAS Institute.

Scannapieco, F. A., Yu, J., Raghavendran, K., Vacanti, A., Owens, S. I., Wood, K., & Mylotte, J. M. (2009). A randomized trial of chlorhexidine gluconate on oral bacterial pathogens in mechanically ventilated patients. *Critical Care, 13*(4), R117.

Schacht, A., Bogaerts, K., Bluhmki, E., & Lesaffre, E. (2008). A new nonparametric approach for baseline covariate adjustment for two-group comparative studies. *Biometrics, 64*(4), 1110–1116.

Schisterman, E. F., Faraggi, D., Browne, R., Freudenheim, J., Dorn, J., Muti, P., ... Trevisan, M. (2001). TBARS and cardiovascular disease in a population-based sample. *Journal of Cardiovascular Risk, 8*(4), 219–225.

Sen, P. K. (1967). A note on asymptotically distribution-free confidence bounds for P {X < Y}, based on two independent samples. *Sankhyā: The Indian Journal of Statistics, Series A, 29*, 95–102.

Senn, S. (2006). Cross-over trials in *Statistics in Medicine*: The first '25' years. *Statistics in Medicine, 25*(20), 3430–3442.

Serfling, R. J. (1980). *Approximation theorems of mathematical statistics.* New York, NY: John Wiley & Sons.

Shanno, D. F. (1970). Conditioning of quasi-Newton methods for function minimization. *Mathematics of Computation, 24*(111), 647–656.

Sheather, S. J., & Jones, M. C. (1991). A reliable data-based bandwidth selection method for kernel density estimation. *Journal of the Royal Statistical Society. Series B (Methodological), 53*, 683–690.

Silverman, B. W. (1986). *Density estimation for statistics and data analysis* (Vol. 26). Boca Raton, FL: CRC Press.

Stedinger, J. R. (1983). Estimating a regional flood frequency distribution. *Water Resources Research, 19*(2), 503–510.

Stein, C. (1956). Inadmissibility of the usual estimator for the mean of a multivariate normal distribution. In *Proceedings of the Third Berkeley symposium on mathematical statistics and probability* (Vol. 1, No. 399, pp. 197–206). Berkeley: University of California Press.

Su, J. Q., & Liu, J. S. (1993). Linear combinations of multiple diagnostic markers. *Journal of the American Statistical Association, 88*(424), 1350–1355.

Sweeting, T. J. (1995). A framework for Bayesian and likelihood approximations in statistics. *Biometrika, 82*(1), 1–23.

Szabó, B., van der Vaart, A. W., & van Zanten, J. H. (2015). Frequentist coverage of adaptive nonparametric Bayesian credible sets. *The Annals of Statistics, 43*(4), 1391–1428.

Szymczak, S., Igl, B. W., & Ziegler, A. (2009). Detecting SNP-expression associations: A comparison of mutual information and median test with standard statistical approaches. *Statistics in Medicine, 28*(29), 3581–3596.

Takeshi, A. (1984). Tobit models: A survey. *Journal of Econometrics, 24*, 3–61.

Thomas, D. R., & Grunkemeier, G. L. (1975). Confidence interval estimation of survival probabilities for censored data. *Journal of the American Statistical Association, 70*(352), 865–871.

Tierney, L., & Kadane, J. B. (1986). Accurate approximations for posterior moments and marginal densities. *Journal of the American Statistical Association, 81*(393), 82–86.

Tierney, L., Kass, R. E., & Kadane, J. B. (1989). Fully exponential Laplace approximations to expectations and variances of nonpositive functions. *Journal of the American Statistical Association, 84*(407), 710–716.

Tobin, J. (1958). Estimation of relationships for limited dependent variables. *Econometrica: Journal of the Econometric Society, 26*, 24–36.

Turnbull, B. W. (1976). The empirical distribution function with arbitrarily grouped, censored and truncated data. *Journal of the Royal Statistical Society. Series B (Methodological), 38*, 290–295.

Vexler, A., Deng, W., & Wilding, G. E. (2013a). Nonparametric Bayes factors based on empirical likelihood ratios. *Journal of Statistical Planning and Inference, 143*(3), 611–620.

Vexler, A., & Gurevich, G. (2010). Empirical likelihood ratios applied to goodness-of-fit tests based on sample entropy. *Computational Statistics & Data Analysis, 54*(2), 531–545.

Vexler, A., & Gurevich, G. (2011). A note on optimality of hypothesis testing. *Journal Mesa, 2*, 243–250.

Vexler, A., Gurevich, G., & Hutson, A. D. (2013b). An exact density-based empirical likelihood ratio test for paired data. *Journal of Statistical Planning and Inference, 143*(2), 334–345.

Vexler, A., & Hutson, A. D. (2018). *Statistics in the health sciences: Theory, applications, and computing.* New York: Chapman and Hall/CRC Press.

Vexler, A., Hutson, A. D., & Yu, J. (2014a). Empirical likelihood methods in clinical experiments. In N. Balakrishman (Ed.), *Methods and Applications of Statistics in Clinical Trials: "Encyclopedia of Clinical Trials."* Newark, NJ: John Wiley & Sons.

Vexler, A., Liu, A., Eliseeva, E., & Schisterman, E. F. (2008a). Maximum likelihood ratio tests for comparing the discriminatory ability of biomarkers subject to limit of detection. *Biometrics, 64*(3), 895–903.

Vexler, A., Liu, A., Schisterman, E. F., & Wu, C. (2006). Note on distribution-free estimation of maximum linear separation of two multivariate distributions. *Nonparametric Statistics, 18*(2), 145–158.

Vexler, A., Liu, S., Kang, L., & Hutson, A. D. (2009). Modifications of the empirical likelihood interval estimation with improved coverage probabilities. *Communications in Statistics-Simulation and Computation, 38*(10), 2171–2183.

Vexler, A., Liu, S., & Schisterman, E. F. (2011a). Nonparametric-likelihood inference based on cost-effectively-sampled-data. *Journal of Applied Statistics, 38*(4), 769–783.

Vexler, A., Schisterman, E. F., & Liu, A. (2008b). Estimation of ROC curves based on stably distributed biomarkers subject to measurement error and pooling mixtures. *Statistics in Medicine, 27*(2), 280–296.

Vexler, A., Shan, G., Kim, S., Tsai, W. M., Tian, L., & Hutson, A. D. (2011b). An empirical likelihood ratio based goodness-of-fit test for Inverse Gaussian distributions. *Journal of Statistical Planning and Inference, 141*(6), 2128–2140.

Vexler, A., Tanajian, H., & Hutson, A.D. (2014). Density-based empirical likelihood procedures for testing symmetry of data distributions and k-sample comparisons. The *STATA Journal, 14*(2), 304–328.

Vexler, A., Tao, G., & Chen, X. (2015). A toolkit for clinical statisticians to fix problems based on biomarker measurements subject to instrumental limitations: From repeated measurement techniques to a hybrid pooled–unpooled design. In D. Armstrong (Ed.), *Advanced Protocols in Oxidative Stress III* (pp. 439–460). Berlin: Springer.

Vexler, A., Tao, G., & Hutson, A. D. (2014b). Posterior expectation based on empirical likelihoods. *Biometrika, 101*(3), 711–718.

Vexler, A., Tsai, W. M., Gurevich, G., & Yu, J. (2012a). Two-sample density-based empirical likelihood ratio tests based on paired data, with application to a treatment study of attention-deficit/hyperactivity disorder and severe mood dysregulation. *Statistics in Medicine, 31*(17), 1821–1837.

Vexler, A., Tsai, W. M., & Hutson, A. D. (2014). A simple density-based empirical likelihood radio test for independence. *The American Statistician, 68*, 158–169.

Vexler, A., Tsai, W. M., & Malinovsky, Y. (2012b). Estimation and testing based on data subject to measurement errors: From parametric to non-parametric likelihood methods. *Statistics in Medicine, 31*(22), 2498–2512.

Vexler, A., & Wu, C. (2009). An optimal retrospective change point detection policy. *Scandinavian Journal of Statistics, 36*(3), 542–558.

Vexler, A., Wu, C., & Yu, K. F. (2010a). Optimal hypothesis testing: From semi to fully Bayes factors. *Metrika, 71*(2), 125–138.

Vexler, A., & Yu, J. (2011). Two-sample density-based empirical likelihood tests for incomplete data in application to a pneumonia study. *Biometrical Journal, 53*(4), 628–651.

Vexler, A., Yu, J., & Hutson, A. D. (2011c). Likelihood testing populations modeled by autoregressive process subject to the limit of detection in applications to longitudinal biomedical data. *Journal of Applied Statistics, 38*(7), 1333–1346.

Vexler, A., Yu, J., & Lazar, N. (2017). Bayesian empirical likelihood methods for quantile comparisons. *The Journal of Korean Statistical Society, 46*, 518–538. http://dx.doi.org/10.1016/j.jkss.2017.03.002.

Vexler, A., Yu, J., Tian, L., & Liu, S. (2010b). Two-sample nonparametric likelihood inference based on incomplete data with an application to a pneumonia study. *Biometrical Journal, 52*(3), 348–361.

Vexler, A., Zou, L., & Hutson, A. D. (2016). Data-driven confidence interval estimation incorporating prior information with an adjustment for skewed data. *The American Statistician, 70*(3), 243–249.

Vexler, A., Zou, L., & Hutson, A. D. (2017). An extension to empirical likelihood for evaluating probability weighted moments. *Journal of Statistical Planning and Inference, 182*, 50–60.

van Gelder, P. H. A. J. M., & Pandey, M. D. (2005). An analysis of drag forces based on L-moments. *Advances in Safety and Reliability, 1*, 661–668.

Wallis, J. R., & Wood, E. F. (1985). Relative accuracy of log Pearson III procedures. *Journal of Hydraulic Engineering, 111*(7), 1043–1056.

Wang, J. (2006). Quadratic artificial likelihood functions using estimating functions. *Scandinavian Journal of statistics, 33*(2), 379–390.

Wang, Q. H., & Jing, B. Y. (2001). Empirical likelihood for a class of functionals of survival distribution with censored data. Annals of the Institute of Statistical Mathematics, 53(3), 517–527.

Wang, Q. H., & Jing, B. Y. (2003). Empirical likelihood for partial linear models. *Annals of the Institute of Statistical Mathematics*, 55(3), 585–595.

Wang, Q., & Rao, J. N. K. (2002a). Empirical likelihood-based inference in linear errors-in-covariables models with validation data. *Biometrika, 89*(2), 345–358.

Wang, Q., & Rao, J. N. K. (2002b). Empirical likelihood-based inference under imputation for missing response data. *The Annals of Statistics, 30*(3), 896–924.

Wang, S., Qian, L., & Carroll, R. J. (2010). Generalized empirical likelihood methods for analyzing longitudinal data. *Biometrika, 97*(1), 79–93.

Watson, G. S. (1964). Smooth regression analysis. *Sankhyā: The Indian Journal of Statistics, Series A*, 359–372.

Wedderburn, R. W. (1974). Quasi-likelihood functions, generalized linear models, and the Gauss—Newton method. *Biometrika, 61*(3), 439–447.

Wener, M. H., Daum, P. R., & McQuillan, G. M. (2000). The influence of age, sex, and race on the upper reference limit of serum C-reactive protein concentration. *The Journal of Rheumatology, 27*(10), 2351–2359.

Wieand, S., Gail, M. H., James, B. R., & James, K. L. (1989). A family of nonparametric statistics for comparing diagnostic markers with paired or unpaired data. *Biometrika, 76*(3), 585–592.

Wilcox, R. R. (1998). The goals and strategies of robust methods. *British Journal of Mathematical and Statistical Psychology, 51*(1), 1–39.

Wilcoxon, F. (1945). Individual comparisons by ranking methods. *Biometrics Bulletin, 1*(6), 80–83.

Wilks, S. S. (1938). The large-sample distribution of the likelihood ratio for testing composite hypotheses. *The Annals of Mathematical Statistics, 9*(1), 60–62.

Winter, B. B. (1979). Convergence rate of perturbed empirical distribution functions. *Journal of Applied Probability, 16*(1), 163–173.

Wood, A. T., Do, K. A., & Broom, B. M. (1996). Sequential linearization of empirical likelihood constraints with application to U-statistics. *Journal of Computational and Graphical Statistics, 5*(4), 365–385.

Wu, C., & Rao, J. N. K. (2006). Pseudo-empirical likelihood ratio confidence intervals for complex surveys. *Canadian Journal of Statistics, 34*(3), 359–375.

Wu, J., Wong, A. C. M., & Jiang, G. (2003). Likelihood-based confidence intervals for a log-normal mean. *Statistics in Medicine, 22*(11), 1849–1860.

Wu, X., & Ying, Z. (2011). An empirical likelihood approach to nonparametric covariate adjustment in randomized clinical trials. *arXiv preprint arXiv:1108.0484*.

Wylie, K. P., Tanabe, J., Martin, L. F., Wongngamnit, N., & Tregellas, J. R. (2013). Nicotine increases cerebellar activity during finger tapping. *PLoS One, 8*(12), e84581.

Yang, S., & Zhao, Y. (2007). Testing treatment effect by combining weighted log-rank tests and using empirical likelihood. *Statistics & Probability Letters, 77*(12), 1385–1393.

Yates, F., & Grundy, P. M. (1953). Selection without replacement from within strata with probability proportional to size. *Journal of the Royal Statistical Society. Series B (Methodological), 15*, 253–261.

Ye, Y. (1987). *Interior algorithms for linear, quadratic, and linearly constrained non-linear programming* (PhD Thesis). Department of EES, Stanford University.

Yee, J. L., Johnson, W. O., & Samaniego, F. J. (2002). Asymptotic approximations to posterior distributions via conditional moment equations. *Biometrika, 89*(4), 755–767.

You, J., Chen, G., & Zhou, Y. (2006). Block empirical likelihood for longitudinal partially linear regression models. *Canadian Journal of Statistics, 34*(1), 79–96.

Yu, J., Liu, L., Collins, R. L., Vincent, P. C., & Epstein, L. H. (2014a). Analytical problems and suggestions in the analysis of behavioral economic demand curves. *Multivariate Behavioral Research, 49*(2), 178–192.

Yu, J., Vexler, A., & Tian, L. (2010). Analyzing incomplete data subject to a threshold using empirical likelihood methods: An application to a pneumonia risk study in an ICU setting. *Biometrics, 66*(1), 123–130.

Yu, J., Vexler, A., Hutson, A. D., & Baumann, H. (2014b). Empirical likelihood approaches to two-group comparisons of upper quantiles applied to biomedical data. *Statistics in Biopharmaceutical Research, 6*(1), 30–40.

Yu, J., Vexler, A., Kim, S. E., & Hutson, A. D. (2011). Two-sample empirical likelihood ratio tests for medians in application to biomarker evaluations. *Canadian Journal of Statistics, 39*(4), 671–689.

Yu, J., Yang, L., Vexler, A., & Hutson, A. D. (2016). A generalized empirical likelihood approach for two-group comparisons given a U-statistic constraint. *Statistics, 50*(2), 435–453.

Yuan, A., He, W., Wang, B., & Qin, G. (2012). U-statistic with side information. *Journal of Multivariate Analysis, 111*, 20–38.

Zeger, S. L., & Diggle, P. J. (1994). Semiparametric models for longitudinal data with application to CD4 cell numbers in HIV seroconverters. *Biometrics, 50*, 689–699.

Zhao, H., & Tian, L. (2001). On estimating medical cost and incremental cost-effectiveness ratios with censored data. *Biometrics, 57*(4), 1002–1008.

Zhao, Y., & Wang, H. (2008). Empirical likelihood inference for the regression model of mean quality-adjusted lifetime with censored data. *Canadian Journal of Statistics, 36*(3), 463–478.

Zhong, X., & Ghosh, M. (2016). Higher-order properties of Bayesian empirical likelihood. *Electronic Journal of Statistics, 10*(2), 3011–3044.

Zhou, M. (2005). Empirical likelihood ratio with arbitrarily censored/truncated data by EM algorithm. *Journal of Computational and Graphical Statistics, 14*(3), 643–656.

Zhou, M., & Li, G. (2008). Empirical likelihood analysis of the Buckley–James estimator. *Journal of Multivariate Analysis, 99*(4), 649–664.

Zhou, W., & Jing, B. Y. (2003a). Adjusted empirical likelihood method for quantiles. *Annals of the Institute of Statistical Mathematics, 55*(4), 689–703.

Zhou, W., & Jing, B. Y. (2003b). Smoothed empirical likelihood confidence intervals for the difference of quantiles. *Statistica Sinica, 13*, 83–95.

Zhou, X., & Reiter, J. P. (2010). A note on Bayesian inference after multiple imputation. *The American Statistician, 64*(2), 159–163.

Zhou, X. H., McClish, D. K., & Obuchowski, N. A. (2009). *Statistical methods in diagnostic medicine* (Vol. 569). Hoboken, NJ: John Wiley & Sons.

Zhou, Y., & Liang, H. (2005). Empirical-likelihood-based semiparametric inference for the treatment effect in the two-sample problem with censoring. *Biometrika, 92*(2), 271–282.

Zhu, L., & Xue, L. (2006). Empirical likelihood confidence regions in a partially linear single-index model. *Journal of the Royal Statistical Society: Series B (Statistical Methodology), 68*(3), 549–570.

Zhou, X. H., & Qin, G. (2005). Improved confidence intervals for the sensitivity at a fixed level of specificity of a continuous-scale diagnostic test. *Statistics in Medicine, 24*(3), 465–477.

Zou, K. H., Hall, W. J., & Shapiro, D. E. (1997). Smooth non-parametric receiver operating characteristic (ROC) curves for continuous diagnostic tests. *Statistics in Medicine, 16*(19), 2143–2156.

Zou, K. H., Liu, A., Bandos, A. I., Ohno-Machado, L., & Rockette, H. E. (2011). *Statistical evaluation of diagnostic performance: Topics in ROC analysis*. Boca Raton, FL: CRC Press.

Name Index

Subject Index

Note: Page numbers in italic and bold refer to figures and tables respectively.